Disorders of the Oral Cavity

Editor

VITTORIO CAPELLO

VETERINARY CLINICS OF NORTH AMERICA: EXOTIC ANIMAL PRACTICE

www.vetexotic.theclinics.com

Consulting Editor
JÖRG MAYER

September 2016 • Volume 19 • Number 3

ELSEVIER

1600 John F. Kennedy Boulevard • Suite 1800 • Philadelphia, Pennsylvania, 19103-2899
http://www.vetexotic.theclinics.com

VETERINARY CLINICS OF NORTH AMERICA: EXOTIC ANIMAL PRACTICE Volume 19, Number 3
September 2016 ISSN 1094-9194, ISBN-13: 978-0-323-46269-3

Editor: Patrick Manley
Developmental Editor: Meredith Clinton

Veterinary Clinics of North America: Exotic Animal Practice (ISSN 1094-9194) is published in January, May, and September by Elsevier, Inc., 360 Park Avenue South, New York, NY 10010-1710. Subscription prices are $260.00 per year for US individuals, $438.00 per year for US institutions, $100.00 per year for US students and residents, $305.00 per year for Canadian individuals, $528.00 per year for Canadian institutions, $340.00 per year for international individuals, $528.00 per year for international institutions and $165.00 per year for Canadian and foreign students/residents. To receive student/resident rate, orders must be accompanied by name of affiliated institution, date of term, and the *signature* of program/residency coordinator on institution letterhead. Orders will be billed at individual rate until proof of status is received. Foreign air speed delivery is included in all *Clinics* subscription prices. All prices are subject to change without notice. **POSTMASTER:** Send address changes to *Veterinary Clinics of North America: Exotic Animal Practice*, Elsevier Health Sciences Division, Subscription Customer Service, 3251 Riverport Lane, Maryland Heights, MO 63043. **Customer Service: Telephone: 1-800-654-2452** (U.S. and Canada); **1-314-447-8871** (outside U.S. and Canada). **Fax: 1-314-447-8029. E-mail: journalscustomerservice-usa@elsevier.com (for print support); journalsonlinesupport-usa@elsevier.com (for online support)**.

Reprints. For copies of 100 or more of articles in this publication, please contact the Commercial Reprints Department, Elsevier Inc., 360 Park Avenue South, New York, New York 10010-1710. Tel.: 212-633-3874; Fax: 212-633-3820; E-mail: reprints@elsevier.com.

Veterinary Clinics of North America: Exotic Animal Practice is covered in *MEDLINE/PubMed (Index Medicus)*.

Contributors

CONSULTING EDITOR

JÖRG MAYER, Dr.med.vet, MSc
Diplomate American Board of Veterinary Practitioners (Exotic Companion Mammals); Diplomate European College of Zoological Medicine (Small Mammals); Diplomate American College of Zoological Medicine; Associate Professor of Zoological Medicine, Department of Small Animal Medicine and Surgery, College of Veterinary Medicine, University of Georgia, Athens, Georgia

EDITOR

VITTORIO CAPELLO, DVM
Diplomate, European College of Zoological Medicine (Small Mammal); Diplomate, American Board of Veterinary Practitioners-Exotic Companion Mammals; European Veterinary Specialist in Zoological Medicine (Small Mammal), Clinica Veterinaria S. Siro; Clinica Veterinaria Gran Sasso, Milano, Italy

AUTHORS

VITTORIO CAPELLO, DVM
Diplomate, European College of Zoological Medicine (Small Mammal); Diplomate, American Board of Veterinary Practitioners-Exotic Companion Mammals; European Veterinary Specialist in Zoological Medicine (Small Mammal), Clinica Veterinaria S. Siro; Clinica Veterinaria Gran Sasso, Milano, Italy

THOMAS M. DONNELLY, BVSc
Diploma in Veterinary Pharmacy; Diplomate of the American College of Laboratory Animal Medicine; Diplomate of the American Board of Veterinary Practitioners-Exotic Companion Mammals; Diplomate of the European College of Zoological Medicine - Small Mammal; Exotic Animal Service, Centre Hospitalier Universitaire Vétérinaire d'Alfort, École Nationale Vétérinaire d'Alfort, Maisons-Alfort, France

JOANNA HEDLEY, BVM&S
Diploma in Zoological Medicine (Reptilian); Diplomat of the European College of Zoological Medicine (Herpetology); Member of the Royal College of Veterinary Surgeons; Head, RVC Exotics Service, Royal Veterinary College, London, United Kingdom

VLADIMIR JEKL, MVDr, PhD
Diplomate of the European College of Zoological Medicine (Small Mammal); Associate Professor, Avian and Exotic Animal Clinic, Faculty of Veterinary Medicine, University of Veterinary and Pharmaceutical Sciences Brno, Brno, Czech Republic

CATHY A. JOHNSON-DELANEY, DVM
Board of Directors, Washington Ferret Rescue & Shelter, Kirkland, Washington

LOIC LEGENDRE, DVM, FAVD
Diplomate AVDC; DEVDC; West Coast Veterinary Dental Services Ltd, Vancouver, British Columbia, Canada

ANGELA M. LENNOX, DVM
Diplomate of the European College of Zoological Medicine (Small Mammal); Diplomate of the American Board of Veterinary Practitioners-Avian; Exotic Companion Mammal; Avian and Exotic Animal Clinic, Indianapolis, Indiana

ELISABETTA MANCINELLI, DVM, CertZooMed
Diplomate of the European College of Zoological Medicine (Small Mammal); Bath Referrals, Rosemary Lodge Veterinary Hospital, Bath, Somerset, United Kingdom

CHRISTOPH MANS, Dr med vet
Diplomate of the American College of Zoological Medicine; School of Veterinary Medicine, University of Wisconsin-Madison, Madison, Wisconsin

YASUTSUGU MIWA, DVM, PhD
Veterinary Medical Center, School of Veterinary Medicine, The University of Tokyo; Miwa Exotic Animal Hospital, Tokyo, Japan

LAUREN VIRGINIA POWERS, DVM
Diplomate of the American Board of Veterinary Practitioners (Avian Practice); Diplomate of the American Board of Veterinary Practitioners (Exotic Companion Mammal Practice); Avian and Exotic Pet Service, Carolina Veterinary Specialists, Huntersville, North Carolina

HELEN E. ROBERTS-SWEENEY, DVM
Elma Animal Hospital, Williamsville, New York

BRIAN SPEER, DVM
Diplomate of the American Board of Veterinary Practitioners (Avian Practice); Diplomate of the European College of Zoological Medicine (Avian); The Medical Center for Birds, Oakley, California

DAVID VELLA, BSc, BVSc (Hons)
Diplomate of the American Board of Veterinary Practitioners-Exotic Companion Mammals; Sydney Exotics and Rabbit Vets, Crows Nest, New South Wales, Australia

Contents

Ornamental fish represent the largest and most diverse group of exotic
animals kept as pets. The specific oral anatomy of each family or selected
species has evolved to suit the natural environment, feeding behaviors,
food or prey type, and location of the food/prey in the water column.
The anatomy can change over the life of the animal, from fry to adult.
The oral cavity of fish is susceptible to many problems including infectious
and parasitic diseases, trauma, and neoplasia. Diagnosis may involve wet
mount preparations of exfoliative cytology from the lesion, histopathology,
and bacterial or fungal culture.

A wide variety of disorders may be seen affecting the reptile and
amphibian oral cavity. Owners can easily miss problems until they are at
an advanced stage because of the difficulty of examining the oral cavity
at home. Because many problems are secondary to an inappropriate
environment or diet and may be related to systemic disease, a full history
and clinical examination is always required. Treatment of oral disorders
also requires a holistic approach including correction of any predisposing
factors in order for long-term successful resolution of the problem.

Cranial kinesis of the avian beak is complex; particularly in birds with prokinetic beak movement, such as psittacine birds. A number of diseases
can result in damage to the bony and soft tissue structures of the beak
and can lead to secondary pathology, such as beak deviation, abnormal
rhamphothecal growth and wear, and opportunistic infections. A solid
understanding of species-specific anatomic variations is essential before
attempting rhamphothecal restoration or surgical repair. Many diseases
of the oral cavity can appear similar on initial clinical evaluation and therefore warrant appropriate diagnostic testing.

The first part of this review focuses on the anatomy and physiology of the
rabbit mouth. Practical understanding is critical to comprehend the

dynamic pathologic changes of dental disease, which is one of the most common presenting problems in rabbits. The major theories of the etiopathogenesis of dental disease are presented. The second part focuses on non-dental oral disorders, which encompass only a small incidence of stomatognathic diseases when compared with dental disease. These diseases are primarily composed of infections (treponematosis, oral papillomatosis), neoplasia (frequently involving calcified tissue proliferation), and congenital abnormalities (mandibular prognathism, absent peg teeth, supernumerary peg teeth).

Diagnostic imaging techniques are of paramount importance for dentistry and oral disorders of rabbits, rodents, and other exotic companion mammals. Aside from standard radiography, stomatoscopy is a complementary tool allowing a thorough and detailed inspection of the oral cavity. Computed tomography (CT) generates multiple 2-dimensional views and 3-dimensional reconstructions providing superior diagnostic accuracy also useful for prognosis and treatment of advanced dental disease and its related complications. MRI is a diagnostic imaging technique additional to CT used primarily to enhance soft tissues, including complex odontogenic abscesses.

The intraoral treatment of dental disease in pet rabbits follows a complete clinical examination, intraoral inspection under general anesthesia, and diagnostic imaging. It also implies thorough knowledge of dental disease in this species. The most common intraoral procedures are extraction of incisor teeth, coronal reduction, and extraction of cheek teeth. These dental procedures require specific instruments and equipment. They should be performed in conjunction with supportive and medical treatment followed by appropriate nutrition.

Odontogenic facial abscesses associated with periapical infections and osteomyelitis of the jaw represent an important part of the acquired and progressive dental disease syndrome in pet rabbits. Complications such as retromasseteric and retrobulbar abscesses, extensive osteomyelitis of the mandible, and empyemas of the skull are possible sequelae. Standard and advanced diagnostic imaging should be pursued to make a detailed and proper diagnosis, and plan the most effective surgical treatment. This article reviews the surgical anatomy, the pathophysiology, and the classification of abscesses and empyemas of the mandible, the maxilla, and the skull. It also discusses surgical techniques for facial abscesses.

Loic Legendre

Acquired dental disease represents the most common oral disorder of guinea pigs. Most patients are presented with nonspecific clinical signs and symptoms, such as weight loss, reduced food intake, difficulty chewing and/or swallowing. The physical examination must be followed by standard radiography and/or computed tomography, and thorough inspection under general anesthesia. Several complications may follow, including periodontal disease, subluxation of the temporomandibular joint, periapical infection, and abscessation. The dental treatment is aimed to restore the proper length and shape of both the incisor and cheek teeth, associated with medical and supportive treatment. Abscesses should be surgically addressed by complete excision.

Christoph Mans and Vladimir Jekl

Dental disease is among the most common causes for chinchillas and degus to present to veterinarians. Most animals with dental disease present with weight loss, reduced food intake/anorexia, and drooling. Degus commonly present with dyspnea. Dental disease has been primarily referred to as elongation and malocclusion of the cheek teeth. Periodontal disease, caries, and tooth resorption are common diseases in chinchillas, but are missed frequently during routine intraoral examination, even performed under general anesthesia. A diagnostic evaluation, including endoscopy-guided intraoral examination and diagnostic imaging of the skull, is necessary to detect oral disorders and to perform the appropriate therapy.

Elisabetta Mancinelli and Vittorio Capello

The order *Rodentia* comprises more than 2000 species divided into 3 groups based on anatomic and functional differences of the masseter muscle. Myomorph and sciuromorph species have elodont incisors and anelodont cheek teeth, unlike hystrichomorph species which have full anelodont dentition. Diseases of incisors and cheek teeth of rat-like and squirrel-like rodents result in a wide variety of symptoms and clinical signs. Appropriate diagnostic testing and imaging techniques are required to obtain a definitive diagnosis, formulate a prognosis, and develop a treatment plan. A thorough review of elodontoma, odontoma, and pseudo-odontoma is provided, including treatment of pseudo-odontomas in prairie dogs.

Cathy A. Johnson-Delaney

Exotic companion carnivores such as ferrets, skunks, fennec foxes, coatimundis, raccoons, and kinkajous presented in clinical practice share similar dental anatomy, function, and diseases. The domestic ferret serves

VETERINARY CLINICS OF NORTH AMERICA: EXOTIC ANIMAL PRACTICE

RELATED INTEREST

Veterinary Clinics of North America: Small Animal Practice
September 2016 (Vol. 46, Issue 6)
Small Animal Obesity
Amy Farcas and Kathy Michel, *Editors*

THE CLINICS ARE NOW AVAILABLE ONLINE!
Access your subscription at:
www.theclinics.com

Preface

New Perspectives on Dentistry and Oral Disorders of Exotic Companion Animals

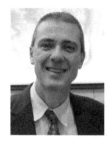

Vittorio Capello, DVM
Editor

Oral disorders are a frequent problem in several groups of exotic animals, such as rabbits, rodents, and to a lesser extent, reptiles. However, they are also encountered in carnivores and other pet species (hedgehogs, sugar gliders, miniature pigs, fish), and even among species lacking teeth entirely, such as birds and chelonians.

Because of increased education of pet owners resulting in the demand for comprehensive diagnosis and treatment, many aspects of dental disease syndrome in exotic mammals have advanced vastly over the past decade. This is especially true with regards to diagnostic imaging and surgery. Furthermore, distinguishing features of dental disease in rabbits and even between different species of rodents are now described separately.

These were the concepts kept in mind when I developed this issue focused on oral disorders, 13 years after another comprehensive issue edited by Dr David Crossley in 2003. That publication covered a broader range of zoological medicine (including nonhuman primates, zoo and wild animals, and invertebrates) and has been a valuable resource for more than a decade. This issue is focused in more detail on exotic companion animals, including ornamental fish; therefore, its goal is not to replace the earlier issue. While the range of species is a bit narrower, the topic is slightly different and broadened. These important species, or groups of species, are now each represented by a dedicated review article. Dentistry and oral disorders of pet rabbits are revisited and updated in four separate articles. Although dental disease actually represents the most common problem of the mouth of rabbits and rodents, we chose to not only include dentistry, but also oral disorders.

Whereas there are other important textbooks and articles featuring this topic, we hope this issue of the *Veterinary Clinics of North America: Exotic Animal Practice* will represent a useful and practical resource for the veterinary practitioner. One specific

Vet Clin Exot Anim 19 (2016) xi–xii
http://dx.doi.org/10.1016/j.cvex.2016.06.001
1094-9194/16/$ – see front matter © 2016 Published by Elsevier Inc.

vetexotic.theclinics.com

goal was to place a special emphasis on illustrations, and the collaborative effort of all the contributors resulted in 550 illustrations combined in over 200 figures.

My warmest thanks goes to the contributors, who made this issue feasible, because they are among the most renowned authors for both the selected species and the topic. Several articles feature two authors, for a total of 13, with contributions from all over the world, including the Unites States, Canada, United Kigndom, other European countries, Japan, and Australia. I was honored to receive such enthusiastic feedback to my invitation, despite their numerous concurrent ongoing projects.

Last, but not least, a special acknowledgment goes to Dr Melissa Kling, for her invaluable support during the revision of this issue.

Vittorio Capello, DVM
Clinica Veterinaria S.Siro
Via Lampugnano 99
Milano 20151, Italy

Clinica Veterinaria Gran Sasso
Via Donatello 26
Milano 20134, Italy

E-mail address:
capellov@tin.it

Anatomy and Disorders of the Oral Cavity of Ornamental Fish

Helen E. Roberts-Sweeney, DVM

KEYWORDS

- Fish • Infectious disease • Oral anatomy • Feeding behavior • Neoplasia

KEY POINTS

- Oral anatomy in fish varies greatly by taxonomic family, feeding behavior, life stage, and natural habitat; failure to provide the appropriate husbandry and diet type can result in fish disease and deaths.
- An oral examination should always be included as part of the minimum database when examining fish.
- The oral cavity is subject to infectious diseases, trauma, and neoplasia.
- In-house exfoliative cytology is a quick, easy tool to use as an aid in the diagnosis of oral cavity diseases.
- Differentiation of lesions that seem similar helps determine effective treatments rather than using a polypharmacy approach.

INTRODUCTION

Pet (or ornamental) fish represent the largest and most diverse group of exotic animals kept as pets. It is estimated there are more than 4500 species of freshwater fish and 1450 species of marine ornamentals traded[1] to be kept in captivity privately, or displayed, worldwide. There is an immense variety of anatomic adaptations in fish.

ANATOMY AND PHYSIOLOGY OF THE ORAL CAVITY IN FISH

The oral anatomy of each family or a single species has evolved to best suit the local natural habitat or environment, feeding behaviors, food or prey type, location of the food or prey in the water column, and as an aid in reducing interspecific competition for food within a habitat. The function of the oral cavity is not only for the prehension and ingestion of food but can also include raising offspring (mouthbrooding) and as an

The author has nothing to disclose.
Elma Animal Hospital PC, 3180 Transit Road, West Seneca, NY 14224, USA
E-mail address: elmavets@gmail.com

Vet Clin Exot Anim 19 (2016) 669–687
http://dx.doi.org/10.1016/j.cvex.2016.04.001
1094-9194/16/$ – see front matter
vetexotic.theclinics.com

aid in the detection of environmental chemical changes. The anatomy can change or be fixed over the life of the animal, from fry to adult.

Skeletal Structure of the Oral Cavity

The skeletal components of fish vary according to the phylogenetic changes from less advanced fish, the cartilaginous fishes, including elasmobranches (*Chondrichthyes*), to the bony fish (*Actinopterygia*). In general, the fish oral cavity is composed of the lower jaw, the upper jaw, the palate (dorsally), and the hyoid apparatus ventrally (**Fig. 1**).

In contrast to terrestrial animals, the upper jaw consists of the premaxilla and the maxilla (caudal to the premaxilla) in most fish.[2] The caudal portion of the maxilla is often more mobile in comparison with other vertebrates, contributing to the complex series of muscle and skeletal movements required to produce an effective gape (open mouth) for food prehension. During feeding, the premaxilla protrudes rostrally to provide the dorsolateral aspect of the gape. In most fish, this movement enhances the suction required for feeding. Ventral and posterior movement of the mandible passively enables premaxillary protrusion by the presence of a ligament connecting the caudal aspect of the premaxilla to the caudal end of the dentary bone of the mandible.[3]

One study found a specialized adaptation of the *adductor mandibulae* muscle in some cyprinodontiform fish (*Fundus, Gambusia,* and *Poecilia* sp.).[3] This adaptation enables the premaxilla to actively retract producing a forceps like control of the upper and lower jaws giving more dexterity to the mouth.[3] Instead of using suction feeding methods, these fish pick the prey from the water column or graze on substrate. In some species of loricariid and synodontid (*Siluriformes*) catfish, this adaptation works very well for algal scraping from substrates, the preferred feeding mode of these fish.[3]

The lower jaw, the mandible, consists of 3 bones: the more anteriorly placed dentary bone, the central angular bone, and the articular bone. Some fish have an intramandibular joint (IMJ) between the dentary and fused angular-articular bones.[2,4,5] Interestingly, fish species that have an IMJ have better dexterity in feeding; these fish commonly feed by removing food attached to a substrate or by biting pieces off sessile structures.[2,3] A common freshwater aquarium fish, *Helostoma temminckii*

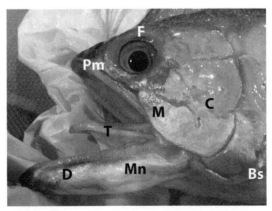

Fig. 1. Skeletal structure of the head. Bs, branchiostegal membrane; C, cheek; D, dentary bone; F, frontal bone; M, maxilla; Mn, mandible; Pm, premaxillary bone; T, tongue. (*Courtesy of* Helen Roberts-Sweeney, DVM, Williamsville, NY; with permission.)

(kissing gourami), is an example of one species with an IMJ.[2,3] The IMJ allows full 360° contact of the mouth on a substrate during a scraping or biting motion to obtain diatoms and microalgae, components of *Helostoma*'s diet in the wild.[2,3] The cost of this anatomic feature is a reduced ability to produce an effective suction, the method most fish use for feeding.[4]

Syngnathidae (seahorses, sea dragons, pipefishes, sea moths, and shrimpfishes) possess a tubular-shaped mouth whereby only the lower jaw is protractile.[6–8] The cranium is connected mechanically to the hyoid apparatus. Prey is captured by simultaneously elevating the head, rapidly depressing the hyoid apparatus, and opening the mouth.[7] Suction is created in the oral cavity by this movement, allowing water (and prey) to enter the small mouth.[7,8]

The parasphenoid bone, located ventrally to the cranium, represents the dorsal aspect of the oral cavity. This bone functions as the hard palate in most fish. Posterior to this bone is the basioccipital bone. Koi (*Cyprinus carpio*) and goldfish (*Carassius auratus*) have lower pharyngeal teeth that grind food against a hard, cartilaginous pad, known as the carp stone, located ventral to the basioccipital bone.[8,9] In koi, molarlike upper pharyngeal teeth are embedded in the pharyngeal pad and shed periodically.[8] To the joy of their owners, these teeth are often seen on the floor of a lined pond, white against the black color of the pond liner, or found in skimmer boxes.

The hyoid apparatus, located on the ventral midline, provides support to the tongue, connects to the mandible, and generates suction in the buccal cavity when depressed ventrally during feeding.[10] In one study, it was found that in addition to the cranial muscles providing some muscle power, it was estimated that the hypaxial and epaxial muscles contributed more significant muscle power for maximum hyoid depression to create the high suction power required for feeding in largemouth bass (*Micropterus salmoides*).[11,12] One study demonstrated the axial musculature may actually contribute 95% of the power for suction feeding in the largemouth bass.[12]

One skeletal structure of importance in the hyoid apparatus is the branchiostegal rays, flat bars that support the branchiostegal membrane.[8] This membrane stretches from the ventral aspect of the opercular flap (a hard bony flap that covers and protects the gills) to the midline of the pharynx and functions as a gasket to help close the operculum when the pharynx is expanded by water intake during suction feeding.

Dentition in Fish

Dentition in fish varies tremendously. Possible combinations include no teeth, small teeth, multiple rows of teeth, pharyngeal teeth (upper only or both upper and lower), platelike teeth, and teeth on gill rakers.

Members of the Osteoglossidae (bonytongues) family have a toothlike bony structure on the floor of the mouth. This structure has teeth and can be used to bite prey when pressed against the dorsal aspect of the mouth (**Fig. 2**).

Soft Tissue of the Oral Cavity

The oral cavity of most fish is lined by stratified epithelium containing numerous mucous cells.[13] Mucus serves to lubricate the surface of the mouth and may provide protection from abrasions.[14] Numerous taste buds are distributed throughout the oral cavity and also appear on barbells.[8,13] Taste bud density can be as much as 1600/cm^2 in some fish.[8] Taste buds in the oral cavity are innervated by the vagus nerve. Fish that ingest and spit out undesirable objects, such as goldfish that possess a high density of taste buds in the oral cavity, have enlarged vagal lobes of the brain.[8]

Many, but not all, fish have a ventrally placed tongue, also populated with taste buds.

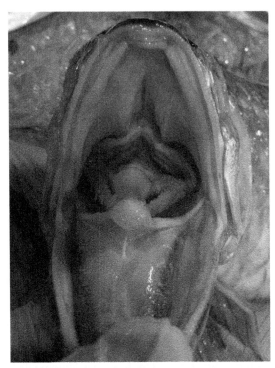

Fig. 2. Open mouth view of Asian Arowana (*Scleropages formosus*) showing bony tongue. (*Courtesy of* Helen Roberts-Sweeney, DVM, Williamsville, NY; with permission.)

Feeding Behaviors

Suction feeding is the most common type of feeding behavior in fish.[2–5,14,15] Suction is created by opening the mouth when the food is close, expanding the mouth laterally, and, simultaneously, lowering the floor of the mouth (primarily by hyoid depression). This movement creates negative pressure and allows water and food to be sucked into the oral cavity (**Fig. 3**).

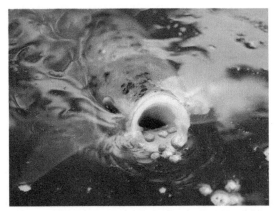

Fig. 3. *Leuciscus idus* (golden orfe) showing gape (open mouth) and food entering mouth via suction created. (*Courtesy of* Helen Roberts-Sweeney, DVM, Williamsville, NY; with permission.)

Once the jaws are closed, oral valves help to prevent food from escaping out of the mouth via the gills with the exiting flow of water.[13] The hyoid apparatus is raised and the sides of the mouth contract, forcing trapped water out of the mouth through the gills. Gill rakers, found on the medial aspect of the gill arch, help strain any food from the outflowing water, keeping it in the oral cavity until it is swallowed.[8]

Other types of feeding behaviors include ram or lunge feeding (forward swimming over prey), suction of tiny crustaceans (syngnathids), biting encrusted algae, ambush attacks, rotational feeding (the fish clamp down on the prey, tearing large chunks off while spinning the its body), suspension feeding (or filter feeding), and scraping/substrate grazing of algae.[3,14] Most of these can be grouped into suction feeding or biting behaviors. Ram feeders actively chase their prey. Fish that use the biting technique swim towards their prey, often opening their mouths while still distant from the food. Grazing or substrate feeders use biting type methods in feeding. In most fish, there is a combination of feeding methods used, with suction feeding predominating.

Failure to provide appropriate substrate or proper food sources for captive fish species may lead to numerous problems, including chronic stress, nutritional deficiencies, starvation, and general debilitation, leading to secondary infections and immune suppression. Environmental enrichment feeding goals should address the natural feeding behaviors of fish.[16]

Mouthbrooding

At least 8 families of fishes practice mouthbrooding (also known as oral or buccal incubation) of the eggs and fry (recently hatched fish).[17–19] The most well-known ornamental fish are members of the Cichlidae family (freshwater tropical cichlids) and Apogonidae (marine cardinal fish).[19] Strategies vary and include biparental, female-only, and male-only mouthbrooding.[18] It is hypothesized that mouthbrooding evolved from biparental substrate guarding.[18,19] Mouthbrooding fish can experience difficulty in hypoxic conditions.[18] Hypoxic conditions increased the need for increased ventilation. Increasing ventilation can be difficult with a large brood of eggs occupying a large volume of the oral cavity. Filial cannibalism or eggs being spit out can occur when hypoxic conditions require increased ventilation because of the large volume the egg mass occupies in the oral cavity.[18] One study demonstrated one species of cardinal fish, *Apogon fragilis*, spat out eggs more readily in response to hypoxia than another cardinal fish, *Apogon leptacanthus*.[18] The primary reason seems to be because *A fragilis* males tend to hold a larger egg mass in their mouths, up to 26% of their body weight compared with *A leptacanthus*, whose egg mass was only 14% of body weight.[19] In cases of continued loss of egg masses by mouthbrooding fish, checking water-quality parameters, particularly dissolved oxygen, would be a crucial part of the case workup.

It is also worth noting that temperature has been shown to affect sex of the offspring in one species of farmed mouthbrooding cichlids, *Oreochromis niloticus*, (Nile tilapia).[20] Male fish are preferred because they grow faster, reaching marketable size sooner. This fact may have future commercial applications but is not the current practice today; the current method includes exposure to $17,\alpha$ methyltestosterone, as fry causes females to become phenotypically male.[21]

In a fish version of size matters, the female Banggai cardinal fish, (*Pteragon kauderni*), produced heavier, larger eggs when paired with large males compared with small clutches when paired with small males.[22] Banggai cardinal fish are obligate paternal mouthbrooders, so choosing a larger male for commercial or home spawning may yield higher numbers of viable offspring.

Studies indicate fry from mouthbrooding parents may receive passive immunity to aid in the prevention of some disease outbreaks. Fry of the maternal mouthbrooding *Oreochromis aureus*, blue tilapia, were protected by passive transfer of protective immunity from mothers vaccinated against *Ichthyophthirius multifiliis*.[23]

Many hobbyists keep species that originate from the same natural environment or geographic area. The colorful, engaging African cichlids are a very common group that is kept in a multi species tank. Freshwater species of the African Great Lakes (Lake Malawi, Lake Victoria, and Lake Tanganyika) are commonly kept in community or cichlid tanks by hobbyists with other species. One popular addition to these African Rift lake tanks is the *Synodontis* sp catfish, also native to Africa. One species in this group, *Synodontis multipunctatus*, is a known brood parasitic catfish.[24] *S multipunctatus* is attracted by spawning cichlids (presumably by smell) and spawns at the same time and in the same location as the spawning cichlid pairs. The cichlids will take up the eggs of this catfish and buccal incubate them with their own eggs. The catfish fry typically hatch earlier than the cichlid fry and will eat the cichlid fry as they hatch inside the female's mouth. The female cichlid will care for and protect them while they are vulnerable. A great video example of this behavior can be found online.[25]

CLINICAL DISORDERS OF THE ORAL CAVITY

Both a good history and physical examination are of paramount importance for effective diagnosis of disease in all animals, and fish are no different. There are several textbooks that discuss how to perform a thorough history[26–28] and complete physical examination in fish.[29–33] Sedation will help facilitate an examination and should always be used if the fish is fractious or has the potential to cause injury to itself and the practitioner. A standard otoscope or small rigid endoscope can be used to illuminate the oral cavity for examination in small fish (**Fig. 4**A).

Oral examinations on larger fish can be accomplished with a direct illumination into the open mouth (see **Fig. 4**B) using a flashlight or an endoscope. A thorough understanding of the normal anatomy of the species is necessary to diagnose or differentiate an actual lesion from a normal anatomic structure. In most cases, bilaterally symmetric structures are normal, such as the rough oral pads seen in the tiger shovel-nosed catfish (*Pseudoplatystoma* sp) shown in **Fig. 4**B. Examination of a noninfected cohort of the same species can also help identify normal anatomic structures.

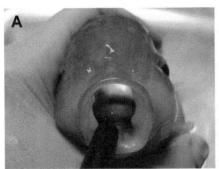 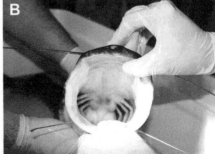

Fig. 4. (*A*) Illumination of the mouth of a goldfish (*Carassius auratus*) with an otoscope. (*B*) Open mouth of tiger shovel-nosed catfish (*Pseudoplatystoma sp*) illuminated by flashlight. (*Courtesy of* Helen Roberts-Sweeney, DVM, Williamsville, NY; with permission.)

This article placees emphasis on infectious, neoplastic, traumatic, and toxic disorders of the oral cavity in fish.

The oral cavity of fish has direct access to the external environment resulting exposure to environmental pollutants and pathogens. In addition, captive fish are subject to issues relating to poor husbandry techniques and management practices.

Infectious Diseases

In captive fish populations, most infectious disease is related to a failure to quarantine new animals. Rapid transmission can occur in closed, recirculating systems, especially if husbandry and water quality are marginal. Viral diseases in fish usually have a specific viral permissive temperature range. It is important to quarantine susceptible species within this temperature range for an adequate length of time. For example, quarantining koi (C carpio) at 16°C to 28°C is recommended to allow for clinical signs of koi herpesvirus (cyprinid herpesvirus 3).[34] Quarantine is one example of the necessary, but often ignored, biosecurity practices necessary to keep infectious disease to a minimum in a stable population.

Viral diseases of concern affecting the oral cavity

1. Cyprinid herpesvirus 1 (carp pox) causes hyperplastic, papillomatous, smooth, candle wax–appearing cutaneous lesions, primarily in cooler water (<20°C/68°F). These lesions can regress in warmer water. Oral lesions typically involve the lips (**Fig. 5**) but the lesions can appear anywhere on the skin. Koi hobbyists are primarily concerned over the cosmetic appearance if they are involved in showing their fish. The virus has been shown to be lethal in koi fry but is not typically a problem in adult fish.[35]
2. Lymphocystis is the most common viral disease seen in pet fish.[35,36] The causative agent is an iridovirus, and the disease affects marine and freshwater species with varying susceptibility. The virus causes dermal fibroblasts to hypertrophy, up to 10,000 times their normal size.[35] A typical clinical sign is the appearance of multiple focal gray or white masses. Wet mounts of skin scrapings will demonstrate the hypertrophied cells. Lesions often regress over time, especially with stress-reduction techniques and careful handling practices.[35,36] If the lesions are located in, on, or

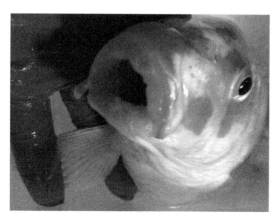

Fig. 5. The lips of a koi (*Cyprinus carpio*) affected by carp pox. (*Courtesy of* Helen Roberts-Sweeney, DVM, Williamsville, NY; with permission.)

around the mouth, they may interfere with eating. These lesions can be surgically reduced but may reappear at a later time.

3. Angelfish lip fibromas may be associated with a viral cause. Multiple clinically affected fish can be found in one tank; retroviral-like particles have been found on electron microscopy, but attempts to reproduce the disease have not been successful.[35,36] Depending on the reference, lip fibromas may be classified as a viral disease, neoplasia, or retroviral-associated neoplasia.[35,37–39] The masses can interfere with feeding and can be surgically excised.

4. Less common viruses[39,40] causing oral disease in fish are listed in **Table 1**.

Bacterial diseases of concern affecting the oral cavity

1. *Flavobacterium columnare*, previously known as *Flexibacter columnaris*, is a gram-negative, orange-to-yellow pigmented, colony-forming bacteria and the etiologic agent of columnaris disease (fin rot, cotton-wool mouth).[36,41] Columnaris disease affects many species of fish, both wild and captive.[41,42] A common presentation in tropical fish is the development of oral ulcerations that may develop secondary fungal infections giving rise to the terms *cotton wool disease*, *mouth rot*, and mouth fungus.

    Clinical signs are not pathognomonic and include fluffy cutaneous patches or cutaneous ulceration on the fins/tail, mouth (necrotic stomatitis), periocular region, and the dorsal aspect (saddleback disease).[41–43] Infections involving the gills will cause respiratory signs (dyspnea, piping, gasping, and so forth).[43] The disease is often secondary to poor water quality, overcrowding, poor husbandry, and other stressors in the environment.[43,44]

    Diagnosis can be made in the clinic by evaluating wet mount preparations from the lesions. The wet mount prep examination reveals long, thin rods that may glide or flex or are arranged in a haystack appearance.[36,41,43]

    Experimentally induced infection in koi (*C carpio*) was shown to significantly reduce packed cell volume, cause marked hyponatremia, hypochloridemia (due to loss of osmoregulatory capacity), and hyglycemia.[41] Significant increases in alkaline phosphatase, aspartate aminotransferase, lactate dehydrogenase, and creatine kinase were also reported.[41]

    In addition to correcting any underlying contributing factors, bath treatments can be used to treat columnaris disease (**Table 2**). For severe infections, systemic antimicrobials may be necessary.

2. *Flavobacterium psychrophilum* (bacterial cold-water disease, peduncle disease, saddleback disease) has been shown to cause pyogranulomatous and necrotic

Table 1 Less common viruses affecting the oral cavity in fish		
Virus	**Species Affected**	**Lesions Seen**
Oncorhyncus masu virus (Salmonid herpesvirus 2)	Masu, coho, chum and kokanee salmon, rainbow trout	Epithelial tumors (cutaneous carcinomas) on the mouth and jaw
White sturgeon herpesvirus	White sturgeon	Oral, epidermal hyperplasia
Tiger puffer virus (white mouth disease, kuchihiro-sho)	Tiger puffer, grass puffer, fine-patterned puffer, panther puffer, pagrus sea bream, Schlegel black rockfish	Oral and snout ulcerations

Table 2
Bath treatments for superficial bacterial diseases such as columnaris

Copper sulfate	1–4-h bath treatment 100 mg/L 0.2 mg/L free copper ion for prolonged immersion	*Always observe fish during treatment.* Measure alkalinity before calculating dose. Reduced alkalinity and low pH increases toxicity of copper. It is immunosuppressive and can cause gill toxicity.
Diquat[1,3]	2–18 mg/L 4-hour baths	Monitor fish during treatment. Repeat daily for 3–4 treatments.
Hydrogen peroxide	3.1 mg/L for 1-h bath treatment	Monitor fish during treatment.
Oxytetracycline	750–3780 mg per 10 gallons for 6–12 h, repeat daily for 10 d (dose will depend on hardness of water)	It is not very effective in hard water or seawater.
Potassium permanganate	2 mg/L prolonged immersion	Levels are reduced by high levels of organic matter in the water. Treatment can be stopped by adding hydrogen peroxide to water.

Adapted from Roberts HE, Palmeiro B, Weber ES. Bacterial and parasitic diseases of pet fish. Vet Clin North Am Exot Anim Pract 2009;12:615; with permission.

lesions in the cartilage and bone of the snout, vertebrae, and surrounding tissues, sometimes referred to as "dissolving head disease."[44,45] Antimicrobials, as for columnaris disease, may be used in addition to correcting husbandry and management deficiencies.[44]

3. *Tenacibaculum maritimum* (formerly known as *Flexibacter maritimus*) is a gram-negative bacteria that causes lesions similar to *F columnare* or columnaris disease in marine species, primarily young fish.[36,42]

4. Enteric redmouth disease is caused by the gram-negative rod, *Yersinia ruckeri*.[36,42,46] The disease is seen in salmonid species, such as rainbow trout (*Oncorhynchus mykiss*), and can cause significant economic losses in the industry.[46] Subcutaneous hemorrhages of the mouth, gums, and tongue are typically seen, giving the disease its name. The disease condition can be anywhere from acute with high mortalities, especially in young fish, to chronic, low-level mortalities in older fish. Diagnosis is made by culture or serologic testing.[46] Treatment involves the use of antimicrobial therapy, adding probiotics, and vaccination, and improved sanitation and biosecurity practices.[36,46] In food fish, antimicrobial options are limited to a few approved drugs, including oxytetracycline and oxolinic acid.

5. Oral lesions are often seen associated with or secondary to systemic bacterial infections. In the author's practice, lip lesions are noted in koi with systemic aeromonad infections (**Fig. 6**). Erosions, ulcerations, and severe osteomyelitis can be seen in the mouth and surrounding tissue. These infections are often secondary to severe parasitism, poor water quality, and other immunosuppressive conditions. More about systemic aeromonad infections and treatment recommendations has been previously reported.[43]

6. Mycobacteriosis is the most common chronic bacterial disease in aquarium fish.[47,48] The most often identified species causing mycobacteriosis in fish include *Mycobacterium marinum*, *M fortuitum*, and *Mycobacterium chelonae*.[43,48]

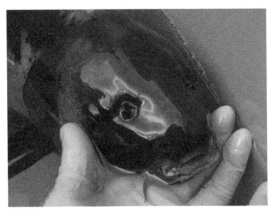

Fig. 6. Linear ulceration on the dorsal lip of a koi (*Cyprinus carpio*). (*Courtesy of* Helen Roberts-Sweeney, DVM, Williamsville, NY; with permission.)

Mycobacteria are slow-growing, acid-fast-staining bacteria and are ubiquitous in the aquatic environment.[43,48] Mycobacteriosis is also a zoonotic disease (fish handler's disease or fish tank granuloma) and causes ulcerative or raised granulomatous nodules.[47] The lesions are typically located on the extremities because of the temperature preferences of *Mycobacterium* spp.[47] The most common clinical signs seen in fish affected with mycobacteriosis are granulomas located in internal organs, although granulomas can also form inside the oral cavity.

In one publication,[49] *M chelonae* was found associated with tumorlike skin and oral masses in Russian sturgeons, *Acipenser gueldenstaedii. M chelonae* was considered a secondary to trauma and increased stress in the sturgeons.[49] Lesions developed in areas on the fish susceptible to chronic traumatic injury. It was theorized these traumatic lesions developed dystrophic calcification, then subsequent granuloma formation in response to the foreign body, calcium.[49] The lesions were subsequently colonized by the opportunistic, ubiquitous *M chelonae.*[49] None of the typical internal granulomas were seen in the fish, making mycobacteriosis unlikely to be the primary cause of the oral and skin masses.[49]

7. *Vibrio spp*, a marine gram-negative bacteria, causes disease in a wide variety of marine fish species.[43,47,48] Clinical signs are similar to those found in aeromonad infections in freshwater fish species, including cutaneous ulcerations and systemic infections. *Vibrio splendidus* infections have been reported to cause lesions in the jaw and oral cavity of farmed turbot.[42] *Vibrio vulnificus* is the most reported *Vibrio* spp cultured in zoonotic infections in humans.[47]

8. A less commonly seen pathogen, Sekiten-byo (*Pseudomonas anguilliseptica*) causes petechiae around the mouth, operculum, and ventrum of Japanese and European eels.[48] Experimentally induced infections can be seen in common carp, bluegills, goldfish, ayu, and crucian carp.[48]

Parasitic diseases affecting the oral cavity
Many common external parasites can be found in and around the oral cavity in addition to the rest of the external body. A few in particular favor the oral cavity and surrounding tissues.

1. Parasitic isopod infestations often involve the oral cavity of wild, marine fish.[36] These crustacean parasites are grossly visible and are manually removed if present in a few numbers or treated with bath medications, including organophosphates.[36] One of the largest isopod families, Cymothoids, contains members that specifically target the oral and buccal cavity of fish.[36,50,51] One member, *Cymothoa exigua*, the tongue eating isopod, causes degenerative changes in the tongue of the host fish, a common food fish (rose snapper).[52] It then replaces and functions as the tongue by attaching to the remaining stub.[52]

2. Myxosporeans, spore-producing parasites with complex life cycles, have a world-wide distribution and infect a variety of fish species.[43] Not all species are pathogenic. A Myxobolus sp was found to cause an oral deformity in a goldfish, *C auratus*.[53] The goldfish presented respiratory difficulty, flared opercula on one side, unilateral exophthalmia, and anorexia. Exploration of the area revealed a pink, nodular mass partially occluding the mouth and associated ventrally with the gill arch[53] (**Fig. 7**). Tentative diagnosis was made based on an impression smear of the mass.[53] Another myxosporean, *Myxobolus oralis* sp, has been associated with infection of the palate of a gibel carp, *Carassius auratus gibelio*.[54] There is no effective treatment of myxozoan infections. Prevention and management is aimed at preventing the presence of the intermediate hosts, oligochaete worms (red worms, black worms, *Tubifex* worms). Unfortunately these are often fed as a live food source to aquarium fish.[55]

3. *Epistylis*, a ciliated sedentary protozoan, is a common secondary pathogen of skin damage caused by bacteria, other primary parasites, and trauma.[36,43] The oral cavity is a common site of infestation. *Epistylis* infestations can appear as white, cottony, fluffy lesions similar to *Flavobacterium* infections (columnaris disease) and fungal infections.[36,43] Wet mount preparations of the lesion examined under direct microscopy will help differentiate. Formalin and salt as baths or prolonged immersion can be helpful in treating *Epistylis*.[36]

4. The ocean sunfish, Mola mola, is often infested by the trematode parasite *Accacoelium contortum*. This parasite attaches itself inside the pharyngeal and gill chambers, causing an extensive inflammatory response.[56] Interestingly, more parasites were found on the right side than the left.[56] The reason was proposed to be due to ocean sunfish behavior of leaning their bodies on the right as they incline when in lateral recumbency.[56] The parasites on the left side would be more exposed to desiccation, heating, and UV exposure.[56]

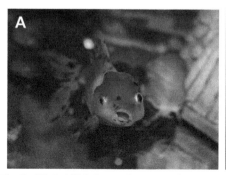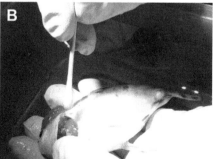

Fig. 7. (*A*) Goldfish (*Carassius auratus*) showing deviation/deformity of the mouth. (*B*) Exploration reveals nodular mass below left operculum. (*Courtesy of* Helen Roberts-Sweeney, DVM, Williamsville, NY; with permission.)

Fungal infections of the oral cavity

Most fungal infections found in the oral cavity of fish are caused by *Saprolegnia*, a common water mold (*Oomycetes*). Water molds are opportunistic and often associated with immunosuppression in fish.[36] Immune suppression can occur with primary infections; poor water quality; rapidly changing water conditions; increased fish density in ponds, tanks, raceways, and aquaria; and other common stressors. Diagnosis of secondary fungal infections should always steer the clinician to search for primary problems on/in the fish or in the environment. Fungal infections appear as white to tan, fluffy, superficial lesions. Diagnosis is made by examination of wet mount preparations taken from the lesions of a live fish. Dead fish will quickly become colonized by saprophytic fungi, so it is critical to evaluate the lesion on live fish. It is important to perform a wet mount preparation to differentiate fungal lesions from columnaris disease and *Epistylis* infections.[36,43] Treatment is aimed at identification and correction of primary stressors. Prolonged immersion in less than 3 parts per thousand noniodized salt can aid in healing. Other treatments, such as malachite green, are not recommended. Malachite green is a known carcinogen and is prohibited from use in food fish.

Neoplasia of the Oral Cavity

Neoplasms in fish reflect the tissue type of the oral cavity. The cause can be genetic mutation, husbandry or environmental stressors, and virally associated or induced. Often the cause is multifactorial involving genetic susceptibility, stress of captivity (overcrowding, poor nutritional status, trauma), and exposure to carcinogenic pollutants in the environment.[37,57] The incidence of virally induced tumors in wild fish often shows a seasonal pattern.[57,58] **Table 3** lists the most common viral-associated tumors in fish.

Spawning, viral permissive temperatures, pollutants, life stage of the fish, water temperature, and weather patterns have all been suggested as contributing factors for the seasonality associated with development of tumors in fish.[37,58,59] In wild fish,

Table 3 Viral-associated neoplasia of the oral cavity in fish			
Carp pox/cyprinid herpesvirus 1	*Cyprinus carpio*	Benign papillomas	—
Onchorhyncus masu virus	Salmonids, including Masu, coho, chum and kokanee salmon, rainbow trout	Epithelial tumors (cutaneous carcinomas) on the mouth and jaw	—
Retroviral-like particles (unidentified)	*Pterophyllum scalare* (freshwater angelfish)	Angelfish lip fibroma/ odontoma	Experiments thus far have failed to isolate the virus.
Retroviral-like particles	*Catostomus commersoni* (white sucker)	Epidermal papillomas, predilection for lips and head[7]	Experiments to isolate the virus have been unsuccessful. Pollution may be a contributing factor.
Virus suspected papillomatosis	*Anguilla anguilla* (European eel)	Oral papillomas, commonly around mouth[6]	Lesions regress with cooler water temperatures or higher salinities.

the presence of polynuclear aromatic hydrocarbon and chlorinated chemical contaminated sediments have been associated with squamous cell carcinomas and papillomas.[37,59–61] In particular, bottom-dwelling fish that scavenge the floor of lakes, streams, and rivers have increased prey contamination, incidence of oral trauma, and exposure to pollutants in sediments.[37,59–61]

Squamous cell carcinoma is a frequent diagnosis of cutaneous neoplasms in koi (*C carpio*) in the author's practice. Lesions can appear anywhere on the body, including the mouth (**Fig. 8**). Masses can interfere with feeding and lead to emaciation, poor condition, and death.

Masses of any kind should be removed or biopsied to determine cell type. Treatment success depends on degree of tissue invasion, condition of the fish, and the level of owner commitment.

Miscellaneous Disorders of the Oral Cavity

1. Traumatic injury of the oral cavity is a relatively common occurrence in captive fishes.[62] Mechanical damage to the mouth results in deformities, hemorrhages, hematomas, tissue erosion, and snout deformation.[62] Traumatic injuries can result in an inability to feed and breath normally.[62] Lightning strikes in ponds, predators, and sudden changes in the environment (inappropriate lighting conditions, sudden presence of light, presence of humans) that trigger the startle reflex result in self-inflicted oral injuries as the fish move rapidly and strike objects, such as the sides of a pond or aquaria with their mouth. These injuries are often accompanied by opercular and spinal trauma.[62] Netting fish can cause trauma to delicate mouthparts in addition to the fins and tail.[62] Oral damage is likely to be painful, and the fish should be treated appropriately with analgesics. Wounds and secondary infections should be treated via debridement (if needed) and appropriate antimicrobials.
2. Nutritional diseases affecting the oral cavity are listed in **Table 4**.[63,64] Nutritional diseases are often caused by inadequate knowledge on the natural diet of the captive species, feeding a diet meant for one species to another, unrelated species (commercial catfish food given to salmonids, the use of outdated food, and the feeding of spoiled or rancid food.
3. Traditionally bottom-feeding fish that ingest and spit out inedible items (stones, small twigs, tank décor), such as goldfish (*C auratus*) and koi (*C carpio*), are

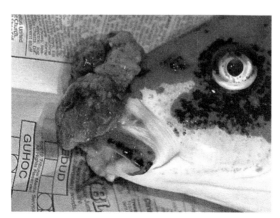

Fig. 8. Squamous cell carcinoma on the rostrum of a koi (*Cyprinus carpio*). (*Courtesy of* Helen Roberts-Sweeney, DVM, Williamsville, NY; with permission.)

Table 4
Nutritional disorders of the oral cavity

Hypovitaminosis C	Short snout, lower jaw deformity, including erosion/ulceration	Vitamin C content in food diminishes quickly. Replacing food every 90 d is suggested.[3]	—
Hypervitaminosis A	Overall increase in mouth deformities, pug headedness	There is an increased incidence due to metabolite and retinoic acid.	—
Niacin deficiency	Hemorrhage and erosion around the mouth	—	—
Leucine excess in diet	Deformed opercula	It is noted in rainbow trout (Onchorhyncus mykiss).	—
Phosphorus deficiency	Cranial deformities	It is noted in carp/koi (Cyprinus carpio).	—
Pantothenic acid deficiency	Deformities of the lower jaw and head	It is noted in channel catfish (Ictalurus punctatus).	Protect food from excessive heat.

susceptible to oral and pharyngeal foreign bodies. The most common foreign body is a piece of gravel or rock substrate (**Fig. 9**). Appropriate-sized substrate should be provided for these fish. Historically, it is not uncommon of the owner to report the fish appear hungry and approach the food but do not ingest it. On examination, these fish may have developed erythema, erosions, or ulceration ventral to the foreign body. Foreign bodies can also be observed in other captive species with a tendency to ingest anything in the search of food. Diagnosis of an oral foreign body is made by direct visualization of the oral cavity. Most items can be removed in the sedated or anesthetized fish via forceps. Occasionally, surgical extraction and repair of the surrounding tissue is necessary. Prophylactic antibiotics, analgesics, and gavage feeding may be necessary in fish with a large degree of trauma to the oral cavity.

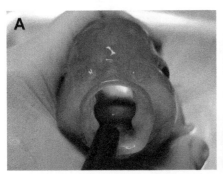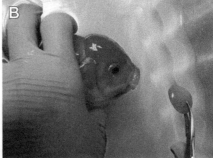

Fig. 9. (A) Open mouth examination of goldfish (Carassius auratus) with pharyngeal foreign body visible (gravel). (B) Gravel removed. Note the size in comparison with the mouth and body size. (Courtesy of Helen Roberts-Sweeney, DVM, Williamsville, NY; with permission.)

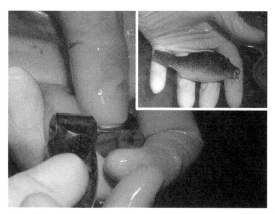

Fig. 10. Sedated puffer fish, lateral aspect showing dental overgrowth (*inset*); and using a dental handpiece with bur to reduce overgrown beak. (*Courtesy of* Helen Roberts-Sweeney, DVM, Williamsville, NY; with permission.)

4. The most common dental abnormality seen in pet fish is overgrowth of the incisor platelike teeth in Tetraodontidae, puffer fish. The incisor teeth of puffer fish are fused and can resemble a beak. These incisor plates continuously grow throughout life and are usually worn down by their natural feeding habits. Failure to provide a source of species-appropriate corals, mollusks, and crustaceans in captivity can result in severe overgrowth and malocclusion. Clinical signs and symptoms include anorexia, inability to close the mouth, severe malocclusion, and death due to an inability to eat. In addition, traumatic injury can occur because of excessively hard food items, leading to fracture of the plates, malocclusion, jaw fractures, and secondary infections. A good oral examination under sedation allows a complete look at the external and inner aspect of the dental plates.

Trimming of the teeth has been described[65] and can readily be performed in a clinical setting with a minimal investment in equipment. Small-animal high-speed dental handpieces equipped with a bur head (**Fig. 10**) or a low-speed device, such as a Dremel tool (Dremel, Racine, WI), equipped with a grinding disc[65] are effective in reducing the teeth to the proper size and alignment. It is important to include client education and suggest husbandry changes to prevent recurrence in these fish. Regular follow-ups are suggested to monitor the teeth.

SUMMARY

Oral disorders in captive fish are fairly common and usually readily identifiable. Clinical signs and symptoms, such as anorexia, food regurgitation, persistent and frequent opercular movements, coughing, rubbing, and identifiable masses and deformities, should be evaluated and treated promptly when possible. Because the oral cavity is essential to proper feeding and respiration, oral disorders may have fatal consequences if not diagnosed and treated early.

ACKNOWLEDGMENTS

The author would like to thank Detective Kevin Sweeney for his continued support and all the pet fish owners that allow us to expand the knowledge base of pet fish medicine. Special thanks to those pictured here: Lucita (**Figs. 1** and **2**), Maggie (**Fig. 7**), Goldie (**Figs. 4**A and **9**), and Mr Cuddles (**Fig. 4**B).

REFERENCES

1. Miller-Morgan TA. Brief overview of the ornamental fish industry and hobby. In: Roberts HE, editor. Fundamentals of ornamental fish health. Ames (IA): Wiley-Blackwell; 2009. p. 25–32.
2. Gibb AC, Staab K, Moran C, et al. The teleost intramandibular joint: a mechanism that allows fish to obtain prey unavailable to suction feeders. Integr Comp Biol 2015;55:85–96.
3. Hernandez LP, Ferry-Graham LA, Gibb AC. Morphology of a picky eater: a novel mechanism underlies premaxillary protrusion and retraction within cyprinodontiforms. Zoology (Jena) 2007;111:442–54.
4. Ferry LA, Konow N, Gibb AC. Are kissing gourami specialized for substrate-feeding? prey capture kinematics of helostoma temminckii and other anabantoid fishes. J Exp Zool A Ecol Genet Physiol 2012;317(9):571–9.
5. Gibb AC, Ferry-Graham LA, Hernandez LP, et al. Functional significance of Intramandibular bending in Poeciliid fishes. Environ Biol Fish 2008;83:507–19.
6. Koldewey H. Syngnathid husbandry manual. Project Seahorse. USDA National Agricultural Library website. 2005. Available at: https://awic.nal.usda.gov/zoo-circus-and-marine-animals/exhibit-animal-species/fish. Accessed November 20, 2015.
7. Bergert BA, Wainwright PC. Morphology and kinematics of prey capture in the syngnathid fishes Hippocampus erectus and Syngnathus floridae. Mar Biol 1997;127:563–70.
8. Evans HE. Anatomy of tropical fishes. In: Gratzek JB, Evans HE, Reinert RE, et al, editors. Fish anatomy, physiology, and nutrition. Morris Plains (NJ): Tetra Press; 1992. p. 19–41.
9. Stoskopf MK. Anatomy. In: Stospkopf MK, editor. Fish medicine. Philadelphia: WB Saunders; 1993. p. 449.
10. Aerts P. Hyoid morphology and movements related to abducting forces during feeding in Astaotilapia elegans (Teleostei: Cichlidae). J Morphol 1991;208(3): 323–45.
11. Camp AL, Brainerd EL. Role of axial muscles in powering mouth expansion during suction feeding in largemouth bass (Micropterus salmoides). J Exp Biol 2014; 217:1333–45.
12. Camp AL, Roberts TJ, Brainerd EL. Swimming muscles power suction feeding in largemouth bass. Proc Natl Acad Sci U S A 2015;112(28):8690–5.
13. Abbate F, Germana GP, DeCarlos F, et al. The oral cavity of the adult zebrafish (Danio rerio). Anat Histol Embryol 2006;35:299–304.
14. Ferry LA, Paig-Tran EM, Gibb AC. Suction, ram, and biting: deviations and limitations to the capture of aquatic prey. Integr Comp Biol 2015;55(1):97–109.
15. Skorczewski T, Cheer A, Cheung S, et al. Use of computational fluid dynamics to study forces exerted on prey by aquatic suction feeders. J R Soc Interface 2010; 7:475–84.
16. Corcoran M. Environmental enrichment for aquatic animals. Vet Clin North Am Exot Anim Pract 2015;18:305–21.
17. Ostlund-Nilsson S, Nilsson GE. Breathing with a mouth full of eggs: respiratory consequences of mouthbrooding in cardinalfish. Proc Biol Sci 2004;271:1015–22.

18. Balshine-Earn S, Earn DJD. On the evolutionary pathway of parental care in mouth-brooding cichlid fish. Proc Roy Soc Lond B Biol Sci 1998;265:2217–22.
19. Goodwin NB, Balshine-Earn S, Reynolds JD. Evolutionary transitions in parental care. Proc Roy Soc Lond B Biol Sci 1998;265:2265–72.
20. Baroiller JF, Chourrout D, Fostier A, et al. Temperature and sex chromosome govern sex ratios of the mouthbrooding Cichlid fish Oreochromis niloticus. J Exp Zool 1995;273(3):216–23.
21. Rakocy JE. Cultured aquatic species information programme. Oreochromis niloticus. Rome (Italy): FAO Fisheries and Aquaculture Department; 2005. Available at: http://www.fao.org/fishery/culturedspecies/Oreochromis_niloticus/en. Accessed December 1, 2015.
22. Kolm N. Females produce larger eggs for large males in a paternal mouthbrooding fish. Proc Biol Sci 2001;268:2229–34.
23. Sin YM, Ling KH, Lam TJ. Passive transfer of protective immunity against ichthyophthiriasis from vaccinated mother to fry in tilapias, Oreochromis aureus. Aquaculture 1994;120:229–37.
24. Sato T. A brood parasitic catfish of mouthbrooding cichlid fishes in Lake Tanganyika. Nature 1986;323:58–9.
25. National Geographic. 2016. Available at: Http://Video.Nationalgeographic.Com/Video/Cichlid_Movingyoung. Accessed January 19, 2016.
26. Noga EJ. Fish disease diagnosis form. In fish disease: diagnosis and treatment, Appendix I. St Louis (MO): Mosby; 1996. p. 327–8.
27. Roberts HE. History. In: Roberts HE, editor. Fundamentals of ornamental fish health. Ames (IA): Wiley-Blackwell; 2009. p. 158–60.
28. Stoskopf MK. Tropical fish medicine. Taking the history. Vet Clin North Am Small Anim Pract 1988;18(2):283–91.
29. Butcher RL. General approach. In: Wildgoose W, editor. BSAVA manual of ornamental fish. 2nd edition. Gloucester (United Kingdom): BSAVA Publications; 2001. p. 63–7.
30. Campbell TW. Performing a basic examination in fish. Vet Med 2005;100(12): 844–55.
31. Roberts HE. Physical examination of the fish. In: Roberts HE, editor. Fundamentals of ornamental fish health. Ames (IA): Wiley-Blackwell; 2009. p. 161–5.
32. Stoskopf MK. Clinical examination and procedures. In: Stoskopf MK, editor. Fish medicine. Philadelphia: WB Saunders Co; 1993. p. 62–78.
33. Weber ES, Innis C. Piscine patients: basic diagnostics. Compend Contin Educ Vet 2007;29(5):276–88.
34. McDermott C, Palmeiro B. Selected emerging infectious diseases of ornamental fish. Vet Clin North Am Exot Anim Pract 2013;16:261–82.
35. Petty BD, Fraser WA. Viruses of pet fish. Vet Clin North Am Exot Anim Pract 2005; 8:67–84.
36. Noga EJ. Problems 11 through 43: diagnoses made by either gross external examination of fish, wet mounts of skin/gills, or histopathology of skin/gills. In: Noga EJ, editor. Fish disease: diagnosis and treatment. 2nd edition. Ames (IA): Wiley-Blackwell; 2010. p. 107–77.
37. Martineau D, Ferguson HW. Neoplasia. In: Ferguson HW, editor. Systemic pathology of fish: a text and atlas of normal tissues in teleosts and their responses in disease. 2nd edition. Ames (IA): Scotian Press; 2006. p. 312–35.
38. Francis-Floyd R, Bolon B, Fraser W, et al. Lip fibromas associated with retrovirus-like particles in angel fish. J Am Vet Med Assoc 1993;202(3):427–9.

39. Noga EJ. Problems 77 through 88: rule-out diagnoses 1(viral infections): presumptive diagnoses is based on absence of other etiologies combined with a diagnostically appropriate history, clinical signs, and/or pathology. Definitive diagnosis is based on presumptive diagnosis combined with confirmation of viral presence. In: Noga EJ, editor. Fish disease: diagnosis and treatment. 2nd edition. Ames (IA): Wiley-Blackwell; 2010. p. 269–303.

40. Spickler AR. Oncorhynchus masou virus disease. 2007. Available at: http://www.cfsph.iastate.edu/Factsheets/pdfs/oncorhynchus_masou_virus_disease.pdf. Accessed October 20, 2015.

41. Declercq AM, Haesebrouck F, Van den Broeck W, et al. Columnaris disease in fish: a review with emphasis on bacterium-host interactions. Vet Res 2013;44:27.

42. Lumsden JS. Gastrointestinal tract, swim bladder, pancreas, and peritoneum. In: Ferguson HW, editor. Systemic pathology of fish: a text and atlas of normal tissues in teleosts and their responses in disease. 2nd edition. Ames (IA): Scotian Press; 2006. p. 169–99.

43. Roberts HE, Palmeiro B, Weber ES. Bacterial and parasitic diseases of pet fish. Vet Clin North Am Exot Anim Pract 2009;12:609–38.

44. Bebak JA, Welch TJ, Starliper CE, et al. Improved husbandry to control an outbreak of rainbow trout fry syndrome caused by infection with Flavobacterium psychrophilum. J Am Vet Med Assoc 2007;231(1):114–6.

45. Koppang EO, Bjerkas E. The eye. In: Ferguson HW, editor. Systemic pathology of fish: a text and atlas of normal tissues in teleosts and their responses in disease. 2nd edition. Ames (IA): Scotian Press; 2006. p. 245–65.

46. Kumar G, Menanteau-Ledouble S, Saleh M, et al. Yersinia ruckeri, the causative agent of enteric redmouth disease in fish. Vet Res 2015;46:103.

47. Lowry T, Smith SA. Aquatic zoonoses associated with food, bait, ornamental, and tropical fish. J Am Vet Med Assoc 2007;231(6):876–80.

48. Noga EJ. Problems 45 through 57: diagnoses made by bacterial culture of the kidney or affected organs. In: Noga EJ, editor. Fish disease: diagnosis and treatment. 2nd edition. Ames (IA): Wiley-Blackwell; 2010. p. 107–77.

49. Antuofermo E, Pais A, Hetzel U, et al. Mycobacterium chelonae associated with tumor-like skin and oral masses in farmed Russian sturgeons (Acipenser gueldenstaedtii). BMC Vet Res 2014;10:18.

50. Brusca RC. A monograph on the Isopoda Cymothoidae (Crustacea) of the Eastern Pacific. Zoo J Linn Soc 1981;73:117–99.

51. Thatcher VE, de Araujo GS, de Lima JT, et al. Cymothoa spinipalpa sp. nov (Isopoda, Cymothoidae) a buccal cavity parasite of the marine fish, Oligoplites saurus (Bloch & Schneider) (Osteichthyes, Carangidae) of Rio Grande do Norte State, Brazil. Rev Bras Zool 2007;24(1):238–45.

52. Dos Santos Costa EF, de Oliveira MR, Chellappa S. First record of Cymothoa spinipalpa (Isopoda: Cymothoidae) parasitizing the marine fish Atlantic bumper, Chloroscombrus chrysurus (Osteichthyes: Carangidae) from Brazil. Marine Biodiversity Records 2010;3(e1):1–6.

53. Nolan MW, Roberts HE, Zimmerman KL, et al. Pathology in practice. Severe, chronic, focal, granulomatous, nodular and ulcerative stomatitis with myxosporidia (Myxobolus sp.). J Am Vet Med Assoc 2010;236(6):631–3.

54. Liu Y, Whipps CM, Nie P, et al. Myxobolus oralis sp. n (Myxosporea: Bivalvulida) infecting the palate in the mouth of gibel carp, Carassius auratus gibelio (Cypriniformes: Cyprinidae). Folia Parasitol 2014;61(6):505–11.

55. Noga EJ. Problems 58 through 76: diagnoses made by necropsy of the viscera and examination of wet mounts or histopathology of internal organs.

In: Noga EJ, editor. Fish disease: diagnosis and treatment. 2nd edition. Ames (IA): Wiley-Blackwell; 2010. p. 107–77.

56. Ahuir-Baraja AE, Padros F, Palacios-Abella JF, et al. Accacoelium contortum (Trematoda: Accacolelidae) a trematode living as a monogenean: morphological and pathological implications. Parasit Vectors 2015;8:540.

57. Coffee LL, Casey JW, Bowser PR. Pathology of tumors in fish associated with retroviruses: a review. Vet Pathol 2013;50(3):390–403.

58. Anders K, Yoshimizu M. Role of viruses in the induction of skin tumours and tumour-like proliferations of fish. Dis Aquat Organ 1994;19:215–32.

59. US Fish and Wildlife Service, Chesapeake Bay Office. Fact sheet: tumors in brown bullhead catfish in the Anacostia and Potomac Rivers. 2013. Available at: www.fws.gov/chesapeakebay/pdf/BrownBullheadTumorsFactSheet%200416 2013.pdf. Accessed August 4, 2015.

60. Poulet FM, Wolfe MJ, Spitsbergen JM. Naturally occurring orocutaneous neoplasms and carcinomas of brown bullheads (Ictalurus nebulosus) in New York State. Vet Pathol 1994;31:8–18.

61. Black JJ, Baumann PC. Carcinogens and cancers in freshwater fishes. Environ Health Perspect 1991;90:27–33.

62. Noble C, Jones HAC, Damsgard B, et al. Injuries and deformities in fish: their potential impacts upon aqua cultural production and welfare. Fish Physiol Biochem 2012;38:61–83.

63. Wimberger PH. Effects of vitamin C deficiency on body shape and skull osteology in Geophagus brasiliensis: implications for interpretations of morphological plasticity. Copeia 1993;2:343–51.

64. Corcoran M, Roberts-Sweeney HE. Aquatic animal nutrition for the exotic animal practitioner. Vet Clin North Am Exot Anim Pract 2014;17:333–46.

65. Lecu A, Lecour F. Teeth trimming in tetraodontidae fish. Exotic DVM 2004;6(6): 33–6.

Anatomy and Disorders of the Oral Cavity of Reptiles and Amphibians

Joanna Hedley, BVM&S, DZooMed (Reptilian), DECZM (Herpetology)

KEYWORDS

• Reptile • Amphibian • Oral • Stomatitis • Neoplasia

KEY POINTS

- A wide variety of disorders may be seen affecting the reptile and amphibian oral cavity.
- Problems can be easily missed by owners until they are at an advanced stage because of the difficulty of examining the oral cavity at home.
- Many problems are secondary to an inappropriate environment or diet and may be related to systemic disease, so a full history and clinical examination are always required.
- Treatment of oral disorders requires a holistic approach including correction of any predisposing factors in order for long-term successful resolution of the problem.

ANATOMY AND PHYSIOLOGY OF THE ORAL CAVITY

The oral cavity in reptiles and amphibians can vary significantly between the different orders and even between species. A clear understanding of the normal anatomy is, therefore, important in order to be able to identify and understand abnormalities that may occur.

The Reptile Oral Cavity

Reptiles are usually divided by their skull structures into 2 groups: either anapsids or diapsids.[1] Anapsids have a simple skull structure lacking true temporal openings, and chelonians are the only extant members of this group. Other reptiles have a diapsid or modified diapsid skull structure with temporal openings, which are particularly well developed in lizards and snakes.

Dentition varies among different families; but if present, teeth are composed of enamel, dentine, and cement similar to those of other vertebrates.[2] However, teeth are typically homodont (the same shape) and lack a periodontal membrane, so instead are directly ankylosed to the surrounding bone. In many species, teeth are reabsorbed and replaced multiple times throughout their life, a process known as polyphyodonty.

The author has nothing to disclose.
RVC Exotics Service, Royal Veterinary College, Royal College Street, London NW1 0TU, UK
E-mail address: jhedley@rvc.ac.uk

Vet Clin Exot Anim 19 (2016) 689–706
http://dx.doi.org/10.1016/j.cvex.2016.04.002   vetexotic.theclinics.com

A new tooth generally appears lingually to the older tooth, which is subsequently shed. Usually this process occurs in waves starting at the back of the oral cavity and progressing to the front. Those snakes and lizards hatching from eggs also possess an egg tooth modified from the premaxillary teeth in order to rupture the shell. Chelonians, crocodilians, and tuatara instead possess an egg caruncle composed of horny tissue, which serves the same purpose. This egg caruncle is lost or reabsorbed soon after hatching.

Skin folds or lips seal the oral cavity in squamates but are absent in chelonians and crocodilians. The oral cavity itself is lined by a mucous membrane consisting of squamous nonkeratinized epithelial cells, ciliated epithelial cells, columnar epithelial cells, and mucous glands.[3] Mucous membranes can vary in color and may be pigmented but should normally be moist. Salivary glands are present but vary between groups of reptiles, and tongue morphology is also variable depending on species. The glottis is located at the base of the tongue in chelonians and most lizards, whereas in snakes it can be easily visualized further rostrally. The palate is incomplete in all reptiles except crocodilians, which have evolved their own unique adaptations to separate the oral and respiratory systems and allow them to hunt underwater. The oral cavity and nasal cavity in other reptiles are linked by a pair of recesses (choanal openings). Eustachian tubes connect the oral cavity to the middle ear in those species in which a middle ear is present.

Chelonians

Chelonians have a relatively simple yet sturdy skull structure and, unlike other reptiles, can only open their mouth by lowering the mandible. They also lack teeth, so cannot chew their food. Instead, they have a keratinized horny beak (rhamphotheca) similar to that of birds, which overlies the osseous jaws. This beak is used for prehension, and ridges in the hard palate are also present in herbivores to help them grip and tear pieces of food. Despite their lack of teeth, the bite of a chelonian can be strong because of the adductor muscles running through a trochlear pulley system increasing their force.[1] Some species, such as snapping turtles (*Chelydra* spp), also have very sharp cutting edges to their jaws, so bites can cause significant damage.

Within the oral cavity, a short fleshy tongue is present with the glottis at its base (**Fig. 1**). The tongue aids with swallowing food, and numerous taste buds are present both on the tongue and elsewhere in the oral epithelium. Simple salivary glands are present, which produce mucus but no digestive enzymes.

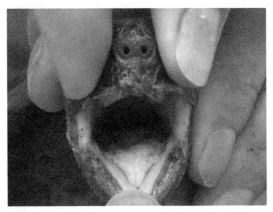

Fig. 1. The normal oral cavity of a tortoise showing the horny beak and short fleshy tongue.

Lizards

Lizards have a more developed kinetic skull, which allows them to both lift their maxilla and lower their mandible simultaneously, resulting in a large gape. They also have a quadrate bone without any firm connection, which can easily move backward and forward. This process is known as streptostyly, which further increases the potential gape of the mandible. This process combined with strong adductor muscles can result in a powerful bite.[1]

Dentition in lizards depends on the species and feeding habits; but unlike chelonians and snakes, lizards can chew their food. Lizard species can generally be split into those that have pleurodont dentition, such as iguanids and varanids, and those that have acrodont dentition, such as agamids and chameleonids.[2] Pleurodont teeth are attached to the lingual side of the jawbone and are shed and replaced regularly throughout the animal's life. In contrast, acrodont teeth are firmly attached to the crest of the jawbone and are rarely replaced, hence, the dental disorders seen in this group of lizards.

The morphology of the tongue also depends on the species; but in general, lizards possess a mobile protrusible tongue with the glottis present at its base (**Fig. 2**). The tongue may be used for catching food, swallowing, lapping water, or to bring scent particles to the Jacobson organ for olfaction. For example, varanids and teiids have a forked tongue resembling that of a snake and seem to use it to collect chemical scents in a similar way. In other lizards, such as the green iguana (*Iguana iguana*), the rostral tip of the tongue is a darker color, which is a completely normal finding.[1] Taste buds seem abundant in those species with fleshy tongues but poorly developed in those with keratinized tongues. Salivary glands are present, and specialized oral glands include the venom glands found in the Mexican beaded lizard (*Heloderma horridum*) and Gila monster (*Heloderma suspectum*).[4] In these species, neurotoxic venom is produced from the sublingual glands in the lateral lower mandible and secreted via ducts on the labial surface. Grooved teeth lie adjacent to these ducts to ensure that venom can be transferred to its target.

Snakes

The snake skull is even more kinetic than the lizard skull, being composed of very flexible mobile bones and a loosely connected quadrate bone, which can move forward and backward freely. Snakes, however, have no mandibular symphysis with the overlying flexible skin allowing an even greater range of movement of the two sides of the

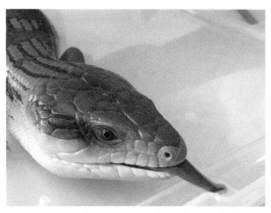

Fig. 2. The normal extensible blue tongue of the blue-tongued skink (*Tiliqua scincoides*).

mandibles than is possible in lizards. Each half of the skull can be moved separately to allow the snake to clamp down on large prey and then gradually advance the jaw forward, one side at a time, to push the prey further back within the oral cavity. After eating, snakes will often be seen to gape widely to reposition the jawbones.[1]

Dentition in snakes is pleurodont, and most species also possess an extra maxillary arcade of teeth[2] (**Fig. 3**). Teeth are long, curved, and point caudally within the oral cavity. Food is not chewed but swallowed whole, so teeth usually function solely for food prehension. Numerous salivary glands are present that produce copious amounts of saliva to aid with swallowing.[4] Venomous species have maxillary teeth modified into fangs, and venom is produced in modified labial salivary glands. Different species have different compositions of venom; but its composition often includes a mixture of collagenases, proteases, and phospholipases. In rear-fanged (opisthoglyphous) species, such as some colubrids, venom is produced in a gland behind the eye and just above the lips called the Duvernoy gland. Venom is transferred from here by modified grooved fangs at the caudal maxilla. In front-fanged snakes, the venom glands are found separate from the labial glands behind the eye and linked by a duct to fangs at the rostral maxilla. In proteroglyphous species, such as elapids, fangs remain erect at all times, whereas in solenoglyphous species, such as viperids, fangs are folded backward within a sheath when the oral cavity is closed. These fangs can then be raised by contraction of the pterygoid muscles when required for striking. The tongue is generally very mobile with a slender, long, forked appearance and kept in a sheath under the glottis. A notch at the rostral aspect of the oral cavity allows the tongue to be protruded even when the mouth is closed. The glottis is very mobile and can be shifted to one side when eating large prey to allow the snake to keep breathing.

Crocodilians

Crocodilians have a true diapsid skull structure with extremely strong adductor muscles able to close the jaws with great force. The muscles which open the mouth are in contrast fairly weak, so the jaws can be easily taped shut for safe handling if examination of the oral cavity is not required.[5] Dentition in crocodilians is different from other reptiles as teeth are embedded within a bony socket similar to mammals but without the periodontal membranes.[2] This arrangement is known as thecodont. Teeth are conical; they are shed and replaced approximately every 2 years (**Fig. 4**). The new tooth develops from germinal tissue within the socket and eventually dislodges the

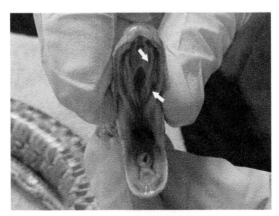

Fig. 3. The normal oral cavity of a corn snake (*Pantherophis guttatus*) showing the extra arcades of teeth (*arrows* pointing to the left arcade).

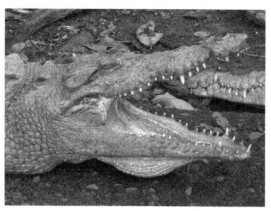

Fig. 4. The normal oral cavity of an American crocodile (*Crocodylus acutus*) showing the conical teeth and large gape.

preexisting tooth. Food is not chewed; instead pieces are swallowed whole. The tongue cannot protrude from the oral cavity because of its strong attachment to the ventral surface and, even within the mouth, is relatively immobile. At the caudal margin, the tongue fuses with a transverse fold separating the oral cavity from the pharynx. This fold overlaps with a transverse fold formed by the end of the palate ensuring complete separation of the oral cavity from the respiratory system and allowing the animal the capability to hold prey underwater without drowning.[5] The tongue, being immobile, cannot aid in swallowing, so the snout must be raised to allow food to fall backward into the pharynx instead.

The Amphibian Oral Cavity

Amphibian skull structures can be highly variable and are often incompletely ossified.[1] However, all adult amphibians are carnivorous and generally have a large, wide oral cavity (**Fig. 5**).

If present, teeth are jointed and composed of a crown loosely attached to a base or pedicel, which is then attached to the jaw. Similar to some reptiles, teeth are shed and

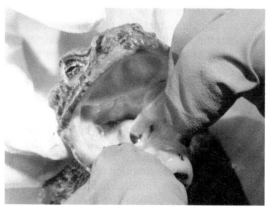

Fig. 5. The normal oral cavity of a cane toad (*Rhinella marina*) post mortem with an endotracheal tube pointing to the glottis.

replaced throughout life and generally pointed caudally. They are not generally used for chewing but simply for prehending food. The layout of teeth depends on species; for example, salamanders, caecilians, and some anurans have one or 2 arcades of maxillary and mandibular teeth, whereas ranid frogs do not have any mandibular teeth. On the roof of the mouth, small groups of teeth may also be present, known as the vomerine and palatine tooth patches. Tongue morphology varies depending on the species but can often be very flexible, extending up to 80% of the total length of the animal to prehend food in some species. Swallowing occurs by the animal raising the floor of the mouth and closing the eyelids to force the globes ventrally and push the food caudally into the pharynx. Most species have salivary glands, but these simply produce mucus rather than aiding in digestion.

DISORDERS OF THE ORAL CAVITY IN REPTILES
Infectious Stomatitis

Stomatitis is a common presentation in captive reptiles and may occur for a variety of reasons. However, it is usually secondary to an underlying deficit in husbandry or diet leading to immunosuppression. Examples include inappropriate environmental temperatures, inappropriate hibernation, or nutritional disease.[6] Stomatitis may also be seen secondary to the disruption of normal oral tissue due to trauma or neoplasia or alternatively in association with concurrent problems, such as renal disease. If left untreated, disease may progress to involve the surrounding bone and respiratory tract and eventually lead to septicemia and death.

Bacterial stomatitis

The normal oropharynx contains a wide range of aerobic and anaerobic microorganisms including both gram-positive and gram-negative bacteria.[7] However, the gram-negative bacteria are usually the most common organisms to overgrow in cases of stomatitis and result in pathologic changes. *Pseudomonas, Aeromonas, Proteus,* and *Escherichia coli* are all commonly isolated from cases of stomatitis.[8] Anaerobic bacteria may also be isolated, including *Bacteroides, Fusobacterium, Clostridium*, and *Peptostreptococcus*.[9] Animals may be presented with nonspecific symptoms, such as reduced appetite and lethargy, or owners may have noticed visible changes in the oral cavity. On clinical examination, the oral mucosa often appears erythematous and swollen with pockets of abscesses (**Figs. 6** and **7**). Lesions should be distinguished from the white tophi deposited in visceral gout, which may also be seen within the oral cavity.

The initial diagnostic approach to stomatitis should include a full history and clinical examination to identify any predisposing factors or systemic disease. Hematology and biochemistry may be indicated if systemic disease is suspected. Radiography of the skull is advised in moderate to severe cases of stomatitis to identify the extent of any potential bone involvement. This imaging will usually need to be performed under general anesthesia to obtain adequate views. Following initial assessment, oral lesions can then be sampled for microbiological culture and sensitivity to help guide selection of appropriate antibiotic therapy. Pending results, third-generation cephalosporins, fluoroquinolones, and aminoglycosides have all been used successfully in the treatment of bacterial stomatitis because of the prevalence of gram-negative bacteria usually seen.[10] General anesthesia may need to be considered to allow debridement, flushing, and initial topical treatments, although follow-up treatments may potentially be performed in the conscious animal. Topical treatments include dilute chlorhexidine, dilute povidone-iodine, and silver sulfadiazine ointment. Analgesia will also be required for this potentially very painful condition. Nonsteroidal antiinflammatories are most commonly used, but it is important to ensure that the animal is well hydrated

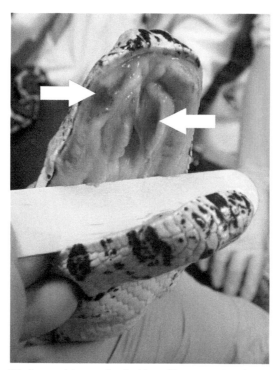

Fig. 6. Mild stomatitis (*arrows*) in a red-tailed boa (*Boa constrictor*).

and there are no concerns with renal function. As many of these animals have been anorexic for a prolonged time period, rehydration and supportive feeding may initially be required.

In the case of chronic nonhealing lesions within the oral cavity, infection with atypical bacteria, such as *Mycobacterium* species, should also be considered.[11] These cases often present as granulomatous or hemorrhagic lesions within the oral cavity (**Fig. 8**). More nonspecific symptoms of mycobacteriosis, such as lethargy

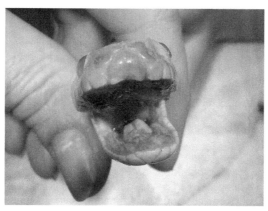

Fig. 7. Severe stomatitis in a corn snake (*Pantherophis guttatus*). (*Courtesy of* Nadene Stapleton, MRCVS.)

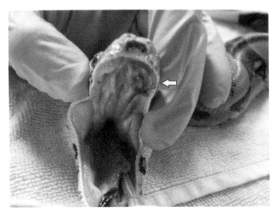

Fig. 8. Mycobacterial lesions can present as chronic granulomas (*arrow*) as seen in this red-tailed boa (*Boa constrictor*).

and weight loss, may also be seen if infection has spread systemically. Treatment is generally unsuccessful; because of the zoonotic implications, euthanasia should be considered.

Viral stomatitis
Viral stomatitis may be seen as either a primary or secondary problem in reptiles. Potential pathogens include herpesviruses in chelonians[12] and lizards[13,14] and ranaviruses in chelonians.[15] Herpesvirus infection in chelonians seems common throughout the captive population, often in association with *Mycoplasma* infection. Animals may be presented for lethargy, reduced appetite, hypersalivation, dysphagia, or sometimes concurrent respiratory signs, including ocular or nasal discharges. On oral examination, yellow diphtheritic lesions may be visualized within the oral cavity. They can be very large, to the point that they impair the animal's ability to eat. Diagnosis can be confirmed by taking an oral swab for polymerase chain reaction. False negatives can, however, occur, as the herpesvirus can lie dormant within the body, only resulting in a clinical problem at times of immunosuppression. Treatment is mainly symptomatic, although oral acyclovir has been trialed at 40 to 80 mg/kg every 8 to 24 hours with variable success.

Fungal stomatitis
Fungal stomatitis usually occurs secondary to inappropriate husbandry and often in association with bacterial stomatitis. Pathogens reported include *Candida albicans, Aspergillus, Sporothrix schenkii*, and *Paecilomyces spp.*[16,17] Diagnosis is based on fungal culture of affected lesions. Treatment with systemic antifungals is usually required in addition to topical agents as infection is often systemic. Treatment may need to be continued for at least 4 to 6 weeks.

Parasitic stomatitis
Parasitic stomatitis is rarely seen, as most parasites carry out their life cycle further within the alimentary system; but occasional parasites may be found encysted within the oral cavity.[18] An example would be the pentastomids (tongue worms), which may be seen in wild-caught reptiles, especially snakes. Animals may be presented for respiratory symptoms or excessive mucus in the mouth. Parasites can be found in the pharynx where they bury deeply into tissues resulting in inflammation and

secondary infection and may need to be physically removed. An intermediate host is required for the parasite to complete its life cycle, so infections are generally self-limiting in captivity. However, these parasites do have zoonotic potential, so care should be taken when dealing with parasitized infected animals.[19]

Infectious Cheilitis

Although primarily a dermatologic problem, infection with the gram-positive rod, *Devriesia agamarum* may result in significant cheilitis in some species, especially spiny-tailed lizards (*Uromastyx spp*)[20] (**Fig. 9**). Unlike bearded dragons (*Pogona spp*), which usually carry this bacterium asymptomatically as part of their normal oral flora,[21] infection in spiny-tailed lizards seems to result in severe hyperkeratotic dermatitis and cheilitis. Infection can normally be confirmed by bacterial culture and can be successfully treated with intramuscular administration of ceftiofur at 5 mg/kg every 24 hours for an average of 12 days in *Uromastyx spp*.[22] If left untreated, however, signs may progress to potentially result in septicemia and death.

Periodontal Disease

Periodontal disease is generally seen in acrodont lizards, such as bearded dragons, and seems to be a disease of captivity.[23,24] Inappropriate diets, such as too many soft fruits or wax worms, are thought to result in the development of plaque, subsequent bacterial colonization, and then gingivitis and calculus formation. Initial bacteria involved are normally gram-positive aerobic cocci; but as the disease progresses anaerobic bacteria, gram-negative bacteria, and spirochetes may also become involved and underlying bone may become affected. The animal may be presented for reduced appetite or lethargy; but often the owner is unaware of the extent of the problem, and periodontal disease is only detected incidentally on clinical examination. Gingival erythema, proliferation, and calculus deposition is normally obvious on oral examination (**Figs. 10** and **11**). In more advanced cases, abscesses and discoloration of the associated bone may also be seen. As in cases of stomatitis, radiography under general anesthesia is recommended to assess the extent of infection. An ultrasonic dental scaler may then be used to remove calculus; an antibacterial solution, such as 0.05% chlorhexidine, can be used to clean and flush the oral cavity. Prevention of periodontal disease involves dietary changes to reduce bacterial buildup and increased removal of plaque.

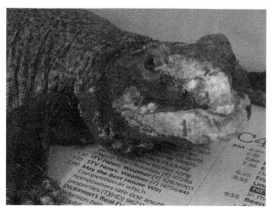

Fig. 9. *Devriesia agamarum* infection may result in significant cheilitis as shown in this Bell's Dabb lizard (*Uromastyx acanthinura*).

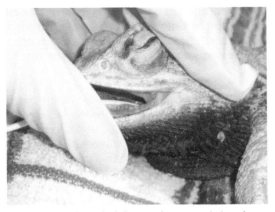

Fig. 10. Periodontal disease in a bearded dragon (*Pogona vitticeps*).

Neoplasia

A variety of tumors have been identified in the oral cavity in reptiles, including squamous cell carcinoma, fibroma, fibrosarcoma, fibropapilloma, melanoma, iridophoroma, and ameloblastoma.[25–31] Tumors may vary widely in appearance and initially often resemble lesions seen in infectious stomatitis. Biopsies are, therefore, strongly recommended for any nonresolving cases of presumed infectious stomatitis. Surgical excision is the preferred option for treatment of oral tumors if complete excision is possible. Radiation therapy has been trialed and is a potential option depending on the location of the tumor.[25,32] Otherwise treatment is generally palliative, including treatment of any secondary infections, analgesia as appropriate, and dietary modifications as necessary. Ultimately if neoplasia is progressing to potentially cause pain or impact on the animal's ability to feed, euthanasia should be considered.

Congenital

Congenital disorders are not uncommonly seen in reptiles, including maxillary brachygnathism, mandibular brachygnathism, and defects of the palate.[33] Causes are often unknown but may include genetic defects or environmental factors during incubation or gravidity, such as inappropriate temperatures or chemical exposure.

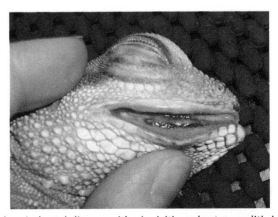

Fig. 11. Advanced periodontal disease with gingivitis and osteomyelitis in a Chinese water dragon (*Physignathus cocincinus*). (*Courtesy of* Marie Kubiak, MRCVS; with permission.)

Many animals can live with mild defects as long as their ability to feed is not compromised. In more severe cases, euthanasia may need to be considered.

Nutritional

Nutritional secondary hyperparathyroidism

Nutritional secondary hyperparathyroidism may result in a range of clinical signs, but oral disorders are generally associated with changes in the facial bones. Mandibles may appear thickened and swollen because of fibrous osteodystrophy. Over time, significant deformities may be seen because of the pressures applied by the attached jaw muscles (**Fig. 12**). Stomatitis may result from constant gingival and mucosal exposure in those animals unable to fully close their mouth. On clinical examination the jaw may feel extremely flexible, and care needs to be taken not to cause iatrogenic mandibular fractures when examining the oral cavity (**Fig. 13**).

Alternatively, in some species, such as chameleons, the muscles of the tongue may be seen to noticeably weaken resulting in difficulties extending and retracting and subsequent damage.[34] Diagnosis is usually based on clinical signs, but radiography will confirm reduced bone density. Other causes of metabolic bone diseases, such as renal hyperparathyroidism, should also be ruled out. Long-term treatment consists of improving diet and supplementation to provide an appropriate level of calcium, phosphorus, and vitamin D in addition to correction of any environmental deficits, such as inappropriate temperatures or UVB light provision. Analgesia should be considered, especially in cases with mandibular fractures. Supportive feeding may also be required. The need for additional feeding and medication should, however, be balanced with the potential pain and stress of opening the oral cavity in these animals. Placement of an esophagostomy tube may, therefore, be preferred in order to avoid excessive handling in some patients. However, euthanasia should be considered for advanced cases, especially if return to normal feeding is not considered likely and the animal's quality of life is judged to be compromised.

Hypovitaminosis C

In most reptiles, vitamin C is synthesized in the kidneys and, therefore, not required in the diet. However, hypovitaminosis C has been reported in boas and pythons and could potentially result in signs of spontaneous gingival bleeding similar to scurvy in other

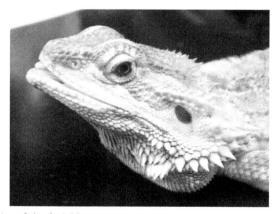

Fig. 12. Deformities of the facial bones are a common consequence of nutritional secondary hyperparathyroidism, as seen in this bearded dragon (*Pogona vitticeps*), which is unable to close its mouth.

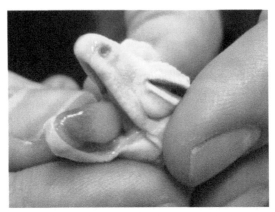

Fig. 13. The mandible can become very flexible as a consequence of nutritional secondary hyperparathyroidism as seen in this leopard gecko (*Eublepharis macularius*).

animals. This deficiency could, therefore, be a potential differential diagnosis for lesions in these species.[33]

Hypovitaminosis E and selenium deficiency

Hypovitaminosis E and selenium deficiency have been suggested to be the cause of a nutritional myopathy seen in a veiled chameleon (*Chamaeleo calyptratus*).[35] The chameleon was presented for a progressive inability to open its mouth and use its tongue. Postmortem examination revealed histopathologic lesions of myodegeneration and myolysis consistent with those seen in other animals with nutritional myopathy. A similar syndrome has also been reported in another veiled chameleon unable to open its mouth, but in this case histopathologic lesions were consistent with a fibrosing myopathy and cause could not be determined.[36]

Trauma

Reptiles can often sustain severe trauma to the oral cavity. In captive animals, one of the most commonly seen examples of this is rostral trauma. This trauma seems especially common in flighty species, such as water dragons (*Physignathus spp*), who often run head first into the sides of their enclosure when startled[34] (**Fig. 14**). Damage to the

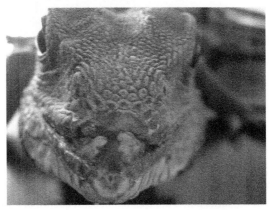

Fig. 14. Rostral abrasions and secondary infection in a Chinese water dragon (*Physignathus cocincinus*). (*Courtesy of* Marie Kubiak, MRCVS; with permission.)

snout may also be seen in some snakes, which may fail to perceive glass barriers and attempt to strike through them. In mild cases with only superficial abrasions, lesions are often self-limiting as long as the environmental cause is corrected. Providing an appropriate quiet secluded environment with plenty of areas to hide should reduce traumatic incidents. Placing opaque material, such as tape, on any glass surfaces should also reduce the risks of a snake not perceiving the glass wall and striking at it. However, with repeated injuries, the underlying tissue may become secondarily infected and both stomatitis and osteomyelitis may result. These cases will need more intensive management with both topical and systemic antibiotics and analgesia as described under treatment of stomatitis.

However, traumatic injuries are not just a result of captivity; skull fractures have been reported in both wild and captive reptiles. These injuries may interfere with oral function (**Fig. 15**). Imaging is required for full assessment of the fracture; advanced imaging modalities, such as computed tomography, can be particularly useful in cases whereby surgical stabilization is to be performed. In one case of a wild Eastern blue-tongued skink (*Tiliqua scincoides scincoides*) with both maxillary and mandibular fractures, successful stabilization was achieved using a combination of nonabsorbable suture material and an intramedullary pin.[37] In another case of a captive Fly River turtle (*Carretochelys insculpta*) with multiple fractures, an external skeletal fixator was used in combination with pins and cerclage wire for successful fracture repair.[38] Alternatively nonsurgical treatment using a tape muzzle and intraoral plate has also been reported to be successful in a blue-tongued skink. In this case, placement of an esophagostomy tube was also required to provide nutrition during the healing process.[39]

Trauma may also occur to soft tissue structures within the oral cavity, such as the tongue. This trauma may happen during ingestion of prey or due to ingestion of inappropriate objects by mistake, such as hair or string. Thermal burns may also be seen, especially in snakes that are fed prey that has been overheated.[10] Lesions should be cleaned, analgesia provided, and secondary infections treated as necessary.

Toxins

The ingestion of toxins usually results in more obvious systemic effects in reptiles, but occasionally stomatitis may be seen. For example, suspected oak (*Quercus*) leaf toxicity has been reported in an African spurred tortoise (*Geochelone sulcata*).[40]

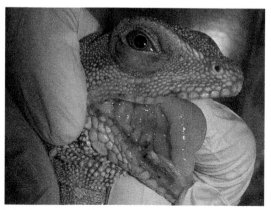

Fig. 15. Fracture of the mandible with disruption of the associated oral mucosa and dental arcade in a Chinese water dragon (*Physignathus cocincinus*).

Post mortem, significant oral mucosal ulcerations were noted, which were attributed to tannin toxicity. Alternatively, local irritation or gingivitis may also occur following accidental ingestion of any caustic food or liquid.

Beak Overgrowth

Beak overgrowth is often seen in captive chelonians in association with accelerated growth due to either the feeding of high-protein food items or alternatively just large quantities of food. However, other factors, such as trauma, congenital defects, hypovitaminosis A, or altered keratin synthesis secondary to hepatic disease or dietary deficiency, should be considered.[41] Deformities may also be seen in association with metabolic bone diseases as discussed earlier. Animals often present with deformed upper and lower beaks, nail abnormalities, and shell abnormalities, such as pyramiding (**Fig. 16**). As a keratinous structure, the beak can be easily trimmed without sedation in most animals; use of a tool, such a Dremel (Dremel, Racine WI) or a professional dental burr, is advised in order to accurately restore normal beak shape (**Fig. 17**). Diet should be fully reviewed to identify and correct any predisposing cause; but once the beak is deformed, regular trims are likely to be necessary. Some investigators consider that lack of abrasive substrate may be a factor; if so, then feeding the animal on an abrasive surface would be recommended to help wear down the beak.[6]

DISORDERS OF THE ORAL CAVITY IN AMPHIBIANS

Amphibians are susceptible to many of the same oral disorders as those seen in reptiles, but a few common problems are discussed next.

Infectious Stomatitis

Stomatitis in amphibians usually occurs secondary to rostral abrasions. Pathogens that may be involved include *Aeromonas hydrophila*, *Citrobacter freundii*, and *Pseudomonas spp;* but a variety of gram-negative bacteria may be isolated.[42] Secondary fungal infection may also occur. There is little soft tissue overlying the bone in this region, so prompt treatment is vital to prevent infection spreading systemically with potential fatal consequences. Lesions should be gently cleaned and debrided with saline solution, and treatment with topical silver sulfadiazine ointment is recommended.

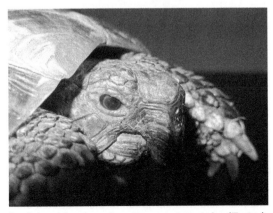

Fig. 16. Overgrowth of the rhinotheca in a Hermann's tortoise (*Testudo hermanni*).

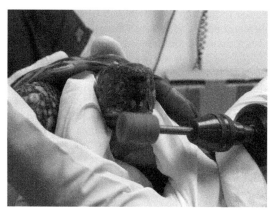

Fig. 17. Tortoise beaks may be burred using a hand power tool, such as a Dremel.

Systemic antibiotics or antifungal therapy may then be initiated, ideally based on cytology or culture results.

Neoplasia

A variety of tumors affecting the oral cavity have been reported in amphibians, including fibroma, lymphosarcoma, and neuroepithelioma of olfactory origin.[43,44] Diagnosis has historically been confirmed post mortem, but surgical excision would be the recommended treatment of choice when detected at an early stage.

Nutritional

Nutritional secondary hyperparathyroidism is commonly encountered in captive amphibians. Signs may include mandibular thickening and protrusion.[45] Although the causes and pathogenesis for metabolic bone diseases are similar to those seen in reptiles, vitamin D3 may play a more significant role. In amphibians, transport of 25-hydroxycholecalciferol relies on availability of lipoproteins.[46] Inappropriate levels of fatty acids and fats in the diet may, therefore, lead to reduced availability of the active vitamin D3 metabolite and the development of metabolic bone disease, despite adequate dietary calcium, phosphorus, and vitamin D3. Otherwise the approach to diagnosis and treatment is similar to that in reptiles.

Hypovitaminosis A is also seen in captive amphibians and has recently been described in association with "short tongue syndrome" in the Wyoming toad (*Anaxyrus baxteri*).[47] The term originated from early observations that the animals were unable to strike successfully at their prey, as their tongue seemed to be too short. Histopathology revealed that the normal nonkeratinizing, glandular, mucus-producing epithelium of the tongue had been disrupted by squamous metaplasia; consequently, the tongue was no longer fully functional. Hypovitaminosis A should be considered in any captive amphibian fed a primarily insectivorous diet. Diagnosis is usually based on history and clinical signs, as sampling is not normally practical in the live animal. Treatment involves supplementation with vitamin A, which can result in resolution of mild lesions. The diet should ideally be modified in the longer-term to prevent further problems.

Trauma

Rostral abrasions are some of the most commonly seen traumatic injuries in captive amphibians, especially in particularly nervous animals, who may collide with the sides of their enclosure similar to the behavior seen in the nervous water dragon. Salamanders and newts have also been reported with stomatitis lesions secondary to burrowing attempts when kept on inappropriate substrate, a syndrome known as atrophic mandibular stomatitis.[42] As discussed earlier, prompt treatment is necessary as lesions can progress quickly with potentially fatal consequences.

Foreign body ingestion and subsequent gastrointestinal impaction is commonly seen in amphibians because of their wide gape, but a slightly more unusual presentation was reported in an American toad (*Anaxyrus americanus*), which presented with a reduced appetite and abnormal vocalization. Examination revealed a firm mass under the tongue, which was removed and found to be composed of keratinocytes and necrotic cell debris consistent with impaction of ingested epidermal shed.[48] Ingestion of shed skin is a normal behavior, and in this case the underlying cause for the impaction was not determined. However, it highlighted abnormal vocalization as an unexpected clinical sign of oral pathology due to pressure on the glottis in this case.

SUMMARY

A wide variety of disorders may be seen affecting the reptile and amphibian oral cavity. Owners can easily miss problems until they are at an advanced stage because of the difficulty of examining the oral cavity at home. Because many problems are secondary to an inappropriate environment or diet and may be related to systemic disease, a full history and clinical examination is always required. Treatment of oral disorders also requires a holistic approach, including correction of any predisposing factors in order for long-term successful resolution of the problem.

REFERENCES

1. O'Malley B. Clinical anatomy and physiology of exotic species. London: Elsevier Saunders; 2005.
2. Edmund A. Dentition. In: Gans C, editor. Biology of the reptilia, volume 1, Morphology A. London: Academic Press; 1970. p. 117–94.
3. Luppa H. Histology of the digestive tract. In: Gans C, Parsons T, editors. Biology of the reptilia, volume 6, Morphology E. London: Academic Press; 1977. p. 225–313.
4. Kochva E. Oral glands of the reptilia. In: Gans C, Gans K, editors. Biology of the reptilia, volume 8, Physiology B. New York: Academic Press; 1978. p. 43–161.
5. Lane T. Crocodilians. In: Mader D, editor. Reptile medicine and surgery. 2nd edition. St Louis (MO): Saunders Elsevier; 2006. p. 100–18.
6. McArthur S. Problem-solving approach to common diseases. In: McArthur S, Wilkinson R, Meyer J, editors. Medicine and surgery of tortoises and turtles. Oxford (United Kingdom): Blackwell Publishing Ltd; 2004. p. 301–77.
7. Dipineto L, Russo T, Calabria M, et al. Oral flora of Python regius kept as pets. Lett Appl Microbiol 2014;58(5):462–5.
8. Draper C, Walker R, Lawler H. Patterns of oral bacterial infection in captive snakes. J Am Vet Med Assoc 1981;179(11):1223–6.
9. Stewart J. Anaerobic bacterial infections in reptiles. J Zoo Wildl Med 1990;21(2): 180–4.
10. Mehler S, Bennett R. Upper alimentary tract disease. In: Mader D, editor. Reptile medicine and surgery. 2nd edition. Malabar: Saunders Elsevier; 2006. p. 924–30.
11. Quesenberry K, Jacobson E, Allen J, et al. Ulcerative stomatitis and subcutaneous granulomas caused by Mycobacterium chelonei in a boa constrictor. J Am Vet Med Assoc 1986;189(9):1131.

12. Soares J, Chalker V, Erles K, et al. Prevalence of mycoplasma agassizii and chelonian herpesvirus in captive tortoises (Testudo Sp.) in the United Kingdom. J Zoo Wildl Med 2004;35(1):25–33.
13. Wellehan J, Nichols D, Li L, et al. Three novel herpesviruses associated with stomatitis in Sudan plated lizards (*Gerrhosaurus major*) and a black-lined plated lizard (*Gerrhosaurus nigrolineatus*). J Zoo Wildl Med 2004;35(1):50–4.
14. Wellehan J, Johnson A, Latimer K, et al. Varanid herpesvirus 1: a novel herpesvirus associated with proliferative stomatitis in green tree monitors (*Varanus prasinus*). Vet Microbiol 2005;105(2):83–92.
15. Johnson A, Pessier A, Wellehan J, et al. Ranavirus infection of free-ranging and captive box turtles and tortoises in the United States. J Wildl Dis 2008;44(5): 851–63.
16. Heatley J, Mitchell M, Williams J, et al. Fungal periodontal osteomyelitis in a chameleon (*Furcifer pardalis*). J Herpetol Med Surg 2001;11(4):7–12.
17. Cheatwood J, Jacobson E, May P, et al. An outbreak of fungal dermatitis and stomatitis in a free-ranging population of pigmy rattlesnakes (*Sistrurus miliarius barbouri*) in Florida. J Wildl Dis 2003;39(2):329–37.
18. Griffiths A, Jones H, Christian K. Effect of season on oral and gastric nematodes in the frillneck lizard from Australia. J Wildl Dis 1998;34(2):381–5.
19. Jacobson E. Parasites and parasitic diseases of reptiles. In: Jacobson E, editor. Infectious diseases and pathology of reptiles. Boca Raton (FL): CRC Press; 2007. p. 571–666.
20. Martel A, Pasmans F, Hellebuyck T, et al. *Devriesea agamarum Gen. Nov., Sp. Nov.*, a novel actinobacterium associated with dermatitis and septicaemia in agamid lizards. Int J Syst Evol Microbiol 2008;58(9):2206–9.
21. Devloo R, Martel A, Hellebuyck T, et al. Bearded dragons (*Pogona Vitticeps*) asymptomatically infected with *Devriesea agamarum* are a source of persistent clinical infection in captive colonies of dab lizards. Vet Microbiol 2011;150(3):297–301.
22. Hellebuyck T, Pasmans F, Haesebrouck F, et al. Designing a successful antimicrobial treatment against *Devriesea agamarum* infections in lizards. Vet Microbiol 2009;139(1):189–92.
23. McCracken H. Periodontal disease. In: Fowler M, Miller R, editors. Zoo and wild animal medicine. 4th edition. Philadelphia: WB Saunders; 1999. p. 252–7.
24. Simpson S. Dragon breath: periodontal disease in central bearded dragons. In: Proceedings of the Association of Reptile and Avian Veterinarians. Orlando, October 18–24, 2014. p. 42.
25. Steeil J, Schumacher J, Hecht S, et al. Diagnosis and treatment of a pharyngeal squamous cell carcinoma in a Madagascar ground boa (*Boa madagascariensis*). J Zoo Wildl Med 2013;44(1):144–51.
26. S de Brot, Sydler T, Nufer L, et al. Histologic, immunohistochemical, and electron microscopic characterization of a malignant iridophoroma in a dwarf bearded dragon (*Pogona henrylawsoni*). J Zoo Wildl Med 2015;46(3):583–7.
27. Thompson K, Campbell M, Levens G, et al. Bilaterally symmetrical oral amelanotic melanoma in a boa constrictor (*Boa constrictor constrictor*). J Zoo Wildl Med 2015;46(3):629–32.
28. Idowu A, Golding R, Ikede B, et al. Oral fibroma in a captive python. J Wildl Dis 1975;11(2):201–4.
29. Comolli J, Olsen H, Seguel M, et al. Ameloblastoma in a wild black rat snake (*Pantherophis alleghaniensis*). J Vet Diagn Invest 2015;27(4):536–9.
30. Salinas E, Arriaga B, Lezama J, et al. Oral fibrosarcoma in a black iguana (*Ctenosaura pectinata*). J Zoo Wildl Med 2013;44(2):513–6.

31. Work T, Balazs G, Rameyer R, et al. Retrospective pathology survey of green tur-tles *Chelonia mydas* with fibropapillomatosis in the Hawaiian Islands, 1993-2003. Dis Aquat Organ 2004;62:163–76.

32. Bishop T, Cumming B. Treatment of a squamous cell carcinoma in a bearded dragon (Pogona vitticeps) using radiation therapy. In: Proceedings of Assoc Avian Vet (AC) & Unusual/Exotic Pets. Cairns, Australia, April 22–24, 2014.

33. Frye F. 2nd edition. Biomedical and surgical aspects of captive reptile husbandry, vols. I and II. Malabar: Krieger Publishing Co; 1991.

34. McArthur S, McLellan L, Brown S. Gastrointestinal system. In: Girling S, Raiti P, editors. BSAVA manual of reptiles. 2nd edition. Gloucester (United Kingdom): BSAVA; 2004. p. 210–29.

35. Rowland M. Fibrosing myopathy of the temporal muscles causing lockjaw in a veiled chameleon (*Chamaeleo calyptratus*). Vet Rec 2011;169(20):527.

36. Cole G, Rao D, Steinberg H. Suspected vitamin E and selenium deficiency in a veiled chameleon (*Chamaeleo calyptratus*). J Herpetol Med Surg 2008;18(3–4):113–6.

37. Scheelings T. Surgical management of maxillary and mandibular fractures in an eastern bluetongue skink, *Tiliqua scincoides scincoides*. J Herpetol Med Surg 2008;17(4):136–40.

38. Tuxbury KA, Clayton LA, Avian D, et al. Multiple skull fractures in a captive fly river turtle (*Carretochelys insculpta*): diagnosis, surgical repair, and medical manage-ment. J Herpetol Med Surg 2010;20(1):11–9.

39. Köchli B, Schmid N, Hatt J, et al. Nonsurgical treatment of a bilateral mandibular fracture in a blue-tongued skink. Exot DVM 2008;10(2):25–8.

40. Rotstein D, Lewbart G, Hobbie K, et al. Suspected oak *Quercus* toxicity in an African spurred tortoise, *Geochelone sulcata*. J Herpetol Med Surg 2003;13(3):20–1.

41. Chitty J, Raftery A. Essentials of tortoise medicine and surgery. Chichester (United Kingdom): Wiley Blackwell; 2013.

42. Wright K. Trauma. In: Wright K, Whitaker B, editors. Amphibian medicine and captive husbandry. Melbourne (Australia): Krieger Publishing Co; 2001. p. 233–8.

43. Balls M. Spontaneous neoplasms in amphibia: a review and descriptions of six new cases. Cancer Res 1962;22(10):1142–54.

44. Brunst V, Roque A. Tumors in amphibians. I. Histology of a neuroepithelioma in Siredon mexicanum. J Natl Cancer Inst 1967;38(2):193–204.

45. Antwis R, Browne R. Ultraviolet radiation and vitamin D 3 in amphibian health, behaviour, diet and conservation. Comp Biochem Physiol Part A Mol Integr Phys-iol 2009;154(2):184–90.

46. Hay A, Watson G. The plasma transport proteins of 25-hydroxycholecalciferol in fish, amphibians, reptiles and birds. Comp Biochem Physiol Part B 1976;53(2): 167–72.

47. Pessier A. Short tongue syndrome and hypovitaminosis A. In: Mader D, Divers S, editors. Current therapy in reptile medicine & surgery. St Louis (MO): Elsevier Saunders; 2014. p. 271–6.

48. Selig M. Subglossal impaction in an American toad (*Anaxyrus americanus*). J Herpetol Med Surg 2011;21(1):3–4.

Anatomy and Disorders of the Beak and Oral Cavity of Birds

Brian Speer, DVM, DABVP(Avian Practice), DECZM(Avian)[a],[*],
Lauren Virginia Powers, DVM, DABVP(Avian Practice),
DABVP(Exotic Companion Mammal Practice)[b]

KEYWORDS

- Avian • Beak • Cranial kinesis • Rhamphotheca • Keratin • Oral cavity

KEY POINTS

- Cranial kinesis of the avian beak is complex, particularly in birds with prokinetic beak movement, such as parrots.
- Imaging of the avian facial and neurocranial bones can be valuable in identifying beak lesions and in planning corrective techniques. Micro–computed tomography is an emerging diagnostic modality useful for evaluation of beak disorders.
- Developmental beak deviations are common in birds and can be corrected with ramp orthotics or tension band devices.
- Any disease that affects rhamphothecal growth or abrasion (wear) can result in excessive rhamphothecal thickness or tomial elongation and necessitate periodic rhamphothecal corrective procedures.
- Many diseases of the oral cavity have similar clinical appearance, such as hypovitaminosis A, candidiasis, avian pox, trichomoniasis, and capillariasis, warranting appropriate diagnostic testing.

INTRODUCTION

The anatomy and function of the heads and beaks of birds have some shared common features and a large number of unique adaptations specific to species groups and their unique niche functions. Similarly, disorders of the head and beak and the oral cavity also share common characteristics and some species-specific features. This article reviews anatomy, form and function, and disease conditions of the beak and the

The authors have nothing to disclose.
[a] The Medical Center for Birds, 3805 Main Street, Oakley, CA 94561, USA; [b] Avian and Exotic Pet Service, Carolina Veterinary Specialists, 12117 Statesville Road, Huntersville, NC 28078, USA
[*] Corresponding author.
E-mail address: avnvet@aol.com

Vet Clin Exot Anim 19 (2016) 707–736
http://dx.doi.org/10.1016/j.cvex.2016.04.003   **vetexotic.theclinics.com**

oral cavity, with an emphasis on those of the more commonly kept companion and aviary species.

ANATOMY AND FUNCTION
General Gross Anatomic Terminology

Anatomic and topographic terms and their synonyms for the beak are depicted in **Table 1**. The bill, or beak, of birds is known anatomically as the rostrum. It includes the bones of the upper and lower jaws and their horny sheaths. The upper component of the bill is the maxillary rostrum (rostrum maxillare) and the lower component is the mandibular rostrum (rostrum mandibulare).[1,2] The upper and lower beaks of birds are covered by a hard epidermal structure derived from keratin, which covers the rostral parts of the upper and lower jaws.[2] Synonyms for this keratin covering are the horny bill, or rhamphotheca. Synonyms for the upper and lower horny sheaths are the maxillary rhamphotheca (or rhinotheca), and the mandibular rhamphotheca (or gnathotheca).[2]

Musculoskeletal Anatomy

Bones, joints, and cranial kinesis

In most birds, the upper jaw functions as a rigid triangular block that can be elevated or depressed.[1,3] The upper jaw hinges at the flexible junction of the upper jaw with

Table 1
Anatomic terms and common synonyms used to describe avian beak topography

Anatomic Term	Synonyms
Rostrum	Bill or beak
Maxillary rostrum	Upper bill or beak
Mandibular rostrum	Lower bill or beak
Rhamphotheca	Keratin sheath of the beaks, horny bill
Rhinotheca	Maxillary rhamphotheca, keratin sheath of the upper bill
Gnathotheca	Mandibular rhamphotheca, keratin sheath of the lower bill
Tomium (singular), tomia (plural)	Rostral and lateral cutting edges of the rhamphotheca
Maxillary tomium, tomia	Rostral and lateral cutting edges of the maxillary rhamphotheca
Mandibular tomium, tomia	Rostral and lateral cutting edges of the mandibular rhamphotheca
Midline beak profile terms	
Culmen	Mid-dorsal profile of the maxillary rhamphotheca
Gonys	Mid-ventral profile of the mandibular rhamphotheca
Other topographic terms	
Gape	The entire opening of the mouth
Rictus	Caudal part of the oral opening, beginning at the caudal end of the tomia and ending caudally at the angle of the mouth
Inter-ramal region	Inter-ramal space, zone of soft tissue beginning at the caudal end of the gonys, extending between the mandibular rami as far as the end of the mandible
Gular region	Caudal portion of the inter-ramal space
Naris (singular), nares (plural)	Nostril and nostrils

the neurocranium at the craniofacial hinge (nasofrontal hinge). In parrots, this is a synovial joint, and is also known as the ginglymus. The form of cranial kinesis in which the movement of the jaw occurs at the junction of the jaw and the neurocranium (**Table 2**) is termed "prokinesis."[1,3] The osteology of cranial kinesis of a scarlet macaw (*Ara macao*) is depicted in **Fig. 1**. Prokinetic movement of the upper beak requires the movement of 4 pairs of bones: the jugal arch and the pterygoid, palatine, and quadrate bones.[1,3] Another form of cranial kinesis, termed "rhynchokinesis," occurs through independent motion of the upper beak. Movement of the upper jaw is made possible in rhynchokinetic species by the presence of flexible elastic zones in the nasal bony bars.[1] The 2 mandibular rami are joined in the rostral midline at the rostrum (symphysis) mandibulae.[1] The quadrate bone forms the primary link between the lower jaw and the neurocranium.[1,3] In psittacine birds, the pterygoid bone articulates rostrally with the rostral portion of the palatine bone and caudally with the quadrate bone in a synovial hinge joint.[1,3] The jugal arch articulates rostrally with the maxilla, and caudally it forms a ball and socket joint with the quadrate bone.[1,3] The jugal arch consists of 3 bones fused together; from rostral to caudal, the jugal process of the maxillary bone, the jugal bone, and the quadratojugal bone.[1,3] There is no true zygomatic bone in birds. The quadrate bones are immensely mobile and function as the key elements in most of the movement of the upper and lower jaws in the prokinetic beak: articulating with the lower jaw, the neurocranium, the jugal arch, and the pterygoid bone.[3] The joint formed between the quadrate bone and the neurocranium is a double articulation.[4] All of these bony elements are coupled mechanically; hence, force applied at any point in the system either internally by muscle contraction or via external factors will be transmitted throughout the system and cause deflection of the system in one or the other direction.[1,3] The convention is to consider the quadrate bone as the starting point and to describe all movements as initiated from it.[1]

Muscles and motor innervation
Muscles involved with prokinesis are depicted in **Table 3**. In most avian species, 7 pairs of muscles act on the upper and lower jaws.[1] Parrots have 2 unique pairs of muscles and lack 1 of this original pair of 7. Parrots do not have *pseudotemporalis profundus*, which is common in other bird species groups.[1,5] The mandibular nerve provides the primary motor innervations for the muscles of mastication, with the exception of the *depressor mandibulae*, which is supplied by the facial nerve.[6]

Table 2
Terms used to describe avian cranial kinesis and examples of avian species that demonstrate different methods for cranial kinesis

Term	Definition	Species Examples
Rhynchokinesis	The ability to flex the upper beak, either upward or downward, independently of other cranial structures.	Cranes, shorebirds, swifts, and hummingbirds
Prokinesis	Movement of the upper beak through rotation around a hinge at the junction between the beak and the neurocranium. Movement of the upper beak is dependent on the movement of other cranial structures.	Psittacine birds, songbirds

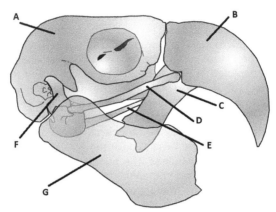

Fig. 1. Illustration of the skull anatomy of a scarlet macaw (*Ara macao*): A, neurocranium; B, premaxilla; C, palatine; D, jugal arch; E, pterygoid; F, quadrate; G, mandible. (*From* Abramson J, Speer BL, Thomsen JB, editors. The large macaws. Fort Bragg (CA): Raintree Publications; 1995; with permission.)

Table 3	
Muscles and their function in prokinetic avian cranial kinesis (eg, psittacine birds)	
Muscle Name	**Function**
Protractor pterygoidei et quadrati	Raises the upper jaw (serving with the depressor mandibulae to open the mouth)
Depressor mandibulae	Lowers the lower jaw (serving with the protractor pterygoidei et quadrati to open the mouth)
Pterygoideus	Functions with the depressor mandibulae to close the upper and lower jaws. In parrots, functions in lower beak protraction and in lowering the lower jaw during chewing. Flexes the quadrate-mandibular joint
Pseudotemporalis profundus	Functions with the pterygoideus to close the upper and lower jaws
Adductor mandibulae externus Pseudotemporalis superficialis Adductor mandibulae caudalis	Function together to raise the lower beak
Ethmomandibularis	Closes and protracts the lower jaw in parrots through flexion of the quadrate-mandibular joint
Pseudomasseter	Raises the lower jaw in parrots through flexion of the quadrate-mandibular joint
Protractor quadrati Pseudotemporalis superficialis Adductor mandibulae caudalis Adductor mandibulae externus	Function together to rotate the quadrate bone rostrally to open the upper beak
Depressor mandibulae	Opens the lower jaw through extension of the quadrate-mandibular joint
Pseudotemporalis profundus	Closes the lower jaw through flexion of the quadrate-mandibular joint

Soft Tissue Anatomy

Epithelial and dermal structures of the beak

The beak of birds consists of epidermis, dermis, bone, and air spaces. The horny bill resembles skin. The dermis is closely attached to the periosteum. The epidermis is modified in 2 ways: the *stratum corneum* is very thick, and the cells of the stratum corneum contain free calcium phosphate and orientated crystals of hydroxyapatite. These modifications, when combined, provide the horny bill with its typical hardness.[5,7] Keratin arises from the Malpighian cells of the bird's epidermis, growing from plates at the base of each bill.[7] Keratin is also produced by the underlying dermis of the beak with varying contributions from the cere.[7] Keratin normally migrates rostrally along the surface of the beak and laterally from its vascular bed.[7] These surfaces are worn continuously through use and mechanical abrasion, and the degree of wear may vary due to foraging styles within individuals, seasons, and within populations.[5,8] Both keratin surfaces are made up of a covering-type (very thin) and a pressure-bearing type (very thick) of keratin. Covering-type keratin is located on the outer and lateral surfaces of the upper and lower beak. Pressure-bearing–type keratin is located on the undersurface of the upper bill, the piercing/shearing point of the upper bill, and at the shearing edges of the upper and lower bills (tomia). The difference in keratin thickness of covering and pressure-bearing types is apparent in **Fig. 2**. In the

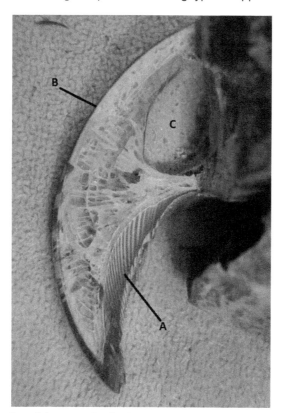

Fig. 2. Sagittal section of the upper beak of the hyacinth macaw (*Anodorhynchus hyacinthinus*): A, pressure-bearing occlusal rhinotheca; B, covering-type keratin of the culmen; C, nasal diverticulum of the infraorbital sinus. (*Courtesy of* Brian Speer DVM, DABVP (Avian Practice), DECZM (Avian), Oakley CA; with permission.)

grey parrot, a keratin monomer of approximately 15,500 Da molecular weight is typical for the harder, pressure-bearing surfaces, and a larger monomer of 25,000 Da is more common with the softer, covering-type keratin structures.[5] Comparatively, solubilized keratinized epithelium in the grey parrot had a molecular weight of 46,000 to 66,000 Da.[5]

Vascular anatomy

The common carotid artery is the primary source of blood to the structures of the beak and oral cavity in birds. This artery divides into internal carotid and vertebral arteries, which ascend the neck and form numerous anastomoses. Areas supplied by the common carotid artery include the lower jaw and its muscles, the palate, oropharynx, upper jaw, larynx nasal cavity, and orbit.[9] The vascular supply to the head and neck of the grey parrot are depicted in **Fig. 3**, and the marked degree of vascularity of the beak, tongue, and other structures can easily be appreciated.

Innervation of the beak

In birds, generally the nerve endings of the upper bill are innervated by the maxillary and ophthalmic divisions of the trigeminal nerve and those of the lower bill by its mandibular division.[6] The ophthalmic nerve supplies the palate, the edge of the upper beak, and the bill tip organ.[6] The maxillary nerve is purely afferent and supplies receptor endings to the lateral tomia of the upper bill. The mandibular nerve is both somatic afferent and efferent, and passes the length of the mandibular canal and provides branches to the skin associated with the lower beak, including the mandibular bill tip organ (**Table 4**).[6]

Thermoregulation

Thermal regulation of excess body heat from the oropharyngeal cavity in some avian species, such as pelicans, is accomplished through evaporative heat loss by thermal tachypnea and gular flutter. Thermal tachypnea involves open mouth breathing or thermal panting, which is associated with an increased respiratory rate, resulting in increased rate of evaporative cooling effect. The gular flutter is characterized by a rapid flutter of the gular region caused by flexure and relaxation of the hyoid

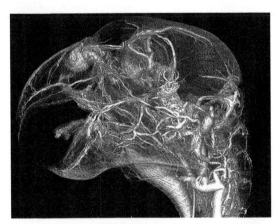

Fig. 3. Micro-CT image of the vascular supply to the head and neck of a grey parrot (*Psittacus erithacus*) cadaver enhanced with BriteVu contrast agent (Scarlet Imaging LLC, Murray, UT). (*Courtesy of* Brian Speer DVM, DABVP (Avian Practice), DECZM (Avian), Oakley CA; with permission.)

Table 4		
Selected key mechanoreceptors of the beak and oral cavity of birds		
Receptor	Location	Function
Herbst	Related to the way the bill is used during feeding. Rhamphothecal tomia of granivores	Sense vibration, up to 1000 Hz
Grandry	Dermis of the bill associated with soft horn in waterfowl, particularly near the sides and tip	Velocity-sensitive
Merkel	Beak and tongue of various nonaquatic birds	Secondary sensory cells

apparatus.[10] In addition to evaporative cooling mechanisms for heat exchange, toucans are capable of heat exchange from their bill, using it as a controllable vascular radiator.[11]

Gastrointestinal Anatomy of the Oral Cavity

The tongue of birds varies extensively among species depending on the forms of adaptation required by an individual species.[12] The tongue is supported by the hyobranchialis (hyoid) apparatus, also known as the *apparatus hyolingualis*.[1,13,14] Psittaciformes is the only taxonomic order that has intrinsic muscles of the tongue that originate and insert on these hyoid bones.[12,13] Adaptive forms for tongues in birds include those for collecting food (eg, woodpeckers), manipulating food (eg, parrots, waterfowl), and swallowing food (eg, domestic fowl).[12] Salivary glands are typically more developed in birds that have a relatively dry type of diet, such as granivorous or insectivorous species. Birds can distinguish tastes, but in general their acuity of the sense of taste is believed to be less than that of mammals. In most species, taste buds are located on the base of the tongue, and are confined to regions in which the epithelium is soft and noncornified, and are more prevalent near the ducts of the salivary glands.[15]

Respiratory Anatomy of the Oral Cavity

The nostrils (nares) and nasal cavity structures are quite variable among species of birds. Generally, the nares are located at the dorsal base of the upper beak. A keratinized flap, termed the operculum, is located dorsal to the nostril in some species (eg, domestic chickens and turkeys), and just within the naris in other species (eg, psittacine birds). The nasal septum is partly bony and cartilaginous, and completely separates the right and left nasal cavity. In some species, it is incomplete rostrally (ducks and grebes), allowing communication between the left and right nasal cavities.[16] The nasal conchae are generally cartilaginous, but may be bony as well. They function to increase the surface area over which inhaled air passes. There are 3 conchae: rostral, middle, and caudal. The combined functions of these nasal cavity structures include olfaction, filtration, water and heat economy, and thermoregulation.[16] Inhaled air passes through these nasal conchae into the rostral aspect of the choana, where it is capable of entering the larynx. The choana is a slitlike opening on the roof of the oral cavity that allows communication between the nasal cavities and oral cavities and permits nasal breathing. Fingerlike mucosal projections line the choanal margins, the choanal papillae, which help prevent food from entering the nasal cavities. The larynx of birds is composed of the laryngeal cartilages, which may be partly ossified. The opening of the larynx is termed the glottis, located between the right and left arytenoid cartilages.[16]

DIAGNOSTIC TESTING
Imaging

Imaging is a useful and important diagnostic modality for evaluating disorders of the beak and oral cavity. It is especially useful to document lesions with a high-quality digital camera, ideally one with excellent macro and lighting features. Standardization of patient position while obtaining these images will help improve methods of comparison when they are evaluated serially. These types of digitally recorded images can facilitate direct comparison of patient status and progression over time, can allow quantitative measurements of lesions or deformities, and photo documentation of current patient status as is described in medical records. With the growing use of digital medical record-keeping systems in veterinary health care, these images are easily embedded in most medical records, allowing rapid access and easier sharing with specialists for further consultation if indicated. **Fig. 4** shows standard lateral and rostrocaudal images being used to document a patient's current condition before corrective grinding of its rhamphothecal overgrowth.

Plain radiography

Radiographic imaging has become a standard and key aspect of the practice of avian medicine by allowing for noninvasive visualization of anatomic features in both health and disease states.[17] Due to the often relatively small body size of many companion bird species, variations in technique and image quality obtained, and the significant overlap of the multiple structures of the head, diagnostic acuity may be more limited as compared with what can be obtained with other imaging studies or plain images of other anatomic regions. Regardless, in the correct clinical situation, these plain radiographic images can offer significant benefit as a component of a diagnostic investigation.[17] Particular problems and diagnostic challenges that may be aided with plain radiographic imagery may include malocclusions with keratin overgrowth, certain skull fractures, and some sinus problems.[17] **Fig. 5** demonstrates a marked rhamphothecal overgrowth in a large macaw, and the use of digital plain radiographs to evaluate and help formulate a restorative rhamphothecal correction strategy.

Computed tomography

Computed tomography (CT) has become an increasingly valuable tool in avian species, with applications that are useful for planning, guiding, and monitoring

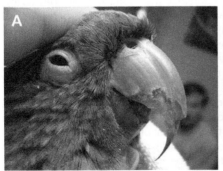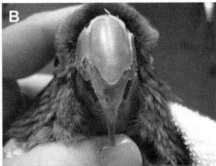

Fig. 4. Marked rhamphothecal overgrowth in a blue crowned conure (*Thectocercus acuticaudatus*). Rostrocaudal (*A*) and lateral (*B*) images. Note the buildup of layers of lateral covering-type keratin of both the rhinotheca and gnathotheca, but normal occlusal surfaces of the maxillary lateral tomia. (*Courtesy of* Brian Speer DVM, DABVP (Avian Practice), DECZM (Avian), Oakley CA; with permission.)

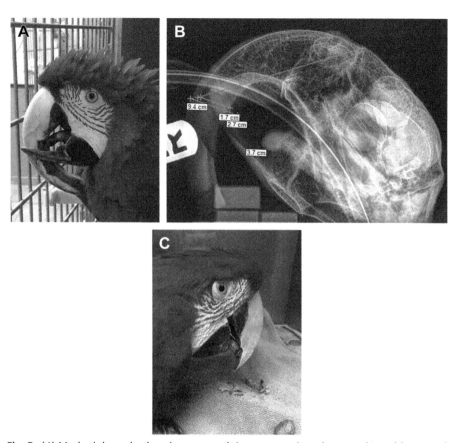

Fig. 5. (*A*) Marked rhamphothecal overgrowth in a green winged macaw (*Ara chloroptera*). Note the scissoring deformity of the gnathothecal rostral and lateral tomia on the bird's left, rhinothecal rostral and lateral tomia on the bird's right, and overgrowth of the occlusal ledge of rhinotheca. (*B*) Lateral projection survey skull radiograph of the bird depicted in A. Measurements of the upper and lower bill allow for strategic calculation of what keratin overgrowth should be trimmed to optimize occlusion and force vector delivery. (*C*) The same patient in A, immediately following a rhamphothecal restorative procedure. Note the apparent improved kinetic function and ability to chew hard foods. Longer term follow-up still is indicated, with a balanced and enriched behavior change strategy focused on increased chewing activities. (*Courtesy of* Brian Speer DVM, DABVP (Avian Practice), DECZM (Avian), Oakley CA; with permission.)

therapy.[17–19] The main advantage of CT imaging compared with standard digital radiography is that there is no interference from superimposition. Thus, despite their lower resolution, both 2-dimensional (2D) serial images and 3-dimensional (3D) renderings obtained through CT imaging enable better visualization of various tissues and structures, including those that would otherwise have remained undetected with conventional radiographs. In general, micro-CT imaging has higher resolution than digital radiography, which is higher than what is seen via standard CT. CT also offers comparatively short investigation times, particularly as compared with MRI.[19] Contrast media may be used to increase the radiodensity of tissues, organs, and/or vascular systems, which helps depict lesions or abnormalities. Soft tissue structures with abnormal vascularization caused by disease (eg, neoplasia, inflammation) will show increased uptake of contrast medium, differentiating it from normal tissue.[19] In areas with significant bone superimposition, CT imaging has been found especially useful. CT has a large range of relevant and practical applications, particularly for the head. CT is considered superior to radiographs for evaluating the nasal cavity, conchae, and sinuses, allowing detailed studies of the various anatomic structures.[19] Limitations of CT are dependent on the spatial resolution of the CT scanner being used and size of the patient. The more modern (helical) multislice CT scanners may produce images of high enough resolution for smaller structures, such as the avian head. Micro-CT scanners may provide even superior imagery as they become more available in the future.[19] **Fig. 6** shows the acuity of imagery that is offered via micro-CT of the head of a macaw cadaver head. **Fig. 7** shows a 3D volume reconstruction of the head of a grey parrot cadaver, using micro-CT imagery.

Other imaging modalities
Other imaging techniques may be useful in specific conditions of the head and oral cavity, such as MRI, nuclear imaging (including PET), and scintigraphy. Because of its characteristics, MRI is primarily used to image and diagnose soft tissue structures. The primary disadvantages associated with MRI may include prolonged imaging procedure times for some studies, and special spatial resolution challenges. With the increased availability of higher-resolution systems, the use and practical implication of MRI in avian medicine is likely to become more prevalent in veterinary practice overall and avian practice.[19]

Cytology and Special Stains

Cytologic evaluation of lesions of the beak or oral cavity can provide great diagnostic value. The normal oropharyngeal cavity is not sterile, and microbes identified at cytology should be carefully interpreted. Cytologic stains that are commonly used include the Romanowski stains and Gram stain. Normal findings typically include low cellularity, squamous epithelial cells, normal mixed bacterial microflora (mixed cocci and bacilli), plant and seed material, occasional or rare yeast, and mucus.[20] Bacteria are usually found on the surface of squamous epithelial cells.[21] A large cocci, *Sarcinia,* can be easily confused with yeast organisms.[22] *Alysiella filiformis*, an aerobic gram-negative filamentous bacterium, also may be confused with bacterial or fungal pathogens.[20] Abnormal cytologic findings include the presence of inflammatory cells and infectious organisms, such as *Candida* yeasts and trichomonads.[20]

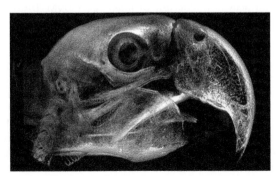

Fig. 6. Micro-CT image of the head of a green winged macaw (*Ara chloroptera*) cadaver head. (*Courtesy of* M. Scott Echols DVM, DABVP (Avian Practice) with permission.)

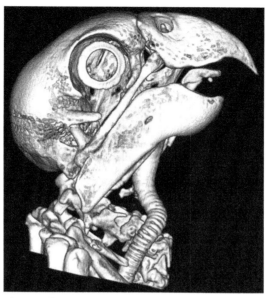

Fig. 7. Micro-CT 3D image of a grey parrot (*Psittacus erithacus*) cadaver head. (*Courtesy of* M. Scott Echols DVM, DABVP (Avian Practice); with permission.)

Microbiology

Aerobic and/or anaerobic bacterial culture and sensitivity testing may provide great diagnostic value in identifying some bacterial and fungal pathogens, as well as selection from treatment options. As noted with cytology, the normal oropharyngeal cavity is not sterile, and microbes identified through microbiologic culture should be carefully interpreted. The presence of a known or potential pathogen does not always correlate with the presence of disease. Furthermore, aerobic culture is not alone a clear means with which to identify all suspected bacterial or fungal agents. For example, *Chlamydia psittaci*, *Mycoplasma* spp, *Bordetella avium*, *Haemophilus somnus*, and other bacteria do not grow under typical aerobic isolation procedures.

BEAK AND ORAL CAVITY DISORDERS AND TREATMENT
Developmental Beak Deviations

Beak deformities in birds are either congenital or acquired. Acquired beak deformities can be secondary to any disease that damages the musculoskeletal components or overlying rhamphotheca. Developmental beak deviations are a result of abnormal development of musculoskeletal beak structures during the rapid growth phase of the immature bird. The etiology of developmental beak abnormalities is poorly understood, but is likely complex, variable, and multifactorial.[23,24] Proposed underlying causes include genetic abnormalities, incorrect egg incubation techniques, malnutrition, mycotoxicosis, improper hand-feeding techniques, and trauma.[21,23,24] Severe cases may result in difficulty in prehending food.[23,24] Beak malalignment often results in abnormal beak wear, requiring periodic corrective rhamphothecal reshaping procedures.[23,24] The 2 most common types of developmental beak disorders in psittacine birds are lateral beak deformity and mandibular prognathism.

Lateral beak deviation (scissors beak)

Lateral beak deformity is most often seen in macaws,[23–25] but can also affect other psittacine species, as well as doves, raptors, and domestic chickens, among others (**Fig. 8**).[24] Lateral beak deformity is characterized by a lateral bowing of the rhinotheca, often along with the underlying maxillary beak facial bones. Deformity generally occurs when there is disrupted or altered growth of the bony structures of the maxillary beak, such as the rictus or the premaxilla, nasal, and frontal bones.[24] As force vectors are repeatedly applied during regular beak use and rhamphothecal growth, this deformity often will become progressively worse, ultimately generating a "scissors effect."[26] Uneven abrasion (wear) results in lateral rhinothecal and gnathothecal tomial elongation.[23,26] Severe deformity may result in difficulty prehending food. Mild disease in immature birds may improve with gentle pressure periodically applied toward a normal direction of alignment. Mildly affected adult birds may do well with periodic rhamphothecal restorative procedures. Corrective surgery may be indicated for severe cases.

Surgical corrective techniques for lateral beak deviation

Surgical correction is most successful in young birds when the beak tissues are ossified but still developing and more pliable than in adult birds.[24,26] There are 2 main types of repair. The first involves building a ramp orthotic device along the lateral wall of the beak to redirect bite forces to a more normal plane. This technique is used more often in immature birds. The second involves applying lateral redirectional forces to the maxillary beak through transfrontal pinning and the use of tension wires or bands.[24]

For the beak ramp orthosis, an extension of the lateral beak wall is created using structural adhesive resins, such as liquid acrylic, epoxy putty, or light-cured dental resin composites.[23,26,27] The device is applied to the mandibular beak on the same side to which the maxillary beak is deviating and redirects bite forces to a more natural plane. Although ramp orthoses are most commonly applied to the mandibular beak, a maxillary beak ramp orthosis was successful in correcting a lateral beak deformity in a 2-year-old striped owl (*Rhinoptynx clamator*).[27] The height of the orthosis must be tall enough to prevent the opposite beak from extending over it.[26] Stainless steel mesh, nylon mesh, cerclage wire, or a combination of materials can be used to support, build, and reinforce the orthosis.[24,27] Anesthesia may not be necessary if rapidly

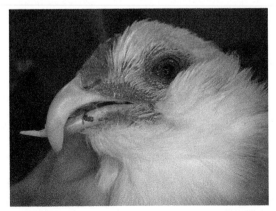

Fig. 8. Lateral beak deformity (scissors beak) of undetermined etiology in an adult female pet domestic chicken (*Gallus gallus domesticus*). Frequent rhamphothecal restoration procedures were required to maintain self-feeding ability. (*Courtesy of* Lauren Powers DVM, DABVP (Avian Practice, Exotic Companion Mammal Practice); with permission.)

setting materials are used, such as dental composites, and if construction of the device does not involve perforation of deeper tissues, such as bone.[24] Lightly notching the rhamphotheca can improve adhesion of the ramp construct to the beak keratin.[24] Extending the orthosis to wrap around the beak to the opposite side also can strengthen the device.[26] If the lateral rhamphothecal tomia are elongated due to uneven wear, the keratin should be reshaped to a more normal appearance to permit improved apposition. Potential complications include malalignment at the mandible-quadrate interface and fracture of the mandible, particularly in immature birds. Correction using a ramp orthotic typically requires 1 to 3 weeks.[26]

Tension band techniques are considered by some to be more effective for severe beak deviations in adult birds, but can be highly effective also in subadult birds.[23,24] An intramedullary pin or Kirschner wire is carefully drilled transversely through the frontal bone caudal to the nasofrontal hinge and caudoventral to the nares.[24] Threaded pins are preferable to nonthreaded pins. The exposed end of the pin on the side of the beak opposite the direction of the deviation is left long and used to construct a connecting rod for tension band placement. The pin can be either left straight and short, or bent at a 90° angle and extended rostrally parallel to the maxillary beak with the end in close apposition to the tip of the maxillary beak.[18,24] An elastic band is then looped around the tip of the maxillary beak at one end and through a loop created in the distal end of the pin at the other, applying gentle lateral tension to the beak tip (**Fig. 9**). Effective correction often can be accomplished in a matter

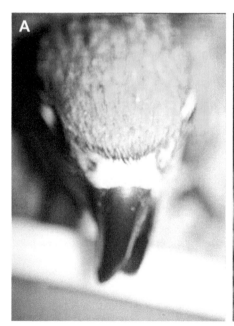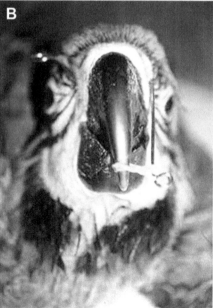

Fig. 9. (*A*) Skyline view of a young blue and gold macaw (*Ara ararauna*) with a lateral beak deviation. Note the rostral and left lateral tomia of the gnathotheca are exposed, and the rostral and right lateral tomia malaligned, leading to functional malocclusion and imbalanced keratin wear. (*B*) Rostrocaudal view of the same blue and gold macaw with a lateral beak deviation from A. Note that occlusion has been restored, with the rhamphothecal tomia in proper alignment. This individual was functionally corrected with 3 days of tension. (*Courtesy of* Brian Speer DVM, DABVP (Avian Practice), DEÇZM (Avian), Oakley CA; with permission.)

of a few days to 2 weeks in most birds.[18,24] Potential complications from this procedure include infection and iatrogenic damage to the frontal bone and sinus, nasofrontal hinge, and maxillary beak structures, particularly in young birds.[23,26]

Mandibular prognathism

Mandibular prognathism is most often seen in cockatoos, but can occur in other avian species.[23] The distal maxillary beak rests caudal to the rostral margin of the mandibular beak, within the oral cavity ("underbite").[23] Mandibular prognathism can be a result of excessive contraction of the muscles that lower the maxillary beak, an abnormally curved or otherwise malformed premaxilla, or excessively elongated mandibles. If recognized early in growing birds, attempts at correction can be made through applying gentle periodic outward pressure to the maxillary beak.[24]

Surgical corrective techniques for mandibular prognathism

As with lateral beak deviation, repair is most successful in young birds when the bony structures are still growing and pliable. There are 2 main methods of repair, one that uses the construction of an extension along the tip of the maxillary beak, and another that involves applying rostral redirectional forces to the maxillary beak through tension wires or bands. Both of these methods apply tension to the *pterygoideus* and *pseudotemporalis profundus* muscles, which are often contracted in affected birds, resulting in abnormal lowering (flexion) of the upper jaw.

The maxillary beak extension orthotic device is similar to the ramp orthosis used for correction of a lateral beak deformity.[23] A functional cap, extending from the cere distally, and encompassing the pressure-bearing marginal rhinotheca, is progressively structured. Careful placement of a sterile pin dorsal to ventral through the tip of the premaxilla may help to stabilize the device (**Fig. 10**). However, pins placed through

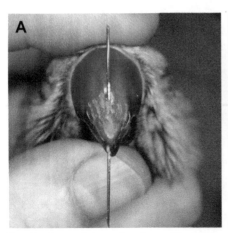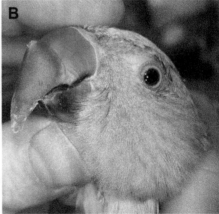

Fig. 10. Successful repair of mandibular prognathism in a 6-month-old male Indian ring-necked parakeet (*Psittacula krameri manillensis*). The beak was repaired with a pin (22-gauge spinal needle stylet) placed dorsal to ventral through the rostral premaxilla and covered with liquid acrylic (Technovit Liquid; Jorgensen Laboratories, Loveland, CO). The rhinotheca was superficially scarified with a dental bur before application of acrylic to improve attachment to the beak. The device was well-tolerated and fell out on its own after 6 weeks. (*A*) Appearance of beak after pin placement and scarification of the rhinotheca. (*B*) Appearance of the beak after orthotic construction was complete. (*Courtesy of* Lauren Powers DVM, DABVP (Avian Practice, Exotic Companion Mammal Practice); with permission.)

the bone of growing birds may result in trauma to the softer, pliable tissues and caution is warranted with their use.

For the tension-band technique, transverse placement of a pin through the frontal bone is similar to that for correction of lateral beak deviation. A second pin is placed in the premaxilla along the mid-culmen at the point where inward rotation of the maxillary beak is most severe.[24] Structural adhesive resins can then be applied to support the second pin.[24] An elastic band is placed from the exposed end of the fontal bone pin to the premaxilla pin. The band can be removed after normal alignment is restored, and the pins removed once this correction is ensured.[24] Caution is warranted with this technique because of the risks of trauma to bony and vascular tissues.

Trauma

Beak trauma is very common in companion and aviary birds, such as bite wounds from other birds and predators and from impact injuries.[21] Foreign objects, such as fishing hooks, quick links and carabiners, and toy parts, can piece the oral mucosa and deeper tissues.[21] Birds should be stabilized and fully evaluated for the extent of the injuries. Patients should receive appropriate supportive care and analgesic therapy.[25]

Beak fractures

Trauma involving the bony structures of the beak is common in birds. Poorly healed fractures can result in beak deviations and uneven rhamphothecal wear.[24] Imaging, such as plain radiography and CT of the skull, can be enormously helpful in planning a surgical repair. When there is outright loss of bone or vascular compromise, the prognosis for return to normal form and function is guarded. An attack by a cat resulted in slight lateral deviation of the mandibular beak and reluctance to open the mouth in an adult double–yellow-headed Amazon parrot (Amazona oratrix).[28] A mandibular fracture and disruption to the joint space between the mandible and quadrate bone were identified by CT. An esophagostomy tube was placed and the injury was allowed to heal without surgical intervention, although the ability to open the beaks remained compromised.[28] A 22-year-old hybrid macaw with a rigid nasofrontal hinge and laterally deviated jugal bone from a dog bite was diagnosed by CT and was successfully treated with surgical removal of the nasal-frontal-braincase and jugal-orbital arch.[18] Other surgical procedures using orthopedic or dental techniques and devices, such as stainless steel plates,[29] intramedullary pins,[30] osteogenic distractors,[31] dental resin composites,[32] and elastic bands,[24] among others, have been described in avian patients (**Fig. 11**).

Mandibular symphyseal diastasis and fracture

Separation (diastasis) and/or fracture of the mandibular symphysis is common in companion birds and is most often a result of an impact injury to the beak. The 2 mandibles are joined in the rostral midline at the rostrum (symphysis) mandibulae but this connection can easily become separated with trauma. Separation of this joint would be properly termed a diastasis, although fractures of the adjacent mandibular bone also can be seen, producing a similar net result. These injuries often have a guarded to poor prognosis for successful repair due in part to the thin nature of vascular dermis and bone in this region.[33,34] If a repair is to be successful, it must be attempted soon after the injury occurs. The exposed rostral ends of each mandible should be aseptically prepared for surgery. The separated ends are realigned and secured. In smaller birds, a bridging construct created from structural adhesive resin may be adequate.[33] In larger birds, reinforcement with transmandibular placement of stainless steel cerclage

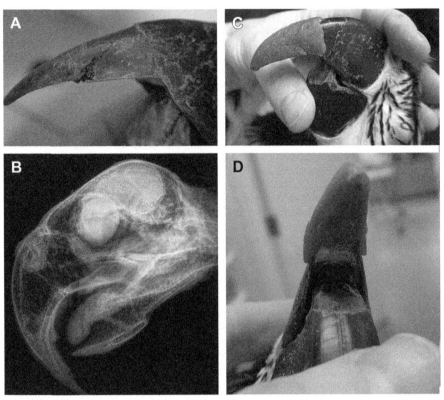

Fig. 11. Fracture of the rostral maxillary beak in a 23-year-old female blue and gold macaw (Ara ararauna) involving the rhinotheca and premaxilla bone (*A*). The rostral premaxilla fracture is visible on a lateral-lateral projection survey radiograph (*B*). The fracture was stabilized with liquid acrylic (Technovit Liquid; Jorgensen Laboratories) placed around the rostral maxillary beak (*C, D*). (*Courtesy of* Lauren Powers DVM, DABVP (Avian Practice, Exotic Companion Mammal Practice); with permission.)

wire or pins is often necessary.[33] The pins can be externally secured to each other by using elastic bands,[24] or with loops of polypropylene or stainless steel suture or wire (**Fig. 12**). Pins and wire can then be covered with adhesive resin for added support and protection.

Palatine bone luxation
Traumatic luxation of the palatine bone has been described in several psittacine birds, most commonly macaws.[24,26,35,36] Luxation occurs when the palatine bone is moved rostrally and then slips dorsally beyond its normal end-point on the mesethmoidal bony ridge at the ventral base of the neurocranium.[26] Luxation results in pathologic hyperextension and inability to close the maxillary beak.[26] The diagnosis is made based on history, examination findings, and radiographic findings.[24,26,35,36] Birds may be able to spontaneously reduce the luxation on their own.[35] If the luxation does not quickly self-correct, surgical intervention is warranted.[24,26] To reduce the luxation, an intramedullary pin or Kirschner wire is driven transversely through the preorbital diverticulum of the infraorbital sinus dorsal to the jugal arch. Downward pressure is applied to the pin and the dorsal margins of the palatine bone while simultaneously extending the maxillary beak, enabling the palatine bone to slide back over the

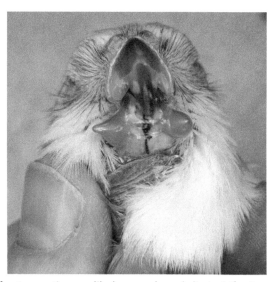

Fig. 12. Repair of a traumatic mandibular symphyseal diastasis/fracture in an adult male cockatiel (*Nymphicus hollandicus*) that resulted from the bird flying into a window in the home. The beak was successfully repaired with a transmandibular pin (hypodermic needle) looped with polypropylene suture and covered with liquid acrylic (Technovit Liquid; Jorgensen Laboratories). (*Courtesy of* Lauren Powers DVM, DABVP (Avian Practice, Exotic Companion Mammal Practice); with permission.)

mesthmoidal ridge and allowing the maxillary beak to return to its normal position.[24,26,37] The pin is then removed from the sinus. Additional stabilization can be provided by passing absorbable suture around the suborbital arch (in those species that possess one) and jugal arch through a lateral surgical approach to the jugal arch.[26,36,37]

Beak avulsion

Traumatic beak avulsion is somewhat common in psittacine birds and waterfowl. In psittacine birds, the injury is almost always a result of a bite from another psittacine bird. Surgical amputation of beak tissues may be indicated for aggressive local disease, such as neoplasia. Ducks and geese are occasionally subjected to bites to the beak from snapping turtles or other predators. Most parrots can adapt and survive traumatic beak avulsion with appropriate wound care, supportive care, and analgesic therapy, and do not require surgical intervention (**Fig. 13**).[21,25,38] Some birds may require assisted feedings or placement of an esophagostomy tube during the initial recovery period. In one case series, 9 of 10 psittacine birds with amputation of the beak survived, and all surviving birds were able to self-feed within 20 days, some much sooner.[38] Psittacine birds that lose most or all of the lateral maxillary tomia often lose the ability to crack seeds and nuts and must be fed a soft diet. Affected birds may require periodic gnathothecal restorative procedures due to inadequate keratin wear from the opposing beak.

Beak prosthetics

Avulsion of the maxillary beak in waterfowl can result in difficulty prehending food and exposure of the tongue. Avulsion of the maxillary beak can also result in difficulty with self-feeding in other avian species, such as ramphastids and storks.[39–41] These birds may benefit from surgical placement of a beak prosthesis. Cosmetic appearance

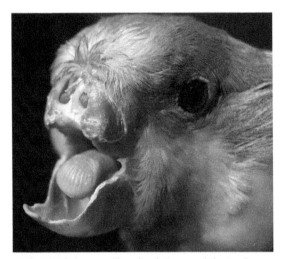

Fig. 13. Traumatic avulsion of the maxillary beak in an adult Quaker parakeet (*Myiopsitta monachus*) several years after the beak was severed from a bite wound from an umbrella cockatoo (*Cacatua alba*). The bird can self-feed on a soft diet, although the mandibular beak requires periodic rhamphothecal reshaping due to chronic overgrowth because of inadequate wear from the maxillary beak. (*Courtesy of* Lauren Powers DVM, DABVP (Avian Practice, Exotic Companion Mammal Practice); with permission.)

should never be the only factor in deciding whether or not to place a beak prosthesis, particularly in psittacine birds. Psittacine birds usually relearn to self-feed,[38] and the powerful forces of the beak and jaw muscles can quickly result in prosthetic failure. There are several reports of prosthetic beak placement in birds. Prosthetic beaks can be constructed from epoxy or acrylic structural adhesive resins applied to intramedullary pins, Kirschner wires, or cerclage wire secured to the trabecular bony structures of the remaining beak (**Fig. 14**). Prosthetic beaks have also been designed and

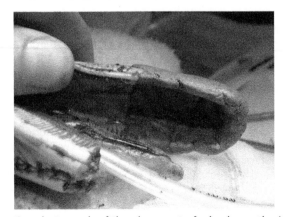

Fig. 14. Intraoperative photograph of the placement of a beak prosthesis on a Pekin duck (*Anas platyrhynchos domesticus*) that had the maxillary and mandibular beak traumatically avulsed. A bite wound from a snapping turtle was the suspected cause of the injury. The prosthetic was constructed from positive profile threaded external skeletal fixation (ESF) pins, cerclage wire, and epoxy putty. The prosthesis lasted approximately 12 months before needing to be replaced. (*Courtesy of* Lauren Powers DVM, DABVP (Avian Practice, Exotic Companion Mammal Practice); with permission.)

constructed using 3D printing for use for a bald eagle (*Haliaeetus leucocephalus*) and a green-billed toucan (*Ramphastos dicolorus*). Regardless of the method of prosthetic beak application, all prostheses will ultimately undergo varying degrees of failure, given that the beak is a living structure composed of light, trabecular bone. Prosthetic beaks must be monitored closely for complications, such as failure and infection, and repaired and managed accordingly.

Lingual Entrapment

Entrapment of the tongue within the sublingual or intermandibular space is occasionally seen in herbivorous waterfowl,[21,42–45] with reports in the Toulouse goose (*Anser anser domesticus*),[45] Chinese goose (*Anser cygnoides*),[44] black swan (*Cygnus atratus*),[42] and Australian shelduck (*Tadorna tadornoides*).[42] This condition is believed to be a result of ingestion, accumulation, and subsequent impaction of dry, fibrous foods within the ventral oral cavity lateral to the frenulum.[21,43–45] Clinical signs include difficulty swallowing and a visible intermandibular swelling.[43] If diagnosed early, the impacted material can be manually removed and affected birds can recover without surgical intervention.[42,43] With chronic or severe disease, a distended pouch often forms within the sublingual or inter-ramal space and entraps the tongue, often requiring surgical reduction. Several surgical techniques have been described, generally involving extraoral resection of redundant skin and resection or tacking of redundant oral mucosa.[43,44] If extensive necrosis or infection is present, tissues can be marsupialized for wound care and allowed to heal by second intention.

Nutritional Disease

Nutritional deficiencies and imbalances can result in pathology of the beak and oral cavity. Malnutrition may result in softening and flaking of the rhamphotheca. Nutritional metabolic bone disease can cause abnormal bone growth in juvenile birds and can potentially result in developmental beak deformities. Hypovitaminosis A can result in blunting of the choanal papillae as well as squamous metaplasia of the oral mucous membranes and epithelium, resulting in erythema and plaque in the oral cavity.[21] Squamous metaplasia of small mucous glands in the oral cavity can cause submucosal nodules that can become large enough to occlude the choanal slit[21] (**Fig. 15**). Secondary bacterial and mycotic infections are common.[21]

Neoplasia

Many neoplasms form visible masses of the beak or oral cavity, whereas others are not directly visible but may distort rhamphothecal growth,[21,46] result in tissue necrosis or hemorrhage,[21] result in difficulty prehending food, or dyspnea.[21,46] Definitive diagnosis generally requires cytology or histopathology.[21]

Squamous cell carcinoma
Squamous cell carcinoma has been described in a number of avian species, including a Buffon macaw (*Ara ambigua*),[47] great hornbill (*Buceros bicornis*),[48,49] and African penguin (*Spheniscus demersus*).[50] Squamous cell carcinoma is often locally invasive with a high rate of local recurrence but a low potential for distant metastasis.[21] Secondary bacterial and mycotic infections are common.[21] Aggressive surgical resection,[47–49] chemotherapy (intralesional cisplatin),[47,50] radiation therapy (cobalt-60),[47] photodynamic therapy,[48] and topical and oral antiangiogenic therapy[49] have been described with mixed success in birds (**Fig. 16**).

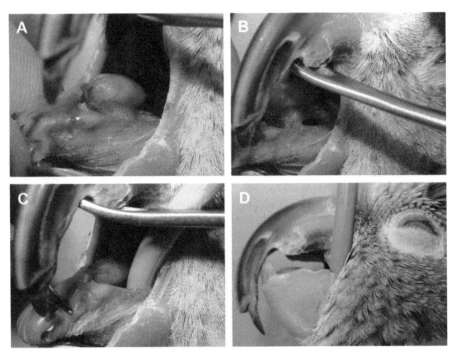

Fig. 15. (*A*) Oral submucosal nodule caused by squamous metaplasia as a result of a vitamin A deficiency in a yellow-crowned Amazon parrot (*Amazona ochrocephala*). The submucosal nodule is just slightly lateral to the base of the tongue. (*B*) The nodule is mobile and partially covers the opening of the glottis. (*C*) An endotracheal tube is placed before surgical removal of the nodule. (*D*) Note the concurrent rhinothecal elongation and thickening and mild gnathothecal elongation. (*Courtesy of* Vittorio Capello, DVM, Milano, Italy; with permission.)

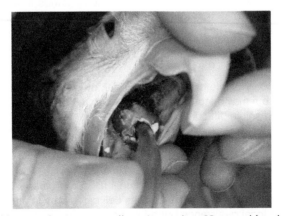

Fig. 16. Oral and laryngeal squamous cell carcinoma in a 23-year-old male double–yellow-headed Amazon parrot (*Amazona oratrix*). Treatments included chemotherapy (intravenous carboplatin) and cryotherapy and resulted in incomplete remission but significant clinical improvement for approximately 12 months. (*Courtesy of* Lauren Powers DVM, DABVP (Avian Practice, Exotic Companion Mammal Practice); with permission.)

Melanoma

Melanoma in generally considered a malignant neoplasm in birds.[21,51] Malignant melanoma of the beak or surrounding tissues has been described in the grey parrot,[52] thick-billed parrot (*Rhynchopsitta pachyrhyncha*),[53] pigeon (*Columba livia*),[54] mandarin duck (*Aix galericulata*),[55] and macaroni penguin (*Eudyptes chrysolophus*).[51] Oral malignant melanoma is uncommon.[21] Not all melanocytic tumors in birds are grossly pigmented, and therefore all suspicious masses should be closely evaluated and sampled for diagnostic testing.[51,55] Reported treatments include surgical excision,[51,54] radiation therapy,[51,53] and oral antiangiogenic therapy.[53] Distant metastasis to the lungs, liver, kidney, spleen, bone marrow, and other organs is common.[21,51–55]

Fibroma and fibrosarcoma

Fibrosarcoma is generally considered to be the most common primary beak tumor in birds.[21,56] Fibrosarcoma is most common in budgerigars (*Melopsittacus undulatus*) and cockatiels (*Nymphicus hollandicus*),[21] although it has also been reported associated with a pathologic fracture and distal avulsion of the maxillary beak in a grey parrot.[56] Fibrosarcomas tend to be locally aggressive with a low risk of distant metastasis, although metastasis has been documented and local recurrence is common after surgical resection.[21] Local invasion into the nares, nasal turbinates, and bone can result in deformation of the beak.[21] Histopathology is generally considered diagnostic.[21,56] Chemotherapy (intralesional cisplatin) and radiation therapy were used in the treatment of a facial fibrosarcoma in a blue and gold macaw (*Ara ararauna*).[57]

Mucosal papillomas

The most common oral neoplasm of New World psittacine birds is mucosal papilloma.[21,58] Lesions also can be found elsewhere in the gastrointestinal tract, most commonly the cloaca.[58] Oral lesions are often found along the choanal margins, larynx, oropharynx, and the base of the tongue.[21,58] Lesions are typically white to pink in color, raised, and often have a cauliflowerlike surface.[21,58] Lesions can wax and wane, often seeming to disappear entirely.[21,58] Secondary bacterial infections are common. Psittacid herpesvirus 1 (PsHV-1) is associated with mucosal papillomas in psittacine birds and is also the cause of Pacheco disease, a rapidly fatal disease of parrots, which is most likely seen in birds not adapted to the specific PsHV-1 genotype exposed.[58] Diagnosis is through histopathology, and testing for PsHV-1 by polymerase chain reaction (PCR) is often positive in affected birds.[58] As lesions often spontaneously regress, surgical excision or debulking is generally not advised unless the lesions interfere with respiratory or gastrointestinal function.[58] Antiviral agents, such as acyclovir also can be used.[58]

INFECTIOUS DISEASES
Viral Diseases

Several viral diseases are associated with damage to the structures of the beak and oral cavity (**Table 5**).

- Psittacine beak and feather disease (PBFD) is caused by a nonenveloped virus in the genus *Circovirus*, family Circoviridae. In the chronic form, beak lesions and feather loss are often observed. Reported beak and oral lesions include rhamphothecal elongation, transverse or longitudinal beak fractures, oral ulceration, and palatine necrosis.[21,59] The rhinotheca may separate from the underlying dermis, potentially resulting in exposure of bone.[21] Diagnosis can be made through PCR and histopathology and demonstration of basophilic intranuclear and intracytoplasmic inclusion bodies.[21,59] Although birds can survive with

Table 5
Infectious diseases of the avian beak and oral cavity, including species and anatomic location most commonly affected

Disease	Species Affected	Beak Lesions	Oral Lesions
Viral diseases			
Poxvirus	Numerous	Uncommon	Yes
Herpesvirus	Numerous, but most notably psittacine birds, such as South American parrots (eg, Amazon parrots, macaws)	No	Yes
Parvovirus	Geese (GPV), ducks (DPV)	Yes (duck)	Yes (ducks and geese)
Polyomavirus	Lady Gouldian finches	Yes	No
Psittacine beak and feather disease (PBFD)	Psittacine birds	Yes	Yes
Bacterial diseases			
"Lockjaw" (*Bordetella avium*)	Cockatiels	No	Yes
Oral spiral bacteria	Cockatiels	No	Yes
Bacterial rhinitis	Numerous, but somewhat common in psittacine birds	Yes	No
Mycotic diseases			
Candidiasis	Numerous, but notably juvenile psittacine birds	Rare	Yes
Cryptococcosis	Reported in Major Mitchell cockatoo	Yes	No
Aspergillosis	Numerous, but reported in Amazon parrots	Yes	Uncommon
Parasitic diseases			
Knemidocoptosis	Budgerigars, finches, other avian species	Yes	No
Capillariasis	Most common in free-ranging avian species	No	Yes
Flukes	Most common in water birds (eg, herons)	No	Yes

supportive care for long periods after developing lesions, immunosuppression and life-threatening opportunistic infections are common.[21,59]

- Avian pox is caused by viruses of the genus *Avipoxvirus* in the family Poxviridae. Pox virus infections are common in avian species but are only occasionally diagnosed in psittacine birds.[21] There are 2 major forms of clinical disease: a dry (cutaneous) or a wet (diphtheroid) form, although a septicemic form also can occur.[21] In the dry form, papules, pustules, nodules, crust, and eschar form on nonfeathered areas of skin, frequently around the eyes, beak commissures, and cere.[21] In the wet form, plaque and diphtheritic membrane form over oral mucus membranes and respiratory mucosa.[21] Lesions can become necrotic and secondarily infected with bacteria and fungi.[21] Diagnosis is generally made through biopsy and histopathology, with demonstration of intracytoplasmic eosinophilic inclusion bodies (Bollinger bodies), although PCR also can be used to demonstrate the presence of virus.[21] Mortality rates are higher with the wet form.[21] Cutaneous lesions will usually spontaneously resolve, and so treatment is primarily supportive.

- Oral mucosal papillomas in psittacine birds associated with PsHV-1 have been discussed previously. Other avian herpesviruses also can result in oral pathology. Pigeon herpesvirus-1 (PHV-1) can cause ulcers and diphtheritic plaques in the oropharynx and on the cere and rictus, particularly in squabs and immunosuppressed young adults.[21]
- Avian polyomavirus (genus *Polyomavirus*, family Polyomaviridae) is often fatal in finches. However, some surviving birds, particularly lady Gouldian finches (*Erythrura gouldiae*), may develop elongation to tubular deformation of the rostral beak tips, and inflammation and necrosis of the beak germinal epithelium.[21]
- Goose parvovirus (genus *Dependoparvovirus*, family Parvoviridae) has been associated with stomatitis in goslings and Muscovy ducks (*Cairina moschata*). "Short-beak syndrome" in mule ducks (Muscovy duck and Pekin duck [*Anas platyrhynchos*] hybrid) is caused by a distinct goose parvovirus.[60]
- A cluster of beak abnormalities in black-capped chickadees (*Poecile atricapillus*) and other avian species has been recently documented in Alaska and elsewhere along the US Pacific Coast.[61–63] Lesions include excessive rhamphothecal growth and elongation with associated epidermal hyperplasia and hyperkeratosis.[61,62] This condition has been termed *avian keratin disorder*. A novel picornavirus, termed poecivirus, was recently identified in clinically affected black-capped chickadees through unbiased metagenomic sequencing.[63] Further screening of affected birds was positive for 19 chickadees, two northwestern crows (*Corvus caurinus*), and two red-breasted nuthatches (*Sitta canadensis*).[63] The authors suggested that this novel picornavirus is the causative agent for avian keratin disorder.[63]

Bacterial Diseases

Primary bacterial infections of the beak are unusual in birds, although secondary bacterial infections are somewhat common.[21,64] Infection with *B avium* in juvenile cockatiels can result in a severe sinusitis and rhinitis with involvement of surrounding prokinetic musculature and bone.[65–68] Some affected birds have reduced ability to open the jaw. Isolated strains of *B avium* from cockatiels have been found to possess a dermatonecrotic toxin gene (DNT)[45,48,49] and to produce osteotoxin.[68,69] Pockets (diverticula) of the infraorbital sinus are closely associated with the quadrate bone and its kinetic joints.[65] Although *B avium* appears susceptible to most antimicrobial agents,[68] treatment should be based on results of culture and sensitivity testing. Once jaw stiffness sets in, the prognosis for recovery is poor, although treatment can still be attempted.[65,70]

Bacterial infections of the oral cavity are usually secondary and often involve opportunistic gram-negative bacteria. Bacterial oral cavity infections may result in mucosal inflammation, ulceration, hemorrhage, and necrosis and often resemble other oral diseases.[21] The diagnosis of bacterial infections is generally made through culture, although additional diagnostics, such as Gram stain and acid-fast stain, can be used to further characterize observed bacteria.[21] Treatment of bacterial infections should be based on results of culture and sensitivity testing and also should include treatment of predisposing and underlying diseases as well as supportive care.

Spirally curved bacteria have reportedly been associated with rhinitis, stomatitis, and pharyngitis in cockatiels and, less commonly, lovebirds.[71] Clinical signs include lethargy, anorexia, sneezing, nasal discharge, inflammation of the choanal papillae, and pharyngeal hyperemia.[71,72] Preliminary results of limited PCR testing suggest the organism may belong to the genus *Helicobacter*.[71] Diagnosis is typically made through cytologic examination of stained choanal or oropharyngeal swabs. Doxycycline in the drinking water and per os is effective in eliminating infections in cockatiels.[71,72]

Mycotic Diseases

Primary mycotic infections of the beak and oral cavity are uncommon in birds, but secondary infections have been reported.[21,73] Sinusitis caused by *Cryptococcus neoformans* var *gattii* in a 7-year-old male Major Mitchell cockatoo (*Cacatua leadbeateri*) was associated with destruction of the rhinotheca.[73] Infection with *Penicillium cyclopium* resulted in rhinothecal necrosis and destruction in a blue and gold macaw (*Ara ararauna*).[22] Topical itraconazole had been ineffective before the diagnosis.[22] *Aspergillus* sp was cultured from an adult yellow-naped Amazon parrot (*Amazona auropalliata*) with sinusitis, radiographic osteolysis of facial bones, and distorted growth of the distal rhinotheca.[74] Fungal mats were observed by histopathology on debrided beak tissues. The bird was treated with itraconazole administered per os.[74]

Oral infection with *Candida albicans* is most often secondary to other diseases. Predisposing factors include viral and bacterial infections and hypovitaminosis A. Oral candidiasis is more common in juvenile birds. Infection often results in thickened oral mucosa with overlying whitish to grayish plaque.[21] Cytology is usually diagnostic.[21] Antifungal agents, such as topical or oral nystatin, are generally effective in eliminating infection.

PARASITIC DISEASES
Ectoparasites

Several ectoparasites can result in damage to the beak and surrounding tissues. Infection with *Knemidocoptes pilae* (scaly face mite; scaly leg mite) is somewhat common in small passerine birds and psittacine birds, such as budgerigars, kākārikis, and *Neophema* and *Polytelis* parrots (**Fig. 17**).[21] The entire life cycle of the mite is spent on the host.[21] Mites are often found along the beak margins but can be found elsewhere on the body, such as the legs, wing tips, and vent.[21] The skin and rhamphotheca can develop a hyperkeratotic and pitted or honeycombed appearance.[21,75–77] Advanced lesions can result in severe distortion of the rhamphotheca.[21,77] Diagnosis is made

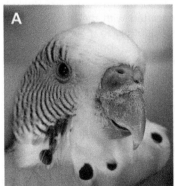 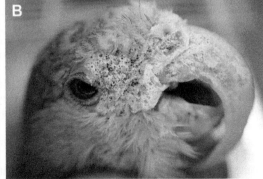

Fig. 17. *Knemidocoptes pilae* (scaly face mite) infection in psittacine birds. (*A*) Adult male budgerigar (*Melopsittacus undulatus*). Note the pitted surface of the rhinotheca and skin adjacent to the beak. (*B*) Adult female Pacific parrotlet (*Forpus coelestis*). Note similar changes to the rhinotheca and skin. (*Courtesy of* Lauren Powers DVM, DABVP (Avian Practice, Exotic Companion Mammal Practice); with permission.)

through direct visualization and microscopic examination of skin or rhamphothecal scrapings.[21,77] Avermectins, such as ivermectin and moxidectin, are commonly used to treat infections and are often administered at 7-day to 10-day intervals until clinical resolution. Ivermectin can be administered orally or applied topically to lesions.[75,77] Weekly topical application of 0.05 mL of a 1 mg/mL solution was effective in eradicating mites within 2 weeks in budgerigars.[75] Systemic treatment is recommended for birds with severe or generalized infections.[76]

Endoparasites

Some parasites that can be found in the oral cavity, such as flukes, are large enough to be visualized without magnification and can be manually removed.[43] Infections with *Capillaria* spp may result in oral lesions. Infections are relatively rare in companion birds unless housed outdoors. Nematode fragments can be observed histologically found within the mucosa.[21]

Trichomoniasis is caused by protozoal parasites in the *Trichomonas* genus, most notably *Trichomonas gallinae*. Infection is common in doves and ornithophagous raptors and is considered an emerging disease of wild passerine birds. In pigeons, the disease is known as "trich," or "canker," and in raptors as "frounce." The disease is rare in psittacine birds.[21] Yellow to white nodules, plaques, and ulcers develop within the oral cavity. Lesions often extend to the esophagus and crop and can be locally invasive. Secondary bacterial infections are common.[21] Lesions can look similar to other oral cavity diseases, such as avian pox, candidiasis, capillariasis, and hypovitaminosis A.[21] Microscopic visualization of wet mount preparations from fresh oropharyngeal or crop swabs is a reliable method of diagnosis.[21] Nitroimidazole drugs such as metronidazole, carnidazole, and ronidazole are most commonly used to treat trichomoniasis in birds.

TOXINS

Mycotoxins such as the tricothene mycotoxin T-2 produced by *Fusarium* spp may result in erosion and plaque involving the palate, tongue, and oropharynx in gallinaceous birds.[21] Beak deformities have been associated with exposure to organic environmental pollutants and selenium in aquatic and fish-eating free-ranging birds.[61]

RHAMPHOTHECAL OVERGROWTH AND DEFORMITY

Elongation and deformation of the beak keratin is common in companion psittacine birds and is most often secondary to uneven rhamphothecal wear from other disease processes.[25,33,63] Any disease that results in uneven growth or abrasion (wear) of the rhamphotheca can result in deformation and overgrowth of the beak keratin. Chronic liver disease appears to be associated with excessive rhinothecal growth and elongation, but the explanation for this association is unknown.

Rhamphothecal Reshaping

Abnormal keratin accumulation is frequently removed from captive parrots and the procedures are often also referred to as "beak trim" procedures; although they do not imply the removal of bone as occurs in poultry. In birds that are maintained in companion or captive settings, the bill is sometimes not subjected to its biologically intended use and resulting wear. This may be the result of the consumption of different food items, a lack of the normal enrichments that would provide such wear, or other factors. A frequent consequence of the lack of normal wear is the perceived or potential need for trimming of these beaks, although this is not necessarily always the case.

Beak trimming is often performed on parrots by veterinarians in private practice for cosmetic purposes and/or to remove excessive keratin that could lead to or is known to be the cause or result of abnormal force vector delivery, abnormal rhamphothecal wear, and progressive development of malocclusion. When trimming the beaks of these birds, it is prudent to describe the deformities carefully, hypothesize the causality despite its potential elusiveness, and strategize an anatomically sound manner of trimming.[78]

Procedural Concepts

Low-stress handling and restraint methods are an essential component of these procedures. The potential for escalating escape and avoidance behaviors, learned fear, increased aggression, generalized fear, or even apathy is very real. These undesired consequences may adversely affect not only the outcome of the procedure itself directly, but the longer-term health and welfare of the bird, as well as the continued strength of the doctor-client relationship. Where appropriate, skilled handling, strategic shaping of the restraint experience, conscious sedation, or even general anesthesia may be indicated. Effectiveness is best judged by assessment of the behavior of the bird during future visits and procedures.

The use of a hobby drill tool (eg, Dremel) or other grinding tools is popular and effective for many keratin-trimming procedures. These tools offer procedural speed, and access to the multiple keratin surfaces that may require attention. The optimal use of this tool requires the selection of the proper size and shaped bits, manual skills in handling and using the tool, and appreciation of the potential for heat that can be generated with excessive pressure or contact time. Not all keratin deformities require the use of a grinding tool, and a variety of other hand-held trimming tools can be used, depending on the patient size, behavior, and the specifics and complexity of the deformities being addressed.

Keratin structures that should be evaluated and shaped in concert with each other include the rostral and lateral rhinothecal tomia, the rostral and lateral gnathothecal tomia, the culmen, and the inner occlusal ledge of the rhinotheca, which functions as the occlusal site for the rostral gnathothecal tomium. With careful assessment, a more focused and effective reshaping procedure can be developed for an individual bird's set of deformities. Where dermal or bony involvement is planned or is known to have occurred, pain management should be incorporated into the procedural plan. In some select cases, preprocedural radiography can help delineate the extent of trimming that may be most appropriate, and general anesthesia can be helpful for some more involved beak corrective trimming procedures.

Following completion of the procedure, a targeted enrichment strategy to result in the functional increased use of these structures in more normal alignment should be contemplated and incorporated as a part of the whole procedure and its follow-up with a goal to reduce the need for and frequency of future procedures, if not eliminate their need completely.

REFERENCES

1. King AS, McLelland J. Skeletomuscular system. In: Birds–their structure and function. 2nd edition. London: Baillière Tindall; 1984. p. 43–51.

2. King AS, McLelland J. External anatomy. In: Birds–their structure and function. 2nd edition. London: Baillière Tindall; 1984. p. 9–10.

3. Bock WJ. Kinetics of the avian skull. J Morphol 1964;114(1):1–41.

4. Baumel JJ, Raikow RJ. Arthrologia. In: Baumel JJ, Kings AS, Breazile JE, et al, editors. Handbook of avian anatomy: nomina anatomica avium. 2nd edition. Cambridge (MA): Nuttall Ornithological Club; 1993. p. 179–90.

5. Carril J, Degrange FJ, Tambussi CP. Jaw myology and bite force of the monk parakeet (Aves, Psittaciformes). J Anat 2015;227(1):34–44.

6. King AS, McLelland J. Nervous system. In: Birds–their structure and function. 2nd edition. London: Baillière Tindall; 1984. p. 258–60.

7. King AS, McLelland J. Integument. In: Birds–their structure and function. 2nd edition. London: Baillière Tindall; 1984. p. 23–6.

8. Hulscher JB. Growth and abrasion of the oystercatcher bill in relation to dietary switches. Neth J Zool 1985;35:124–55.

9. King AS, McLelland J. Cardiovascular system. In: Birds–their structure and function. 2nd edition. London: Baillière Tindall; 1984. p. 214–28.

10. Yahav S. Regulation of body temperature: strategies and mechanisms. In: Scanes CG, editor. Sturkie's avian physiology. 6th edition. London: Academic Press; Elsevier; 2015. p. 869–905.

11. Tattersall GJ, Andrade DV, Abe AS. Heat exchange from the toucan bill reveals a controllable vascular thermal radiator. Science 2009;325(5939):468–70.

12. King AS, McLelland J. Digestive system. In: Birds–their structure and function. 2nd edition. London: Baillière Tindall; 1984. p. 84–109.

13. Baumel JJ, Witmer LM. Osteologia. In: Baumel JJ, Kings AS, Breazile JE, et al, editors. Handbook of avian anatomy: nomina anatomica avium. 2nd edition. Cambridge (MA): Nuttall Ornithological Club; 1993. p. 80–1.

14. Vanden Berge JC, Zweers GA. Myologia. In: Baumel JJ, Kings AS, Breazile JE, et al, editors. Handbook of avian anatomy: nomina anatomica avium. 2nd edition. Cambridge (MA): Nuttall Ornithological Club; 1993. p. 202–5.

15. King AS, McLelland J. Special sense organs. In: Birds–their structure and function. 2nd edition. London: Baillière Tindall; 1984. p. 284–314.

16. King AS, McLelland J. Respiratory system. In: Birds–their structure and function. 2nd edition. London: Baillière Tindall; 1984. p. 110–8.

17. Krautwald-Junghanns ME, Kostka VM, Dörsch B. Comparative studies on the diagnostic value of conventional radiography and computed tomography in evaluating the heads of psittacine and raptorial birds. J Avian Med Surg 1998;12(3): 149–57.

18. Echols MS, Speer B. Diagnosis and treatment of nasal-frontal hinge joint arthrodesis in a hybrid macaw (Ara macao x Ara ararauna). Int Conf Avian Herp Exot Mamm Med 2013;286.

19. van Zeeland YRA, Schoemaker NJ, Hsu EW. Advances in diagnostic imaging. In: Speer BL, editor. Current veterinary therapy in avian medicine and surgery. St Louis (MO): Elsevier; 2015. p. 531–49.

20. Stacy N, Pendl H. Cytology. In: Speer BL, editor. Current veterinary therapy in avian medicine and surgery. St Louis (MO): Elsevier; 2015. p. 501–22.

21. Schmidt RE, Reavill DR, Phalen DN. Pathology of pet and aviary birds. 2nd edition. Ames (IA): Wiley-Blackwell; 2015.

22. Bengoa A, Briones V, Lopez MB, et al. Beak infection by Penicillium cyclopium in a macaw (Ara ararauna). Avian Dis 1994;38:922–7.

23. Schnellbacher RW, Stevens AG, Mitchell MA, et al. Use of a dental composite to correct beak deviation in psittacine species. J Exot Pet Med 2010;19(4):290–7.

24. Martin D, Ritchie W. Orthopedic surgical techniques. In: Ritchie WR, Harrison JG, editors. Avian medicine: principles and application. Lake Worth (FL): Wingers Publishing; 1994. p. 1139–69.

25. Worell AB. Dermatological conditions affecting the beak, claws, and feet of captive avian species. Vet Clin North Am Exot Anim Pract 2013;16(3):777–99.
26. Speer B, Echols MS. Surgical procedures of the psittacine skull. Proc Assoc Avian Vet 2013;99–109.
27. Fecchio RS, Petri BSS, Fitorra LA, et al. Beak correction in a striped owl. Exotic DVM 2010;12(2):7–9.
28. Ashe CA, Morandi F, Greenacre C, et al. What is your diagnosis? J Am Vet Med Assoc 2009;234(4):455–6.
29. Lejnieks D. Treatment of a mandibular fracture using a steel plate in a lesser sulfur-crested cockatoo. Exotic DVM 2004;6(4):15–7.
30. Chitty J. Beak repair in a red-crowned crane. Proc Assoc Avian Vet 2014;113–5.
31. Carrasco DC, Dutton TAG, Shimuzu NS, et al. Distraction osteogenesis correction of mandibular ramis fracture malunion in a juvenile mute swan. Proc Annu Conf Assoc Avian Vet 2014;339–40.
32. Wade L. Acrylic stabilization for psittacine rhinothecal fractures (the "beak helmet"). Proc Assoc Avian Vet 2015;127–32.
33. Olsen GH. Oral biology and beak disorders of birds. Vet Clin North Am Exot Anim Pract 2003;6(3):505–21.
34. Wheler CL. Orthopedic conditions of the avian head. Vet Clin North Am Exot Anim Prac 2002;5(1):83–95.
35. Klaphake E. What is your diagnosis? J Avian Med Surg 2000;14(2):129–31.
36. Foerster SH, Gilson SD, Bennett RA. Surgical correction of palatine bone luxation in a blue-and-gold macaw (Ara ararauna). J Avian Med Surg 2000;14(2):118–21.
37. Bennett RA. Surgery of the avian beak. Proc Assoc Avian Vet 2011;191–5.
38. Ardisana R, Welle KR. Outcomes of beak amputation in psittacine birds. Proc Assoc Avian Vet 2013;49.
39. Crosta L. Alloplastic and heteroplastic bill prostheses in 2 ramphastidae birds. J Avian Med Surg 2002;16(3):218–22.
40. Fecchio RS, Bodde SG, Meyers MA, et al. Mechanical behavior of prosthesis in toucan beak (Ramphastos toco). World Sm Anim Vet Assoc World Congress. São Paulo, Brazil, July 2009.
41. Morris PJ, Weigel JP. Methacrylate beak prosthesis in a Marabou stork (Leptoptilos crumeniferus). J Assoc Avian Vet 1990;4(2):103–6.
42. Brown D. Possible etiology of submandibular lingual entrapment in herbivorous waterfowl. Exotic DVM 2006;8(4):7–9.
43. Echols MS. Soft tissue surgery. In: Greenacre CB, Morishita TY, editors. Backyard poultry medicine and surgery—a guide for veterinary practitioners. Ames (IA): Wiley-Blackwell; 2015. p. 220–59.
44. Grosset C, Guzman DSM, Waymire A, et al. Extraoral surgical correction of lingual entrapment in a Chinese goose (Anser cygnoides). J Avian Med Surg 2013;27(4):301–8.
45. Levine BS. Observations from the field: Surgical treatment of submandibular lingual entrapment in a Toulouse goose. Exotic DVM 2005;6(6):4–5.
46. Owen HC, Doneley RJ, Schmidt RE, et al. Keratoacanthoma causing beak deformity in a budgerigar (Melopsittacus undulatus). Avian Pathol 2007;36(6):499–502.
47. Manucy TK, Bennett RA, Greenacre CB, et al. Squamous cell carcinoma of the mandibular beak in a Buffon's macaw (Ara ambigua). J Avian Med Surg 1998;12(3):158–66.

48. Suedmeyer WK, McCaw D, Turnquist S. Attempted photodynamic therapy of squamous cell carcinoma in the casque of a great hornbill (Buceros bicornis). J Avian Med Surg 2001;15(1):44–9.

49. Baitchman E, Li VW, Li WW, et al. Treatment of squamous cell carcinoma in a great Indian hornbill (Buceros bicornis). Proc Amer Assoc Zoo Vet 2008;134–5.

50. Ferrell ST, Marlar AB, Garner M, et al. Intralesional cisplatin chemotherapy and topical cryotherapy for the control of choanal squamous cell carcinoma in an African penguin (Spheniscus demersus). J Zoo Wildl Med 2006;37(4):539–41.

51. Duncan AE, Smedley R, Anthony S, et al. Malignant melanoma in the penguin: characterization of the clinical, histologic, and immunohistochemical features of malignant melanoma in 10 individuals from three species of penguin. J Zoo Wildl Med 2014;45(3):534–49.

52. Andre JP, Delverdier M, Cabanie P, et al. Malignant melanoma in an African grey parrot (Psittacus erithacus erithacus). J Assoc Avian Vet 1993;7(2):83–5.

53. Guthrie AL, Gonzalez-Angulo C, Wigle WL, et al. Radiation therapy of a malignant melanoma in a thick-billed parrot (Rhynchopsitta pachyrhyncha). J Avian Med Surg 2010;24(4):299–307.

54. Kajigaya H, Katsutoshi K, Ejima H, et al. Metastatic melanoma appearing to originate from the beak of a racing pigeon (Columba livia). Avian Dis 2010;54(2):958–60.

55. Reid HA, Herron AJ, Hines ME, et al. Metastatic malignant melanoma in a mandarin duck (Aix galericulata). Avian Dis 1993;37:1158–62.

56. Riddell C, Cribb PH. Fibrosarcoma in an African grey parrot (Psittacus erithacus). Avian Dis 1983;27(2):549–55.

57. Ramsay E, Bos JH, McFadden C. Use of intratumoral cisplatin and orthovoltage radiotherapy in treatment of a fibrosarcoma in a macaw. J Assoc Avian Vet 1998;42:408–12.

58. Phalen D. Psittacid herpesviruses and their associated diseases. In: Speer BL, editor. Current veterinary therapy in avian medicine and surgery. St Louis (MO): Elsevier; 2015. p. 47–9.

59. Raidal S. Psittacine beak and feather disease. In: Speer BL, editor. Current veterinary therapy in avian medicine and surgery. St Louis (MO): Elsevier; 2015. p. 51–9.

60. Palya V, Zolnai A, Benyeda Z, et al. Short beak and dwarfism syndrome of mule duck is caused by a distinct lineage of goose parvovirus. Avian Pathol 2009; 38(2):175–80.

61. Handel CM, Van Hemert C. Environmental contaminants and chromosomal damage associated with beak deformities in a resident North American passerine. Environ Toxicol Chem 2015;34(2):314–27.

62. Van Hemert C, Handel CM, O'Hara TM. Evidence of accelerated beak growth associated with avian keratin disorder in black-capped chickadees (Poecile atricapillus). J Wildl Dis 2012;48(3):686–94.

63. Zylberberg M, Van Hemert C, Dumbacher JP, et al. Novel picornavirus associated with avian keratin disorder in Alaskan birds. mBio 2016;7(4):e00874–16.

64. Gartrell BD, Alley MR, Kelly T. Bacterial sinusitis as a cause of beak deformity in an Antipodes Island parakeet (Cyanoramphus unicolor). N Z Vet J 2003;51: 196–8.

65. Fitzgerald SD, Hanika C, Reed WM. Lockjaw syndrome in cockatiels associated with sinusitis. Avian Pathol 2001;30(1):49–53.

66. Clubb SL, Homer BL, Pisani J, et al. Outbreaks of bordetellosis in psittacines and ostriches. Proc Assoc Avian Vet 1994;63–8.

67. Matsuda S, Ohya K, Yanai T, et al. Microbiology and histopathology of cockatiel lockjaw syndrome. J Japan Vet Med Assoc 2009;62(2):143–7.
68. Grespan A, Camera O, Knöbl T, et al. Virulence and molecular aspects of *Bordetella avium* isolated from cockatiel chicks (*Nymphicus hollandicus*) in Brazil. Vet Microbiol 2012;160(3):530–4.
69. Moreno LA, Knöbl T, Grespan AA, et al. Draft genome sequence of *Bordetella avium* Nh1210, an outbreak strain of lockjaw syndrome. Genome Announcements 2015;3(2):1–2.
70. Messenger GA. Successful management of lockjaw in a white-bellied caique. Proc Assoc Avian Vet 2009;47–55.
71. Wade L, Simpson K, McDonough P, et al. Identification of oral spiral bacteria in cockatiels (*Nymphicus hollandicus*). Proc Annu Conf Assoc Avian Vet 2003;23–5.
72. Evans EE, Wade LL, Flammer K. Administration of doxycycline in drinking water for treatment of spiral bacterial infection in cockatiels. J Am Vet Med Assoc 2008; 232(3):389–93.
73. Raidal SR, Butler R. Chronic rhinosinusitis and rhamphothecal destruction in a Major Mitchell's cockatoo (*Cacatua leadbeateri*) due to *Cryptococcus neoformans* var *gattii*. J Avian Med Surg 2001;15(2):121–5.
74. Mans C. What is your diagnosis? J Avian Med Surg 2007;21:235–8.
75. Hossain MDK, Sanderson D, Nahar K, et al. Dose titration, efficacy and safety of "drop on" ivermectin for the management of *Knemidocoptes* spp. infestation in budgerigars. J App Pharm 2012;3(4):670–5.
76. Yunker CE, Ishak KG. Histopathological observations on the sequence of infection in knemidokoptic mange of budgerigars (*Melopsittacus undulatus*). J Parasitol 1957;43(6):664–72.
77. Elbal PM, Salido VJ, Murillo JM, et al. Severe beak deformity in *Melopsittacus undulatus* caused by *Knemidocoptes pilae*. Turkish J Vet Anim Sci 2014;38(3): 344–6.
78. Speer BL. Beak deformities: form, function, and treatment methods. Proc Assoc Avian Vet 2014;213–9.

Anatomy, Physiology and Non-dental Disorders of the Mouth of Pet Rabbits

Thomas M. Donnelly, BVSc, DVP, DACLAM, DABVP(ECM), DECZM(SM)[a,*],
David Vella, BSc, BVSc (Hons), DABVP(ECM)[b]

KEYWORDS

- Rabbit • Mouth • Tooth • Oral disorders • Mastication • Neoplasia

KEY POINTS

- The stomatognathic system of rabbits consists of the mouth, teeth, jaws, pharynx, and associated structures, such as the salivary glands, that are involved with eating.
- Numerous research articles are published about different anatomic structures in the rabbit's stomatognathic system, and also on the physiology of leporine mastication; however, no reviews exist that summarize this research for veterinary clinicians.
- In rabbits, the continuous growth of their long-crowned teeth and the steady process of tooth wear results in a dynamic state that leads to complex patterns of acquired dental disease.
- The 2 major theories for the cause of acquired dental disease are inadequate dental wear and metabolic bone disease.
- Nondental diseases of the stomatognathic system are relatively infrequent in rabbits compared with the incidence of dental disease; these diseases are primarily composed of infectious, neoplastic, and congenital abnormalities of the lips, tongue, salivary glands, and jaw.

ANATOMY AND PHYSIOLOGY OF THE RABBIT MOUTH
Dentition

The rabbit dental formula is 2(I2/1 C0/0 PM3/2 M3/3) = 28. It is useful clinically to divide rabbit dentition into 2 groups: the incisor teeth set and *cheek teeth* (CT) set (premolars and molars). The 2 groups form 2 different functional units (**Fig. 1**). There is no anatomic difference between premolars and molars; therefore, they are commonly named CT. Each arcade can be divided in 2 quadrants (maxillary and

The authors have nothing to disclose.
[a] Exotic Animal Service, Centre Hospitalier Universitaire Vétérinaire d'Alfort, École Nationale Vétérinaire d'Alfort, 7 Avenue du Géneral de Gaulle, Maisons-Alfort Cedex 94704, France;
[b] Sydney Exotics and Rabbit Vets, 64 Atchison Street, Crows Nest, New South Wales 2065, Australia
* Corresponding author.
E-mail address: thomas.donnelly@vet-alfort.fr

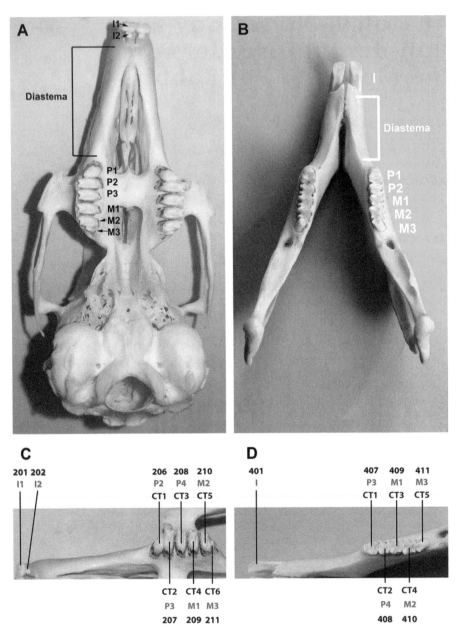

Fig. 1. (*A–D*) Dentition of the rabbit, displaying various numbering methods of teeth. (*A*) Maxillary jaw of a rabbit, ventrodorsal view. (*B*) Mandible of a rabbit, dorsoventral view. The system numbering existing teeth beginning from the rostral (mesial) is displayed in (*A, B*). (*C*) Close up of the left maxillary quadrant and (*D*) close up of the right mandibular quadrant. The modified Triadan system (*black*), the standard system (*brown*), and the practical system numbering the series of cheek teeth are displayed in (*C, D*). (*Courtesy of* Vittorio Capello, DVM; with permission. Photos by Tom Donnelly, DVM (*A, C*) and Vittorio Capello, DVM (*B, D*). Graphics by Vittorio Capello, DVM.)

mandibular on right and left). The rabbit mouth also has a relatively long toothless gap between the incisor teeth and the first cheek tooth known as the *diastema*.

Up to 4 nomenclature systems can be used to identify individual teeth in rabbits. Boarded veterinary dentists prefer to use the modified Triadan system,[1] based on the system introduced by Professor Dent H. Triadan, DMD, in Switzerland.[2] The modified Triadan system provides a consistent method of numbering teeth across different mammal species. The system is based on the permanent dentition of the pig, which has 11 teeth in each quadrant. Teeth are numbered with 3 digits. The first digit represents the quadrant of the permanent dentition (1 = right maxillary; 2 = left maxillary; 3 = left mandibular; 4 = right mandibular). The second and third digits denote the tooth position within the quadrant, with the numbering starting rostrally at the midline (mesially) with fixed landmarks (01 is the mesial incisor, the canine is 04, the premolars are 05–08, the molars are 09–11). According to this numbering system, the right maxillary quadrant of rabbits includes the 101 and 102 incisors; misses 103 to 105 compared with pig's dentition; the remaining 3 premolars are 106 to 108, and the 3 M are 109 to 111. The right mandibular quadrant of rabbits instead includes the 401 incisor; misses 402 to 406 compared with pig's dentition; the remaining 2 premolars are 407 and 408, and the 3 M are 409 to 411.

The other 3 methods do not include identification of the specific quadrant. Two of them differentiate between premolars and molars, by designating with "P" (or "PM") and the latter with "M" respectively. However, 2 types of numbering may be applied to this method. Veterinary dentists prefer to also consider the teeth among the premolar group that have been lost during development. With this method, the most caudal premolar is always numbered P4. Maxillary premolars of the rabbit are therefore labeled as P2, P3, and P4, whereas the mandibular premolars are labeled as P3 and P4.[3–5] A similar but alternative system, used most commonly by general and exotic pet practitioners, numbers the existing teeth beginning from the rostral (mesial) end. Maxillary premolars of the rabbit are therefore labeled as P1, P2, and P3, whereas the mandibular premolars are labeled as P1 and P2. This last method is used in other rodent and rabbit textbooks and this review.[6] Finally, a fourth method does not include identification of the specific quadrant, and does not differentiate between premolars and molars, which are not anatomically different in the rabbit. This method (again used most commonly by exotic pet practitioners), names them generally *molariforms* or CT, numbering maxillary CT CT1 through CT6 from rostral to caudal (ie, from the mesial to the distal end of the quadrant) and mandibular CT from CT1 through CT6[6] (see **Fig. 1**).

Lips

The diastema allows the lips to fold inward (*inflexa pellita*) and come together behind the incisors.[7] The infolding brings fur inside the mouth and effectively forms an antechamber in the rostral part of the mouth. A median cleft of the dorsal lip (harelip) allows easy exposure of the incisors rostrally[7] (**Fig. 2**). This external labial morphology is seen in lagomorphs and rodents.

Jaws

The mandible is narrower than the maxilla, a feature known as anisognathism. Rodent jaws are also anisognathic, but the mandible is wider than the maxilla.[4] Rabbits have no bony union between the 2 mandibles; however, the existence of broad symphyseal plates with highly interdigitating rugosities, united by dense connective tissue, render the symphyseal joint virtually immobile.[8] The rigid symphysis converts the right and left mandibles into a single unit and permits the masticatory muscles on both sides of the head to shift the jaw laterally and generate the force required for grinding.[8] The gape of

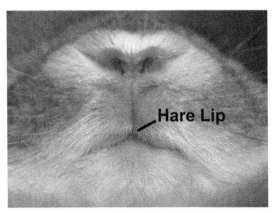

Fig. 2. In lagomorphs and rodents, the *pars supralabialis* (supralabial part) of the *musculus orbicularis oris* (the circular muscle of the mouth) is reduced ventrally and a cleft divides the upper lip. This cleft is called the upper lip cleft or "harelip."

maximal jaw opening in rabbits is only 20° to 25°,[9] compared with rats, which is 40°,[10] or small felids, which is 65° to 70°.[11] These characteristics make examination of the rabbit mouth relatively difficult.

Anatomy and Physiology of the Teeth

Rabbits have only 2 types of teeth, incisors and CT, which are separated by the diastema (see **Fig. 1**). They do not have canines and the premolars are large resembling the molar teeth, whereas the last molars (M3) are diminished (see **Fig. 1**). Unlike rodents, which have only 1 set of teeth (monophyodonty), rabbits have both deciduous and permanent teeth (diphyodonty).[12,13] At birth the mandibular deciduous molars are completely developed and at 4 days their root resorption is initiated.[14] Eruption of the mandibular permanent molars starts at 9 days, and at 23 days for the mandibular permanent premolars. By 32 days all the mandibular permanent CT have erupted.

All the teeth of rabbits are classified as elodont (continuously growing, with no anatomic roots) and hypsodont (long-crowned). The teeth can also be classified as aradicular (no anatomic root). This type of dentition allows for a concurrent increase in teeth size with growth of the animal. It also results in a dynamic state that leads to complex patterns of acquired dental disease.

The standard description of tooth anatomy used for anelodont (truly rooted) teeth is inappropriate for rabbits. In case of anelodont teeth, the crown is the part of the tooth projecting above the gingiva and is covered in enamel; the root is set in the alveolar processes of the jaw and is not covered by enamel. In rabbits there is no distinguishable root and crown. This has led to terms such as "exposed" or "clinical" crown for the part above the gingiva, and "reserve crown," "submerged crown," or "clinical root" for the part below the gum line (**Fig. 3**). The terminology is confusing,[5] and for practical purposes it is easier to divide the tooth, correctly called *anatomic crown*, into the *clinical crown* (the part of the tooth exposed above the gingival margin) and the *reserve crown* (the part of the tooth buried below the gingival margin and within the alveolus). Some clinicians simply use *crown* and *root*, although the terms are anatomically incorrect. In many animals the roots are cone shaped and the term *apex* describes the pointed end of the root. The teeth of rabbits are not conical, but the extremity of the reserve crown is still described as the *apex*, which is open in rabbit teeth.

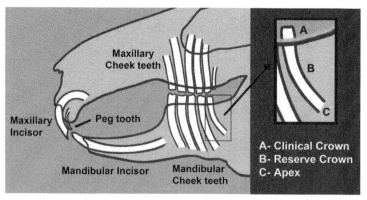

Fig. 3. Cross section schematic of a rabbit skull showing dentition of the mandible and maxilla and of an individual tooth. (*Modified from* Vella D, Donnelly TM. Basic anatomy, physiology, and husbandry. In: Quesenberry KE, Carpenter JW, editors. Ferrets, rabbits and rodents: clinical medicine and surgery. 3rd edition. Philadelphia: Elsevier/Saunders; 2012. p. 161; with permission. *Courtesy of* Marise Watson.)

Microanatomy of the Teeth

In recent decades, knowledge of the complex enamel microstructure of mammalian teeth has increased dramatically. A hierarchical system of levels of complexity is now established to enable the comparison of enamel in different mammalian orders.[15] The lowest level of complexity is the crystallite level, followed by the prism level, and then the enamel-type level. Enamel types are defined by the orientation of enamel prisms. Rabbits possess a distinct enamel microstructure known as irregular enamel in which bundles of enamel rods crisscross in an asymmetrical pattern.[15] This enamel microstructure is different from herbivorous ungulates and rodents, and represents an alternative way of achieving resistance to fracture in multiple directions. The irregular enamel gives rabbit teeth (incisor and cheek) a white appearance in contrast to the yellow-orange pigmented incisor teeth of some rodents. Rodent incisors have a thin, iron-rich layer in their enamel that makes it harder than regular enamel.[16] The level of iron in rodent enamel is 10 times greater than rabbit enamel.

The continuous eruption of both incisor and CT leads to unusual features of the periodontal ligament, which have been studied extensively for the incisors. The ligament is weakest in the basal region, where incisor development occurs, and strongest near the crown, where intrusive forces are resisted.[17]

Incisor Teeth

Rabbits (and lagomorphs in general) have a single pair of large chisel-shaped mandibular incisors. The maxillary incisors include a similar pair of large or primary incisors and a pair of much smaller secondary incisors or "peg teeth" located directly behind the primaries. Normally, the mandibular incisors occlude behind the primary maxillary incisors and against the secondary maxillary incisors, which protrude slightly beyond the gingiva (see **Fig. 3**). The mandibular incisors wear at approximately right angles to the secondary incisors, and the primaries wear along the arc, followed by the mandibular incisors (**Fig. 4**). This is because enamel is present only on the labial side of the strongly curved maxillary incisors, whereas the mildly curved mandibular incisors have enamel on both the labial and lingual aspects of the teeth.[18] Thus, a chisel-like, sharp cutting edge is found at the labial surface of upper primary maxillary and the mandibular incisors (see **Fig. 4**). Rabbits also periodically "grind" their teeth to

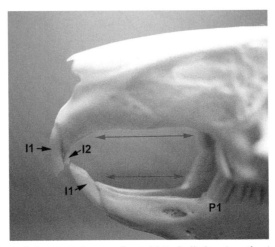

Fig. 4. Lateral view of the rostral part of a rabbit skull showing the incisors (I1, I2) and *diastema (red double point arrows)*. The mandibular incisors wear at approximately right angles to the maxillary secondary incisors (peg teeth), and the maxillary primary incisors wear along the arc followed by the mandibular incisors. P1 is the first premolar (according with the numbering of existing teeth).

help shape their incisor tips.[19] Pet rabbits can survive without incisors if they rely on food provided by the owner.

The maxillary primaries grow slower than the mandibular incisors, at rates of 2.0 and 2.4 mm/wk, respectively,[20] which is 2 to 3 times faster than the CT. On an annual basis, this is approximately 4 inches for each maxillary incisor and 5 inches for each mandibular incisor.[20] In addition, the rate of teeth growth can be influenced by age, pregnancy, and diet.[21] The attrition rate of maxillary incisors primarily depends on the growth of the antagonist mandibular incisors in the lower jaw, and not on the hardness of feedstuffs.[22]

Incisors have a single pulp cavity. In normal occlusion of the jaw, the mandibular incisor tips lay just caudal to the main maxillary incisors, in the space between the primary maxillary incisors and the peg teeth.[23] The tips of the mandibular incisors in occlusively normal rabbits make contact with the peg teeth.

Cheek Teeth

The CT have a single pulp chamber at the tooth apex, which diverges into 2 chambers toward the clinical crown. The smaller maxillary CT6 and mandibular CT5 are an exception, with a single pulp chamber. The CT are longitudinally straighter and somewhat "folded" on the buccal side in cross section (**Fig. 5**). This formation creates an increase in the proportion of enamel on the occlusal surface of the tooth (providing increasing grinding efficiency and aiding in reduction of wear rate). The more heavily calcified alveolar bone surrounding each tooth socket is termed the *lamina dura*.

The CT of the rabbit undergo extensive wear to obtain a functioning crown shape. Most investigators assumed that growth and wear of CT are strikingly lower than that of incisors, and report a growth rate of 3 to 4 mm per month[24] or 0.5 to 0.7 mm/wk[10]; however, 2 studies have reported faster growth rates of mandibular CT: 1.1 to 1.3 mm/wk[25] and 1.37 to 3.23 mm/wk.[10] The different findings highlight the adaptability of rabbit teeth growth and that variation in response to wear can be expected.

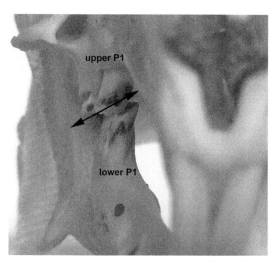

Fig. 5. The CT are longitudinally straighter and somewhat "folded" on the buccal (toward the cheek) side in cross section. This formation creates an increase in the proportion of enamel on the occlusal surface of the tooth (providing increasing grinding efficiency and aiding in reduction of wear rate). The continual attrition that occurs due to tooth-food and tooth-tooth abrasion maintains this file-like occlusal plane on each arcade, and provides an excellent grinding surface. This figure uses the numbering of existing teeth (P1).

The margins of each tooth, and the ridges across the occlusal surface of each tooth, are composed of enamel. Abrasion removes cementum and thin enamel from the cusp tips of the newly erupted molar crown, creating a series of enamel crests on the crown surface.[13] As enamel wears at a slower rate than dentin, the enamel crests eventually project above the adjacent dentin. Further wear results in ridges across the crown, called lophs, which are highly contoured and form a series of transverse ridges and valleys. This results in a series of interlocking transverse ridges and valleys and gives a characteristic zigzag pattern of CT occlusion seen on lateral radiographs of the skull.

The maxilla is wider than the mandible, so when the CT are in occlusion, the mandibular CT rest with their buccal edges occluding with the lingual edges of the maxillary CT. When mastication occurs, each maxillary and mandibular CT contacts 2 opposite CT, except for the first and last maxillary CT which come in contact with only one mandibular CT.[21] This allows the central transverse enamel ridge of each CT to interlock with the opposing interdental space and provide an excellent grinding surface. The continual attrition that occurs due to tooth-food and tooth-tooth abrasion maintains this rasplike occlusal surface of the CT, whereas the continuous growth of the permanent incisors and CT compensates for their occlusal wear.[13]

Mastication

Rabbits in the wild selectively eat young succulent greens and roots, when available.[26–28] Food is detected by sensitive vibrissae on the lips, as rabbits cannot see objects directly in front of the mouth.[29] The lips are highly mobile, and rabbits use their incisors to crop short pieces of vegetation.[12] Rabbits primarily use a vertical action to cut foliage with their incisors.[23] They then use the CT to grind or crush their food. Mastication is dominated by the superficial masseter muscle. Its mechanical advantage is improved by elevation of the mandibular condyle and expansion of the mandibular angle (**Fig. 6**).

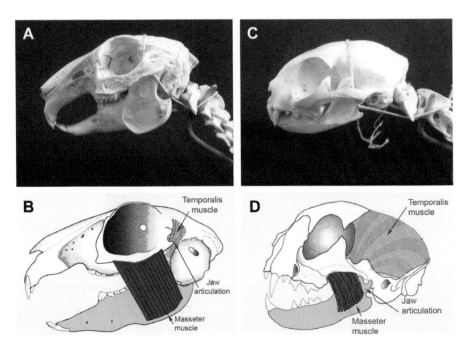

Fig. 6. Skulls of a rabbit (*A, B*) and a domestic cat (*C, D*). Chewing in rabbits involves grinding vegetation, and maximal force is achieved by a large superficial masseter muscle (*A, B*). In contrast, eating in carnivores involves biting into flesh, and maximal force for this action is achieved by a large *temporalis* muscle (*C, D*).

Once plant material is in the mouth, it is masticated primarily in a horizontal or lateral plane by only one side of the CT at a time.[19] This is an important consideration, as dietary factors have been shown to affect a rabbit's normal chewing process.[10] Interestingly, unilateral paralysis of the masseter muscle in rabbits using *Botulinum* toxin does not prevent the animals from chewing on both sides, possibly because of the inclined plane of their occlusion is sufficient to control movement.[30]

There are 2 different modes of the power stroke (ie, the muscle contraction) when observing rabbits consuming hay, pellets, or carrots: a crushing movement where the jaw maintains a rotation to the working side (occurs in carrots and frequently in pellet mastication), and a shearing movement where the jaw rotates back to the midline, with an occasional slight overrotation to the balancing side (occurs in hay and sometimes in pellet mastication).[9] Vegetation, such as grass or hay, complements a standard horizontal chewing action of the CT, whereas harder and thicker food items (such as pellets, grains, or carrots) encourage more vertical and less horizontal chewing movements.[9] Up to 120 jaw movements per minute have been reported during mastication of food.[31] Too little horizontal chewing or too much vertical movement can lead to a reduction in tooth wear and also potentially increase forces on teeth in the vertical plane, producing increased pressure on the growing apex of the tooth.[6] For readers seeking more information, Watson and colleagues[32] have written an outstanding review of mastication in the rabbit.

The processes of tooth wear are still not well understood. Wear of teeth can be caused by both tooth-to-tooth contact (ie, attrition), and by abrasion due to internal abrasives, such as microscopic silica in grasses, or external abrasives such as dust or grit.[10] Muller and colleagues[10] found that food intake rate, as a proxy for chewing activity, is a significant factor for maxillary incisor wear, but not for CT or mandibular incisor wear.[10] They found CT wear occurs in the rabbit independently when fed a pelleted diet, but increases slightly with the degree of dietary abrasiveness, such as microscopic silica in vegetation to sand in the feed.[10] The investigators concluded that tooth growth and wear is more influenced by tooth-to-tooth contact from the type of diet (eg, hay, vegetation) and not so much by abrasiveness of the diet. The natural diet of wild rabbits entails the consumption of large volumes of abrasive high-fiber foods, which results in standard horizontal chewing movement. Clinically, as rabbits are selective feeders, they will choose to consume the more luscious parts of vegetation, such as succulent leaves and shoot tips that complement the standard horizontal chewing movements. However, the eating of fruiting bodies, seeds, roots, and other high-energy storage parts of plants can be seen as purely opportunistic, as it results in vertical chewing movements.

Etiopathogenesis of Dental Disease

The major causes of dental disease are congenital or developmental anomalies affecting the incisor teeth, and acquired dental disease (ADD) affecting the CT and incisors. Congenital and developmental causes can include maxillary brachygnathism, mandibular prognathism, and jaw or teeth malformation.[3,22] ADD accounts for most dental disease seen in pet rabbits. It is a syndrome[6] in which the clinical signs and symptoms follow improper mastication and ineffective dental wear, and that progresses to derangement of the shape, position, and structure of the teeth and associated supported structures causing related (or further) complications. The causes of ADD are much debated and an analysis of these causes is beyond the scope of this review. For readers seeking more information, the review by Jekl and Redrobe (2013)[24] is recommended. The 2 major working causational theories are inadequate dental wear and metabolic bone disease. Rare reports describe neoplasia of the jaw causing ADD,[23,33,34] and malocclusion of teeth is possible after traumatic fractures as well.

One theory suggests that the effects of "insufficient wearing" of the teeth have the greatest impact on the formation of dental disease in rabbits.[6,23,35,36] This interpretation is supported by the assumption that most pet rabbits are fed inappropriate diets that do not mimic the abrasive nature of a natural grass diet.[23,37] Consequently, offering pet rabbits concentrate feeds reduces the amount of typical horizontal masticatory movements and significantly reduces the time spent chewing.[38,39] The result is insufficient wear, especially on the CT, followed by coronal elongation of both the clinical and the reserve crown. Tooth elongation and increased curvature reduces masticatory capacity and/or efficacy. Both coronal spikes that create additional lingual and/or buccal lesions, and increased pressure applied to elongated reserve crowns and the surrounding cortical bone elicits pain that further affects mastication.

This insufficient wear theory partly relies on the premise that the maxillary and mandibular CT are not in contact when at rest.[23,40] The theory assumes that as the CT become elongated, their normal occlusal position changes. Instead of being separated at rest, the maxillary and mandibular CT now come in contact at their occlusal surfaces. Gradually, this is believed to lead to a widening of the normal "closed" mouth position and eventually, resting jaw tone prevents further tooth eruption.[40] A slowing of apical reserve crown growth coupled with a lack of eruption and increased pressure then leads to intrusion of the apices into underlying apical jaw bone.[40] Apical elongation and increased pressure applied to the germinative tissue affect the blood supply and lead to deterioration of the tooth structure of both the reserve and the clinical crown.

Yet another hypothesis, the metabolic bone disease (MBD) theory, proposes that MBD plays a major role in the development of ADD.[21,41,42] Harcourt-Brown[21,41,42] found certain metabolic bone diseases, such as nutritional secondary hyperparathyroidism (NSHP), to be a possible factor in formation of ADD in pet rabbits. These studies suggest that the early loss of supporting alveolar bone (due to underlying NSHP) at the apex of the teeth allow their intrusion into surrounding bone. This can be seen especially in the mandibular CT, in which the teeth apices eventually penetrate the ventral mandibular cortex. The associated weakness of surrounding bone affected by NSHP may lead to distortion of the normal tooth socket. Subsequent alteration in teeth shape (eg, increased curvature) and orientation then leads to CT malocclusion. Further loss of alveolar bone may then initiate loosening of teeth and widening of periodontal spaces, which in turn can initiate the development of secondary infections, subsequent osteomyelitis, and the development of periapical abscessation.

Regardless of the cause of dental disease, the deviation of overgrown CT typically results in apical eruptions of teeth laterally through the associated cortical bone, except for the first and last mandibular CT, which more often tend to erupt medially.[19] Infection and abscessation of the bone and soft tissue follows, and can be caused by endodontic infection, penetrating foreign bodies, trauma to teeth or jaw, and hematogenous spread.[23] The "insufficient wear" theory suggests periodontal pockets are created from loss of periodontal ligaments secondary to periodontitis associated with reduced tooth growth.[23] The MBD theory suggests that accompanying alveolar bone demineralization leads to widening of the periodontal spaces and loosening of the teeth, which then allows bacteria and food particles to enter the periodontal space and cause periodontitis.[21]

Salivary Glands

The rabbit has 4 pairs of major salivary glands: parotid, mandibular (also known as submaxillary or submandibular), sublingual, and zygomatic. There are also many unencapsulated minor salivary glands found throughout the oral mucosa within the *lamina propria*. Von Ebner glands are deep salivary glands found on the dorsal surface of the tongue associated with the *circumvallate vallate* and *foliate papillae*.[43] Saliva is produced continuously by the mandibular glands, and produced in response to food intake by the parotid, mandibular, sublingual, and zygomatic glands.[44] There is a marked taste preference for polycose and its disaccharide constituent maltose, suggesting that these saccharides are likely to add to the taste sensation while feeding on starchy plants.[45] This supposition is supported by the fact that rabbits have been shown to excrete extraordinarily high amounts of amylase, an enzyme that dissociates starch into maltose units, in the saliva produced by their parotid glands. Lipase and urea (prominent in human and ruminant saliva, respectively) are present in only trace amounts in rabbit saliva.[44]

Salivary gland ducts and their openings in the rabbit are not well described, except for the mandibular gland duct, which opens into an elongated sublingual caruncle on the floor of the mouth, under the tongue caudal to the mandibular incisors.[46] Furthermore, in many experimental papers, the ducts are described eponymically (eg, Wharton papilla, Stenson duct). An early German atlas of rabbit anatomy[47] describes the parotid gland duct as opening near the first maxillary premolar, and the ducts of the sublingual and zygomatic glands, which are joined, as opening near the second maxillary molar.

Tongue

The tongue is large for the size of the animal. The large tongue and small mouth make visualization of the epiglottis unrealistic without endoscopic equipment. The dorsal surface is covered by multiple small elevations termed papillae, which give the tongue a roughened surface. The dorsal surface can be divided into 3 parts: the rostral, the middle, and the caudal parts. The rostral part contains the lingual apex and makes up almost half of the tongue. The middle part has a conspicuous lingual prominence (*torus linguae*) located at the intermolar region close to the caudal half area of the tongue[48] (**Fig. 7**). The caudal part is a narrow region located at the lingual root. The presence of a lingual prominence is regarded as a characteristic structure of herbivores. It is an effective structure for grinding food between the tongue and the upper palate. There are large spearheadlike filiform papillae on the rostral edge of the lingual prominence (that occasionally may be mistaken as papillomatous growths) and branched filiform papillae on the caudal area of the prominence. These papillae are not involved in taste, as they serve only to facilitate movement of ingesta within the mouth.[48]

NON-DENTAL DISEASES OF THE MOUTH AND JAWS

Non-dental diseases of the stomatognathic system are relatively infrequent in rabbits. These diseases are primarily represented by infections, neoplasias, and congenital abnormalities of the lips, tongue, salivary glands, and jaw. Traumatic injuries can occur as well.

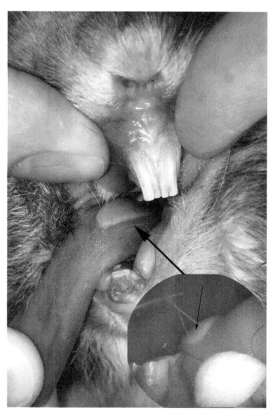

Fig. 7. Rabbits have large tongues. A noticeable prominence known as the *torus linguae* (*black arrow*) is found in the intermolar region and aids in grinding food between the tongue and the upper palate. *Torus linguae* shown on a tongue pulled out of the oral cavity and during endoscopic evaluation (*inset*).

Lips

Facial lesions around the nose, eyelids, and lips are often seen in rabbits with trepone-matosis caused by *Treponema paraluiscuniculi*. Earlier reports of the disease, ranging from the first description more than 100 years ago[49] and up to 30 years ago,[50] describe the most common site of lesions in naturally infected rabbits as the vulva or prepuce,[51] with facial lesions being rare. However, reports in the past 12 years from Asia describe more facial lesions compared with anogenital lesions in infected pet rabbits.[52–54] The range of lesions on the lips was 32% to 60%, on the eyelids was 18% to 19% and on the nose was 57% to 87%.[53,54] Facial lesions were more common in pet rabbits younger than 1 year, and most likely reflect how the disease is acquired. In pet rabbits, maternal transmission is more common,[53,54] but in farm or colony rabbits venereal transmission is more common. Penicillin is the treatment of choice and administered as 3 long-acting injections (benzathine penicillin G/procaine penicillin G 25–50 mg/kg [42,000–84,000 IU/kg]) given subcutaneously 7 days apart.[55]

A mucocutaneous bacterial pyoderma, similar to mucocutaneous pyoderma of dogs, was reported in a 7-year-old rabbit.[56] Clinical signs were severe swelling and erythema of the mucocutaneous junctions of the lips, nares, and vulva. Bilateral, severe periocular dermatitis was also present. Heavy pure growths of a member of the *Staphylococcus intermedius* group were cultured from nasal and aural swabs and skin biopsies. Treatment of the bacterial infection with oral marbofloxacin and topical ofloxacin eye drops together with supportive therapy resulted in resolution of the lesions.

Disseminated histoplasmosis characterized by multiple nodules surrounding the eyes, nose, mouth, and prepuce was reported in a 2.5-year-old male rabbit.[57] The rabbit was treated with micronized griseofulvin (25 mg/kg by mouth every 24 hours) for 12 days but no improvement was seen and the animal was euthanized. Necropsy revealed *Histoplasma capsulatum*, confirmed by positive fungal culture, in the small intestine, skin, penis, rectum, axillary lymph node, and conjunctiva.

Tongue

Oral papillomatosis is widespread among domestic rabbits in Europe and the Americas, particularly young animals.[58] It is caused by rabbit oral papillomavirus, which is distinct from the cottontail rabbit papillomavirus (Shope rabbit papillomavirus). Rabbits present with small (5-mm diameter and 4-mm height), gray-white, filiform or pedunculated nodules that are localized mostly on the underside of the tongue[59] (**Fig. 8**). However, one report describes a conjunctival papilloma.[60] The papillomas usually regress spontaneously within a few weeks to a few months. Lesions typically

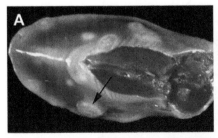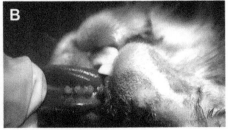

Fig. 8. (*A, B*) Oral papillomatosis. (*A*) A dissected tongue, ventral view. The underside of the tongue shows small, gray-white early lesions of papillomatosis. The blue arrow points to a typical wartlike lesion. (*B*) Incidental finding of lingual papillomas along the ventral midline in a rabbit under general anesthesia for dental treatment. (*Courtesy of* [A] AFIP-Department of Veterinary Pathology; and [B] *Courtesy of* Vittorio Capello, DVM, Milano, Italy; with permission.)

occur in rabbits between 2 and 18 months of age and are found more frequently in young rabbits whose mothers have papillomas and transmission from the mother to offspring during suckling is common.[61] The oral papillomas are not highly contagious and the virus can be recovered from the mouth washings of rabbits having no oral papillomas. The virus is latent in the mouth, and does not proliferate unless the mucous membrane is injured. Most pet rabbit owners do not notice the lesions.

Naturally occurring vesicular stomatitis virus (Rhabdoviridae), a disease of cattle, horses, and pigs, occurred in young rabbits on a rabbit farm in China.[62] The disease caused inflammation and blisters on the tongue, lip, and mouth that later ruptured. The infected rabbits had a temperature of 40° to 41°C and died within 5 to 10 days.

Salivary Glands

A sialocele originating in the duct of the sublingual salivary gland near its opening, close to the lingual frenulum, was observed as a naturally occurring lesion in a laboratory rabbit.[63] The lesion resembled an oral papilloma. However, microscopic examination revealed the lesion to be a sialocele (ranula). Necrotizing sialometaplasia (a non-neoplastic condition of the salivary glands caused by ischemic infarction) has been reported following a traumatic comminuted fracture of the mandible.[64]

Neoplasms

Most of the cases presented involve calcified tissue proliferation, and could be misdiagnosed as a bony lesion potentially related to dental disease. Although rare, it is important to consider neoplasia as a differential diagnosis for dental disease.

Of 22 reported cases of osteosarcomas in rabbits, 7 cases (32%) report the primary site arising in the mandible.[65–71] Another 2 cases arose in the frontal bone[72] and facial bones (nasal, frontal and zygomatic bones, and mandible and maxilla).[73] And yet another case involved an extraskeletal osteosarcoma arising on the right upper lip that spread subcutaneously over the maxilla.[33] An early report by Katase[74] describes 2 rabbits with "round-cell tumors" of the mandible that could have been osteosarcoma. Unfortunately, the tumors are difficult to evaluate, as Katase[74] provided an insufficient description.

Two reports describe odontogenic tumors, an ameloblastoma,[75] and ameloblastic fibroma,[76] in young rabbits presenting with gingival masses. Two cases of mandibular fibrosarcoma extending into the mouth, that radiologically mimicked a mandibular abscess with osteomyelitis, have been reported.[77,78] An ossifying fibroma of the maxilla,[34] a cementoma,[79] and a chondrosarcoma of the mandible (**Fig. 9**) are also described in rabbits.[79]

For soft tissue neoplasms, there is one report of a salivary gland adenocarcinoma.[80] Three cases of a multicystic lesion of the mandible have been reported[81–83]; however, there are opposing views as to what the nature of these lesions is. Gillet and Gunther[82] proposed that the lesions are a mucoepidermoid carcinoma, whereas Gardner and colleagues[81] proposed that the lesions are inflammatory and resemble periodontal (radicular) cysts in human beings, except that they are multilocular.

Congenital Abnormalities

Mandibular prognathism (synonyms: brachygnathia, hypognathia, malocclusion, walrus teeth, buck teeth) is the most common inherited disease in the rabbit. It denotes an abnormally long mandible relative to the length of the maxilla and is inherited as an autosomal recessive trait with incomplete (81%) penetrance.[84,85] Affected animals have reduced length measurements for the skull and the maxillary diastema, without significant deviation from normal length of mandibles.

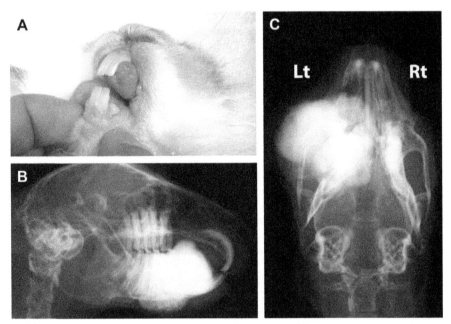

Fig. 9. (*A–C*) Oral neoplasia in pet rabbits. (*A*) Clinical appearance of an osteosarcoma diagnosed at histopathology. (*B, C*) Latero-lateral and dorsoventral projections of a cementoma affecting the left mandible of a 6-month-old rabbit. (*Courtesy of* Yasutsugu Miwa, DVM, Tokyo, Japan; with permission.)

Rabbits with hereditary mandibular prognathism show malocclusion of incisors after 3 weeks of age. Initially, there is an edge-to-edge bite with blunting of incisural cutting edges that rapidly develops into rostral positioning of the mandibular incisors to the maxillary primaries. The maxillary primaries usually curl within the mouth, while the mandibular incisors grow rostrally to protrude from the mouth. The maxillary primaries may pierce the gingival or buccal mucosa, leading to ulceration and/or abscess formation.

The absence of second incisors (ie, peg teeth) occurs in domestic rabbits and occasionally in wild rabbits.[18,86] Inheritance is considered to be dominant. Instead of normal peg teeth, affected animals develop small, rudimentary structures resembling teeth that typically disappear shortly after birth. Dwarf rabbits frequently have an absence of the peg teeth.[18]

A mutation considered less common than the absence of second incisors is that of supernumerary or increased numbers of peg teeth.[86,87] The additional teeth appear between individual members of the first pair of peg teeth and are typically slightly larger than the first pair. Inheritance is considered to be by a single recessive gene with low penetrance.

Mandibulofacial dysostosis characterized by a large mouth has been diagnosed in an inbred line of rabbits.[88] Neonatal rabbits showed papillae at the corners of extremely wide mouths. The rabbits had deformities of the zygomatic bone and zygomatic processes of adjacent bones. Inheritance appears to be due to a single autosomal recessive gene with incomplete penetrance.

Dwarf rabbits may exhibit mandibular prognathism,[36,89] and the condition has been attributed to brachycephaly, a condition in which individuals have short (usually broad) facial profiles due to restricted growth of the skull base.[84,90] In dogs, brachycephaly is associated with mandibular prognathism. In rabbits, the cause is not mandibular prognathism, but maxillary enognathism, a condition in which the maxilla is narrower than normal.[6] It could also be described as a false mandibular prognathism.[91,92] Although malpositioning of the CT in dwarf rabbits is anecdotally attributed to brachycephaly, in one study there was no significant relationship between breed of rabbit and dental disease.[21]

Traumatic Lesions

Rabbits are a laboratory model for bone studies in humans, including studies of healing post experimental fractures of the mandible, and oro-maxillary facial surgery. Although references are plentiful, only those concerning pet rabbits are considered in this discussion.[64]

Primary traumatic fractures of the jaw can occur in rabbits, and may be associated with poor husbandry and improper handling, especially of fractious intact rabbits.

Fractures of the jaws also can be associated with dental disease. Fractures can be secondary pathologic sequela of dental disease, especially to complications such as osteomyelitis (**Fig. 10**A). Risk of fracture also may be higher in rabbits with reduced bone density or bone lysis associated with MBD. Iatrogenic fractures occurring during tooth extraction have been anecdotally reported.

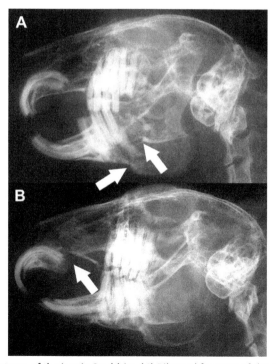

Fig. 10. (*A, B*) Fractures of the jaw in 2 rabbits. (*A*) Bilateral fracture of the mandible (*arrows*) following ADD with periapical infection and osteomyelitis of mandibular CT4 and CT5. The rabbit survived with assisted feeding and conservative treatment. (*B*) Bilateral open fracture of the incisive bones (*arrow*), likely following entrapment of maloccluded incisor teeth in cage bars. (*Courtesy of* Vittorio Capello, DVM, Milano, Italy; with permission.)

Mandibular fractures are more common than those of the maxillary jaw, and may affect one or more of the following: the incisor portion, body, masseteric fossa, branch, and condyles.

Fractures of the maxillary incisive bones or rostral mandible may occur when maxillary or mandibular incisors are trapped in cage bars; this may be more common in rabbits with incisor malocclusion and elongation (see **Fig. 10**B). Fracture of the incisive bones is usually open and bilateral, and may lead to complications such as osteomyelitis and rhinitis. If not already present, these types of fractures will lead to incisor malocclusion.

Unless marked dislocation is present, most fractures of the mandible are relatively stable due to the strength of the masticatory muscle, especially caudal fractures of the masseteric fossa.

Repair of jaw fractures is particularly difficult due to anatomic features, such as long reserve crowns of both incisor and CT, thin bone cortices, and the particularly thin masseteric fossa and branch of the mandible. However, rabbits often heal well with assist feeding, analgesia, and supportive care. Stabilization of the diastasis of the mandible using cerclage wire at the base of the incisor teeth has been anecdotally reported, and may be successful if the fractured portion is still viable.

REFERENCES

1. Floyd MR. The modified Triadan system: nomenclature for veterinary dentistry. J Vet Dent 1991;8(4):18–9.
2. Triadan H. Veterinary dentistry: tooth preservation (cavity therapy with "composite materials" and endodontics) in monkeys. [Tierzahnheilkunde: Zahnerhaltung (Fullungstherapie mit Composite Materials und Endodontie) bei Affen und Raubtieren]. Schweiz Arch Tierheilkd 1972;114(6):292–316 [in German].
3. Verstraete FJ, Osofsky A. Dentistry in pet rabbits. Comp Cont Educ Pract Vet 2005;27(9):671–83.
4. Böhmer E. Dentistry in rabbits and rodents. 1st edition. Chichester, West Sussex: Wiley-Blackwell; 2015.
5. Harcourt-Brown F. Normal rabbit dentition and pathogenesis of dental disease. In: Harcourt-Brown F, Chitty J, editors. Manual of rabbit surgery, dentistry and imaging. 1st edition. Quedgeley (Gloucester): British Small Animal Veterinary Association; 2013. p. 319–36.
6. Capello V, Gracis M, Lennox AM. Rabbit and rodent dentistry handbook. 1st edition. Lake Worth (FL): Zoological Education Network; 2005.
7. Ade M. External morphology and evolution of the rhinarium of lagomorpha. With special reference to the glires hypothesis. Mitt Mus Naturkunde Berl Zoolog Reihe 1999;75(2):191–216.
8. Hirschfeld Z, Michaeli Y, Weinreb MM. Symphysis menti of the rabbit: anatomy, histology, and postnatal development. J Dent Res 1977;56(7):850–7.
9. Weijs WA, Dantuma R. Functional anatomy of the masticatory apparatus in the rabbit (*Oryctolagus cuniculus* l). Neth J Zool 1981;31(1):99–147.
10. Muller J, Clauss M, Codron D, et al. Growth and wear of incisor and cheek teeth in domestic rabbits (*Oryctolagus cuniculus*) fed diets of different abrasiveness. J Exp Zool A Ecol Genet Physiol 2014;321(5):283–98.
11. Emerson SB, Radinsky L. Functional analysis of sabertooth cranial morphology. Paleobiology 1980;6(3):295–312.
12. Hirschfeld Z, Weinreb MM, Michaeli Y. Incisors of the rabbit: morphology, histology, and development. J Dent Res 1973;52(2):377–84.

13. Michaeli Y, Hirschfeld Z, Weinrub MM. The cheek teeth of the rabbit: morphology, histology and development. Acta Anat (Basel) 1980;106(2):223–39.
14. Navarro JA, Sottovia-Filho D, Leite-Ribeiro MC, et al. Histological study on the postnatal development and sequence of eruption of the mandibular cheek-teeth of rabbits (*Oryctolagus cuniculus*). Arch Histol Jpn 1976;39(1):23–32.
15. Koenigswald WV, Clemens WA. Levels of complexity in the microstructure of mammalian enamel and their application in studies of systematics. Scanning Microsc 1992;6(1):195–218.
16. Yanagawa T, Itoh K, Uwayama J, et al. Nrf2 deficiency causes tooth decolouriza-tion due to iron transport disorder in enamel organ. Genes Cells 2004;9(7): 641–51.
17. Komatsu K, Yamazaki Y, Yamaguchi S, et al. Comparison of biomechanical prop-erties of the incisor periodontal ligament among different species. Anat Rec 1998; 250(4):408–17.
18. Taglinger K, Konig HE. Macroscopic-anatomical studies on the teeth of rabbits (Oryctolagus cuniculus). [Makroskopisch-anatomische Untersuchungen der Zahne des Kaninchens (Oryctolagus cuniculus)]. Wien Tierarztl Monatsschr 1999;86(4):129–35 [in German].
19. Harcourt-Brown F. Textbook of rabbit medicine. Oxford (United Kingdom): Butterworth-Heinemann; 2002.
20. Shadle AR. The attrition and extrusive growth of the four major incisor teeth of domestic rabbits. J Mammal 1936;17(1):15–21.
21. Harcourt-Brown FM. Metabolic bone disease as a cause of dental disease in pet rab-bits. London: FRCVS thesis, Royal College of Veterinary Surgeons; 2006. p. 174.
22. Wolf P, Kamphues J. Influence of feeding on the length of incisors in rabbits, chin-chillas and rats. [Untersuchungen zu Fütterungseinflüsse auf die Entwicklung der Incisivi bei Kaninchen, Chinchilla und Ratte]. Kleintierpraxis 1996;41(10):723–32 [in German].
23. Crossley DA. Oral biology and disorders of lagomorphs. Vet Clin North Am Exot Anim Pract 2003;6(3):629–59.
24. Jekl V, Redrobe S. Rabbit dental disease and calcium metabolism—the science behind divided opinions. J Small Anim Pract 2013;54(9):481–90.
25. Koenigswald WV, Golenishev FN. A method for determining growth rates in continuously growing molars. J Mammal 1979;60(2):397–400.
26. Bhadresa R. Food preferences of rabbits *Oryctolagus cuniculus* L. at Holkham Sand Dunes, Norfolk. J Appl Ecol 1977;14(1):287.
27. Marrero P, Martin C. Spring food preferences of rabbits (*Oryctolagus cuniculus* L., 1758) on the Islet of Alegranza (Canarian Archipelago). Z Saugetierkd 2000;65(4):246–50.
28. Martins H, Milne JA, Rego F. Seasonal and spatial variation in the diet of the wild rabbit (*Oryctolagus cuniculus* L.) in Portugal. J Zool 2002;258(3):395–404.
29. Hughes A. Topographical relationships between the anatomy and physiology of the rabbit visual system. Doc Ophthalmol 1971;30(1):33–159.
30. Matic DB, Yazdani A, Wells RG, et al. The effects of masseter muscle paralysis on facial bone growth. J Surg Res 2007;139(2):243–52.
31. Schwartz G, Enomoto S, Valiquette C, et al. Mastication in the rabbit: a descrip-tion of movement and muscle activity. J Neurophysiol 1989;62(1):273–87.
32. Watson PJ, Groning F, Curtis N, et al. Masticatory biomechanics in the rabbit: a multi-body dynamics analysis. J R Soc Interface 2014;11(99) [pii:20140564].
33. Renfrew H, Rest JR, Holden AR. Extraskeletal fibroblastic osteosarcoma in a rabbit (*Oryctolagus cuniculus*). J Small Anim Pract 2001;42(9):456–8.

34. Whitten KA, Popielarczyk MM, Belote DA, et al. Ossifying fibroma in a miniature Rex rabbit (*Oryctolagus cuniculus*). Vet Pathol 2006;43(1):62–4.
35. Capello V. Diagnosis and treatment of dental disease in pet rabbits and rodents: a review. J Exotic Mammal Med Surg 2004;2(2):5–12.
36. Reiter AM. Pathophysiology of dental disease in the rabbit, guinea pig, and chinchilla. J Exotic Pet Med 2008;17(2):70–7.
37. Wolf P, Kamphues J. A critical assessment of commercial supplementary feedstuffs for rabbits, guinea pigs, chinchilla as companion pets. [Kritische Einschatzung kommerzieller Erganzungspraparate fur Kaninchen, Meerschweinchen und Chinchilla]. Prakt Tierarzt 2003;84(9):674–8 [in German].
38. Wolf P, Bucher L, Kamphues J. The feed-, energy- and water intake in dwarf rabbits under feeding conditions of companion pets in the field. [Die Futter-, Energie- und Wasseraufnahme von Zwergkaninchen unter praxisublichen Futterungsbedingungen]. Kleintierpraxis 1999;44(4):263–80 [in German].
39. Wolf P, Kamphues J. Problems in the nutrition of small rodents kept as pet animals. [Probleme der art- und bedarfsgerechten Ernahrung kleiner Nager als Heimtiere]. Prakt Tierarzt 1995;76(12):1088–92 [in German].
40. Crossley DA, Aiken S. Small mammal dentistry. In: Quesenberry KE, Carpenter JW, editors. Ferrets, rabbits, and rodents: clinical medicine and surgery. 2nd edition. St Louis (MO): Saunders; 2004. p. 370–82.
41. Harcourt-Brown FM. Calcium deficiency, diet and dental disease in pet rabbits. Vet Rec 1996;139(23):567–71.
42. Harcourt-Brown FM, Baker SJ. Parathyroid hormone, haematological and biochemical parameters in relation to dental disease and husbandry in rabbits. J Small Anim Pract 2001;42(3):130–6.
43. Toyoshima K, Tandler B. Ultrastructure of von Ebner's salivary glands in the rabbit. J Submicrosc Cytol 1986;18(3):509–17.
44. Davies RR, Davies JA. Rabbit gastrointestinal physiology. Vet Clin North Am Exot Anim Pract 2003;6(1):139–53.
45. Laska M. Gustatory responsiveness to food-associated saccharides in European rabbits, *Oryctolagus cuniculus*. Physiol Behav 2002;76(2):335–41.
46. Madhuri K, Singh NK, Ratnesh K. Histomorphological studies on submandibular salivary gland in rabbit (*Oryctolagus cuniculus*). J Interacad 2011;15(2):282–6.
47. Krause W. The anatomy of the rabbit: in topographic and operative considerations. [Die Anatomie des Kaninchens: In topographischer und operativer Rücksicht]. 2nd edition. Leipzig (Germany): Verlag von Wilhelm Engelmann; 1884 [in German].
48. Nonaka K, Zheng JH, Kobayashi K. Comparative morphological study on the lingual papillae and their connective tissue cores in rabbits. Okajimas Folia Anat Jpn 2008;85(2):57–66.
49. Bayon H. A new species of *Treponema* found in the genital sores of rabbits. Br Med J 1913;2(2757):1159.
50. DiGiacomo RF, Lukehart SA, Talburt CD, et al. Clinical course and treatment of venereal spirochaetosis in New Zealand white rabbits. Br J Vener Dis 1984; 60(4):214–8.
51. Cunliffe-Beamer TL, Fox RR. Venereal spirochetosis of rabbits: description and diagnosis. Lab Anim Sci 1981;31(4):366–71.
52. Kim SH, Lee SE, Song KH, et al. Dermatitis associated with treponematosis in pet rabbits. J Vet Clin 2009;26(6):625–7.
53. Kweon SJ, Kim SH, Park HJ, et al. Seroprevalence and treatment for skin lesions of rabbit syphilis in pet rabbits. J Vet Clin 2014;31(1):15–8.

54. Saito K, Hasegawa A. Clinical features of skin lesions in rabbit syphilis: a retrospective study of 63 cases (1999-2003). J Vet Med Sci 2004;66(10):1247–9.
55. Cunliffe-Beamer TL, Fox RR. Venereal spirochetosis of rabbits: eradication. Lab Anim Sci 1981;31(4):379–81.
56. Benato L, Stoeckli MR, Smith SH, et al. A case of antibacterial-responsive mucocutaneous disease in a seven-year-old dwarf lop rabbit (Oryctolagus cuniculus) resembling mucocutaneous pyoderma of dogs. J Small Anim Pract 2013;54(4): 209–12.
57. Brandao J, Woods S, Fowlkes N, et al. Disseminated histoplasmosis (Histoplasma capsulatum) in a pet rabbit: case report and review of the literature. J Vet Diagn Invest 2014;26(1):158–62.
58. Kerr PJ, Donnelly TM. Viral infections of rabbits. Vet Clin North Am Exot Anim Pract 2013;16(2):437–68.
59. Rdzok EJ, Shipkowitz NL, Richter WR. Rabbit oral papillomatosis: ultrastructure of experimental infection. Cancer Res 1966;26(1):160–5.
60. Munday JS, Aberdein D, Squires RA, et al. Persistent conjunctival papilloma due to oral papillomavirus infection in a rabbit in New Zealand. J Am Assoc Lab Anim Sci 2007;46(5):69–71.
61. Parsons RJ, Kidd JG. Oral papillomatosis of rabbits: a virus disease. J Exp Med 1943;77(3):233–50.
62. Xu B, Sun Y, Lu H. Pathogenic diagnosis of vesicular stomatitis in rabbits. Chin J Rabbit Farm [Zhong Guo Yang Tu] 2005;1(1):8–10 [in Chinese].
63. Weisbroth SH. Sialocele (ranula) simulating oral papillomatosis in a domestic (Oryctolagus) rabbit. Lab Anim Sci 1975;25(3):321–2.
64. Vilano JS, Coope TK. Mandibular fracture and necrotizing sialometaplasia in a rabbit. Comp Med 2013;63(1):67–70.
65. Olafson P. Oral tumors of small animals. Cornell Vet 1939;29(2):222–37.
66. Ozsoy SY, Ozyldz Z. Osteosarcoma in a rabbit. [Bir tavşanda osteosarkom]. Ankara Univ Vet Fak Derg 2008;55(3):211–2 [in Turkish].
67. Walberg JA. Osteogenic sarcoma with metastasis in a rabbit (Oryctolagus cuniculus). Lab Anim Sci 1981;31(4):407–8.
68. Wappler O, Harder A. Osteosarcoma of the maxilla in a rabbit (Oryctolagus cuniculus). [Osteosarkom des Oberkiefers bei einem Kaninchen (Oryctolagus cuniculus)]. Kleintierpraxis 2000;45(9):707–12 [in German].
69. Jacobson SA. The comparative pathology of the tumors of bone. Springfield (IL): Thomas; 1971.
70. Dom P, Ducatelle R, Herdt PD. Osteosarcoma in a young domestic rabbit. [Osteosarcoma bij een juveniel konijn]. Vlaams Diergeneeskd Tijdschr 1992;61(2):50–2 [in Dutch].
71. Weisbroth SH, Hurvitz A. Spontaneous osteogenic sarcoma in Oryctolagus cuniculus with elevated serum alkaline phosphatase. Lab Anim Care 1969;19(2): 263–5.
72. Amand WB, Riser WH, Biery DN. Spontaneous osteosarcoma with widespread metastasis in a belted Dutch rabbit. J Am Anim Hosp Assoc 1973;9(6):577–81.
73. Hoover JP, Paulsen DB, Qualls CW, et al. Osteogenic sarcoma with subcutaneous involvement in a rabbit. J Am Vet Med Assoc 1986;189(9):1156–8.
74. Katase T. Demonstration of various tumors in animals. [Demonstration verschiedener Geschwülste bei Tieren]. Nihon Byori Gakkai Kaishi 1912;2(Verh Jpn Pathol Ges):89 [in German].
75. Volker I, Kammeyer P, Hinzmann B, et al. Peripheral keratinizing ameloblastoma in a dwarf rabbit (Oryctolagus cuniculus f. dom.). [Peripheres keratinisierendes

Ameloblastom bei einem Zwergkaninchen (Oryctolagus cuniculus f. dom.)]. Tierarztl Prax Ausg K Kleintiere Heimtiere 2014;42(5):331–5 [in German].

76. Walter JH, Gobel T, Schauer G. Ameloblastic fibroma in a juvenile rabbit. [Ameloblastisches Fibrom bei einem juvenilen Kaninchen]. Kleintierpraxis 1992;37(9):633–8 [in German].

77. Brower M, Goldstein GS, Ziegler LE, et al. Spontaneous oral fibrosarcoma in a New Zealand rabbit. J Vet Dent 2006;23(2):96–9.

78. Thas I, Dorrestein GM, Cohen-Solal NA. Mandibular fibrosarcoma and bile duct adenoma in a pet rabbit (Oryctolagus cuniculi): a case report. Open J Pathol 2014;4(2):32–40.

79. Miwa Y. Mandibulectomy for treatment of oral tumors (cementoma and chondro-sarcoma) in two rabbits. J Exotic Pet Med 2006;8(3):18–22.

80. Bercier M, Guzman DS-M, Stockman J, et al. Salivary gland adenocarcinoma in a domestic rabbit (Oryctolagus cuniculus). J Exotic Pet Med 2013;22(2):218–24.

81. Gardner DC, Bunte RM, Sawyer DR, et al. Multicystic lesion of the jaw in a rabbit. Contemp Top Lab Anim Sci 1997;36(3):78–80.

82. Gillett CS, Gunther R. Mandibular mucoepidermoid carcinoma in a rabbit. Lab Anim Sci 1990;40(4):422–3.

83. Orr JW. Adamantinoma of the jaw in a rabbit. J Pathol Bacteriol 1936;42(3):703–4.

84. Fox RR, Crary DD. Mandibular prognathism in the rabbit. Genetic studies. J Hered 1971;62(1):23–7.

85. Huang CM, Mi MP, Vogt DW. Mandibular prognathism in the rabbit: discrimination between single-locus and multifactorial models of inheritance. J Hered 1981; 72(4):296–8.

86. Nachtsheim H. Hereditary dental defects in the rabbit. [Erbliche Zahnanomalien beim Kaninchen]. Züchtungskunde 1936;11:273–87.

87. Rohloff R. Developmental studies of hereditary abnormalities of incisors in Oryctolagus cuniculus L. [Entwicklungsgeschichtliche Untersuchungen über erbliche Anomalien der Incisiven bei Oryctolagus cuniculus L]. Berlin (Germany): Faculty of Mathematics and Natural Sciences: Free University of Berlin; 1945. p. 70.

88. Fox RR, Crary DD. Hereditary macrostomus in the rabbit: a model for Treacher Collins syndrome, one form of mandibulofacial dysostosis. J Hered 1979;70(6): 369–72.

89. Wegner W. The problematics of breeding dwarf rabbits. [Zur Problematik der Zwergkaninchen-Zucht]. Dtsch Tierarztl Wochenschr 1997;104(5):181–3 [in German].

90. Crossley DA. Clinical aspects of lagomorph dental anatomy: the rabbit (Oryctolagus cuniculus). J Vet Dent 1995;12(4):137–40.

91. Fisher AK. Some observations on the use of the term prognathism. J Am Dent Assoc 1949;38(5):611–26.

92. Mayoral J. On the classification of dentofacial anomalies. Am J Orthod Oral Surg 1945;31(9):429–39.

Diagnostic Imaging of Dental Disease in Pet Rabbits and Rodents

Vittorio Capello, DVM, DECZM (Small Mammal), DABVP-Exotic Companion Mammal[a,b,*]

KEYWORDS

- Dental disease • Rabbit • Computed radiography • Computed tomography
- Magnetic resonance • Stomatoscopy

KEY POINTS

- Before additional diagnostic imaging, a thorough clinical examination must be performed, including inspection of the oral cavity in the conscious patient.
- Complete radiographic study should include at least 4 projections of good diagnostic quality; additional views are recommended for complete evaluation of dental and bony structures.
- Computed tomography overcomes superimposition of anatomic structures over a single plane, allowing multiple 2-dimensional views in the 3 spatial axes and 3-dimensional surface and volume reconstructions.
- Stomatoscopy is essential for inspection of the oral cavity; it prevents the risk of missing lesions, allows early diagnosis, and facilitates treatment of cheek teeth and other intraoral procedures.
- MRI provides excellent visualization of odontogenic abscesses and their relationship with adjacent anatomic structures, in particular for challenging complications such as retromasseteric and retrobulbar abscesses.

INTRODUCTION

The oral examination and the diagnosis of oral disorders in most exotic companion mammal species are intrinsically difficult (especially in common species such as rabbits and rodents) because of their size and oral anatomy. For these reasons, diagnostic imaging modalities assume particular importance in the evaluation of teeth and surrounding structures.

Aside from traditional radiographs, advanced diagnostic imaging has become popular in exotic mammal medicine. Increased owner education and therefore demand

The author has nothing to disclose.
[a] Clinica Veterinaria S. Siro, Via Lampugnano, 99, Milano 20151, Italy; [b] Clinica Veterinaria Gran Sasso, Via Donatello, 26, Milano 20134, Italy
* Clinica Veterinaria S.Siro, Via Lampugnano, 99, Milano 20151, Italy.
E-mail address: capellov@tin.it

coupled with the availability of referral centers for diagnostic imaging like computed tomography (CT) and MRI, make it both feasible and affordable. In the case of dental disease and other oral disorders (in particular of pet rabbits and selected rodent species), it is of paramount importance for both diagnosis and diagnostic accuracy, for detailed prognosis, and for treatment choice. In the case of extraoral surgical treatment, it is critical to plan the most effective surgical technique or approach.

BEFORE DIAGNOSTIC IMAGING: THE CLINICAL EXAMINATION

Dental disease is a syndrome (in most cases acquired and progressive) and can produce a wide range of clinical signs and symptoms.[1,2] These symptoms may be related specifically to the primary dental problem (reduced food intake, dysphagia, anorexia, changes in fecal quantity and size, weight loss) or to complications associated with dental disease (excessive grooming, excessive salivation and drooling, facial abscesses, epiphora, exophthalmos, nasal discharge, dyspnea). Other signs and symptoms are indicative of diseases or conditions secondary to dental disease (poor general condition, gastrointestinal problems, poor coat and skin diseases, ocular diseases, death).[1–4]

Before the physical examination, a thorough history should be obtained and the diet and feeding habits should be reviewed with the owner. Considering the predisposition of prey species to mask or hide symptoms, the absence of a clear clinical history does not rule out the possibility of dental disease. Reluctance to eat hay, reduced food intake, and abnormal feces in rabbits and rodents are common early symptoms frequently missed by owners. A thick hair coat can hide evident signs such as weight loss or the presence of facial swellings.

After overall inspection, palpation of the external maxillary and mandibular profiles (including the ventral aspect of the mandible and the temporomandibular joint) is performed to detect bony irregularities or swellings consistent with apical elongation of cheek teeth, periapical deformities, or abscesses. The incisor teeth are inspected from both the frontal and lateral aspects. The lateral mobility of the mandible is evaluated to assess the clinical crowns of cheek teeth. With careful and proper restraint, the oral cavity can be inspected with an otoscope in nonsedated rabbits and some large rodents. Even though a complete assessment of the oral cavity using inspection alone is not possible, it is helpful to detect spurs, elongated crowns, and buccal or lingual ulcerations, and to make a preliminary diagnosis. The examination of the eye and periocular structures, including patency of the nasolacrimal duct, should be part of the dental examination in rabbits. When dental disease is a presumptive or a differential diagnosis, the oral examination must be completed with the animal under general anesthesia.[1]

RADIOLOGY

The 2 radiologic imaging techniques used in exotic veterinary practice are radiography and CT.[5] The basic principles of physics are the same for both techniques, as images are generated by x-rays produced by a large diode (the x-ray tube). The most important and practical difference is that CT overcomes the superimposition of imaging that is intrinsic to conventional radiography.[5,6] Although radiography generates images where all tissues in the area of interest are superimposed over a single plane (therefore, multiple, complementary views are necessary to partially bypass this physical limitation), CT generates multiple, parallel cross-sectional images of the tissues of the patient that are elaborated and rendered by computer software.

Radiography

Radiography provides critical information to complement the clinical examination, and represents one of the most important diagnostic tools in veterinary dentistry.[1,2,7] It is also important to consider that the clinical crown, visible above the gingival margin, represents a small portion of the tooth, and that most of the dental structure (the reserve crown of hypsodont/elodont teeth and the root of brachyodont/anelodont teeth) is invisible on clinical inspection. Supporting bone and periapical structures, as well as other parts of the skull, should always be evaluated for diagnosis of dental disease.[1,5]

Digital modalities

Over the past few years, digital radiography (DR) has almost completely replaced conventional film radiography. The basics of radiography on standard films and high resolution films have been reported elsewhere.[5]

Conceptually, digital radiology (DR) is not an advanced technique, and does not necessarily produce higher quality radiographs than good-quality conventional radiographs. Most of the basic principles of traditional radiography on films apply to digital as well. The most important of them is patient positioning to obtain proper diagnostic views. However, some technical features should be considered.

Two digital imaging systems are available: computed radiography (CR) and direct digital radiography (DDR).[5] In the case of CR, detectors are placed in a cassette, which does not include films and intensifying screens. The image plate is processed by a specific scanner, which is a stand alone unit similar to an x-ray film processor, but is faster and does not require a dark room. Data are converted in a digital format image and processed by a computer, with specific software. The greatest advantage of CR is its ability to be coupled with standard radiographic equipment. Ideally, both systems (CR and traditional radiography) can be used with the same x-ray machine, and this is particularly important for the practitioner during the transition between the older system and CR.

DDR sends digital information directly to the computer without the intermediate scanning step. Advantages of DR include no need for x-ray films, dark room, or film storage; an immediate feedback (in case of DDR) and fewer retakes; immediate adjustment of the grayscale; and flexibility of the digital format for storage, recording, and distribution. Nevertheless, some potential advantages may not be so obvious when DR is applied to exotic patients.

The most important concern for use of any digital system in small exotic species is resolution. The area corresponding to the "film" has a fixed number of pixels (usually corresponding with standard resolution of approximately 250 pixels per inch [ppi] with CR, and about 180 ppi with DDR). Higher resolutions plates (commonly named "mammography plates") and scanners able to take and process at double resolution (500 ppi) are available, but they are more expensive and not needed for a standard small animal practice dealing mostly with dog and cat patients.

Reduced time and increased efficiency are well-recognized benefits of DR. However, the exotic patient requires more time for anesthesia, monitoring, and positioning. Therefore, the advantage of reduced time may be less significant with exotic companion mammals.

Teleradiology and increased interactivity with referral clinicians and colleagues is certainly easier with DR. Digitalization of films with a camera results in loss of visual information and altered grayscale. High-quality digital images can be obtained by scanning good quality films, although a scanner for transparencies is required.

Intraoral radiography

The intraoral technique is usually preferred in veterinary medicine over the extraoral technique, because it produces images of optimal resolution and diagnostic quality.[8] Intraoral films or digital plates are nonscreen films that can be placed directly inside the patient's mouth, reducing the object-to-film distance, and therefore minimizing the image size distortion. The use of intraoral film is reported in rabbits and selected rodent species,[9,10] but in the author's experience the correct placement of films within the oral cavity of rabbits and rodents is difficult to suboptimal owing to patient size (and impossible in smaller rodent species). In most patients, intraoral techniques can therefore be used primarily for the evaluation of anatomic structures such as maxillary and mandibular incisor teeth, rostral cheek teeth, and the rostral portion of the maxilla. A dental radiographic unit is preferable to a standard radiographic unit to expose intraoral films, because it can be moved easily, facilitating the positioning of the patient and the use of proper angles to obtain dedicated oblique views.[8]

Intraoral films and plates used extraorally

Larger intraoral films or digital plates and the advantages of mobile dental radiographic units may be coupled to obtain extraoral views using them outside of the oral cavity.[1,8] However, the resulting image is usually not enough to include the entire head of a rabbit or a guinea pig, requiring additional views to obtain the complete picture of the skull. In the author's opinion, this is the most important drawback when using intraoral equipment in an extraoral fashion.

Extraoral radiography

Because of difficulties obtaining good quality intraoral images, in particular of cheek teeth and surrounding structures, the extraoral technique is used most commonly in the evaluation of dental structures in rabbits and rodents by most exotic companion mammal veterinarians.[1,5] Considering the complex dental disease syndrome in rabbits and related complications, such as osteomyelitis of the mandible and other empyemas of the preformed cavities of the skull (nasal cavities, tympanic bullae), radiographic examination of the entire skull is of paramount importance and strongly recommended by this author.

Radiographic projections and normal radiographic anatomy of the head

A complete radiographic study of the head in rabbits and rodents should include 1 or 2 latero-lateral (LL), right-to-left and left-to-right latero-oblique (LO), dorso-ventral (DV; or ventro-dorsal [VD]) and rostro-caudal projections.[1,5,8] Additional views such as LO with a different degree of obliquity, slight LO in the rostro-caudal direction rather than the standard DV, slight obliques from the VD position, VD with the mandible shifted laterally, and intraoral projections may be useful or required for the radiographic study of a specific patient.[5] Also, contrast studies of the nasolacrimal duct may be performed if clinical indications are present. Most authors agree that LL is the most useful view.[1,8] When evaluating a patient for dental disease, the author considers LL, right-to-left and left-to-right LO, and DV views as essential, and recommends additional oblique and rostrocaudal views for assessment of specific areas. With the exception of preliminary test radiographs to obtain an overall evaluation, and in cases of extreme anesthetic risk, general anesthesia is mandatory for accurate patient positioning and to avoid motion artifacts.

Radiographic anatomy of the head of the rabbit, guinea pig, and chinchilla, as well as proper positioning to obtain the 5 standard projections with the extraoral technique, have been described in detail in the literature.[1,5,11,12] The reader is referred to those references on this subject for further details.

Interpretation of radiographs of the skull

Correct positioning and diagnostic quality of the LL view is confirmed by perfect superimposition of bilateral anatomic structures, such as the rostral margin of the right and left orbit, optic foramen, tympanic bullae, mandibular processes, and temporomandibular joints.[1,8,13] The ventral margin of right and left mandibles should appear superimposed. This view should be obtained with the mouth closed and is used to evaluate both the incisor and cheek teeth.

In the rabbit, the mandibular incisor teeth should occlude between the maxillary first and second (accessory) set of incisor teeth. Rodent species are *simplicidentata*, having a single pair of maxillary incisor teeth, and show a functional brachygnathism of the mandible. For these reasons, the mandibular incisor tooth occludes just palatal (caudal) to the maxillary incisor tooth.

In rabbits and chinchillas, the LL projection assesses the occlusal plane of the cheek teeth, but not in the guinea pig because in this species the occlusal plane is angled. Also, the LL projection is critical to evaluate coronal and apical elongation of the cheek teeth, and changes in tooth curvature. To determine abnormalities on one particular side requires oblique views.

The cheek teeth of rabbits form a regular palisade, and their occlusal plane has a zig-zag pattern, owing to the interdigitation of mandibular and maxillary teeth and presence of enamel ridges on their occlusal surface. The dental interproximal spaces of the occlusal surface are virtual, because these teeth are packed together tightly. Mandibular cheek tooth 2 is straight and with the long axis almost perpendicular to the ventral cortex of the mandible. The remaining mandibular cheek teeth show a degree of curvature. Maxillary cheek tooth 1 is curved slightly and the remaining maxillary cheek teeth are almost straight, with slight divergence of the apices. The reserve crowns of maxillary cheek tooth 3 to cheek tooth 6 are located inside a peculiar bony structure of the rabbit skull called the alveolar bulla, which lies cranial, ventral, and medial to the orbital fossa. This anatomic feature plays an important role in formation of retrobulbar and parabulbar abscesses after periapical infection of those maxillary cheek teeth. The apex of maxillary cheek tooth 3 is radiographically slightly dorsal to the apices of the other cheek teeth, following the dome of the alveolar bulla. All mandibular cheek teeth should be at some distance from the ventral cortex of the mandible, which should be visible as a smooth, thick, radiopaque line.

In guinea pigs, the occlusal plane of cheek teeth slopes approximately 30° dorsal to ventral from buccal to lingual side. Because of this angle, the occlusal plane of the cheek teeth cannot be evaluated on an LL view. The mandibular cheek teeth reach close to the ventral mandibular cortex, which should appear smooth.

Clinical crowns of the cheek teeth of chinchillas are short. The occlusal plane is nearly horizontal, so it is easily evaluated on an LL view. The apices of the mandibular cheek teeth are close to the smooth and thin ventral cortex of the mandible, except for the last cheek tooth, which is shorter than the other 3 cheek teeth. The interproximal spaces between cheek teeth are minimal. The ventral cortex of the mandible should be smooth with no deformity.

The LO views are obtained with the animal in lateral recumbency and the head (or the tube head of the x-ray machine) slightly rotated to avoid superimposition between the tooth apices of right and left sides. The rotation should not be excessive to minimize image distortion. Normally a 10° to 20° rotation is sufficient, unless specific oblique views are necessary, in particular to display part of the masseteric fossa. Right-to-left and left-to-right views should always be obtained for comparison, even if dental disease is suspected only on 1 side. Right and left reference structures (tympanic bullae, mandibular processes, and temporomandibular joints) should appear just dorsal and ventral to each other. If the head is incorrectly tilted in rostrocaudal direction as well (eg, lifting the nose too much), these structures will seem to be out of line. A slight oblique projection in the craniocaudal direction may be desired in selected cases. The LO view allows the evaluation of the reserve crowns and apices of the mandibular cheek teeth of one side (usually the side next to the digital plate) and the maxillary cheek teeth of the opposite side. Also, the apex of each incisor tooth can be better visualized than on LL projection.

Symmetry between the right and left sides is critical for proper evaluation of VD or DV projections. These views allow the evaluation of the relationship between the mandible and the skull, and the integrity of the margins of mandibular and maxillary bones. Severe cheek teeth elongation and deformation, bone deformation, and perforation may be visualized. In chinchillas, apical elongation and bone perforation typically occur laterally on the maxilla and the mandible, and are visualized with this projection. In all species, evaluation of the incisor teeth is difficult with this view. A slight oblique projection may be desired in selected cases. Also, the VD projection with the mandible shifted laterally prevents superimposition with part of the maxilla on the contralateral side. This view is useful to evaluate part of the nasal cavity and the maxillary recess.

An adequate rostrocaudal projection is the most difficult to obtain. However, it may give information on cheek teeth before intraoral inspection, including the occlusal plane angle, presence of spikes and spurs, coronal and apical elongation, and cortical perforation by dental apices. This is the only radiographic projection allowing evaluation of the occlusal plane of cheek teeth in guinea pigs. Anisognathism, which is characterized by a narrow mandible and wider maxilla in the rabbit and the opposite in the guinea pig and chinchilla, is easily appreciated with this view.

Common radiographic abnormalities of the skull and teeth of the rabbit (**Figs. 1–7**), rodents, and other exotic mammals have been reported extensively.[1,5,12–14] The reader is referred to those references for further details. Objective interpretation of dental disease in rabbits, guinea pigs, and chinchillas with the use of anatomic reference lines has been described.[10,15] The use of lines may facilitate diagnosis in many cases; however, they should only be applied to optimal projections to be reliable. In rabbits, frequent exceptions do exist depending on morphology of the skull in different breeds.

Computed Tomography

Basic principles

CT is a radiologic technique to obtain multiple, parallel cross-sectional image slices of the tissues of the patient.[1,6,12,16,17] Multiple exposures are made as an x-ray tube within a gantry rotates around the patient as it moves along the gantry on a couch. The final image is generated by a computer. The concept of "slice" imaging originated from the need to overcome superimposition of anatomic structures that is intrinsic to conventional radiography. Actually, the main advantage of CT over radiography is that in the first, all tissues in the area of interest are not superimposed over a single plane. The tissue slice is digitally divided into 3 dimensional tiny blocks named *voxels*. Voxels have length, width, and depth; depth corresponds with the tissue slice and can be less than 1 mm. The computer analyzes the mean attenuation of radiographs of each voxel, producing various shades of grey on the final image. CT scans elaborate images via the standardized, internationally recognized Digital Imaging and Communication in Medicine (DICOM) format.

Imaging exotic patients is a challenge because of their small size. The consequence of smaller patient size is production of a small image that will be of lower resolution

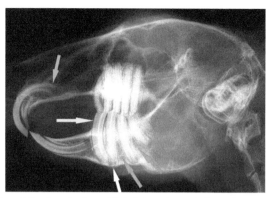

Fig. 1. Radiography of the head of a rabbit, latero-lateral view, demonstrating early stage of acquired dental disease. Overall coronal elongation of both maxillary and mandibular cheek teeth is present. Because both mandibular cheek teeth 1 do not have another tooth rostral to them, they begin to curve, with increasing rostral convexity (*yellow arrow*). Slight deformation of the ventral mandibular cortical bone owing to apical elongation of mandibular cheek tooth 2 is visible (*white arrow*). Owing to the abnormal convexity, the interproximal spaces of mandibular cheek teeth are widened (*orange arrows*). Malocclusion of the incisor teeth is not present at this stage, but apical elongation of a primary maxillary incisor is present (*green arrow*). The zig-zag pattern of the cheek teeth occlusal plane is still normal, but the radiotransparent line is not as discernible when the mandible is at rest. (*Courtesy of* Vittorio Capello, DVM, Milano, Italy; with permission.)

when magnified. Because spiral and multislice scanners offer very thin slices (even <1 mm) and large image matrices (512 × 512 pixels), resolution is superior to that obtained with most single slice scanners. High-resolution CT images can be magnified 1.5 to 2.0 times with computer software allowing better detection of subtle anatomic changes.

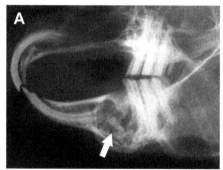
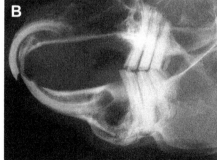

Fig. 2. Radiography of the head of a rabbit, latero-lateral view, demonstrating osteomyelitis of the mandible before (*A*) and after (*B*) surgical treatment. (*A*) A retained reserve crown of mandibular cheek tooth 1 (*arrow*) is visible inside the circular osteolytic area. Severe deformity of the cortical bone and periosteal reaction are visible. Both maxillary cheek tooth 1 and cheek tooth 2 had been extracted previously. Radiotransparency of the surgical site after debridement with extraction of the tooth fragment and necrotic bone tissue. The osteolytic area contained purulent material. (*Courtesy of* Vittorio Capello, DVM, Milano, Italy; with permission.)

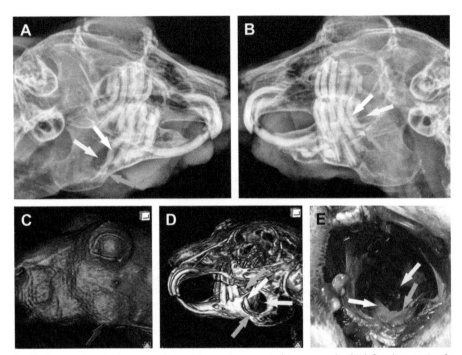

Fig. 3. Comparison between radiography and computed tomography (CT) for diagnosis of a retromasseteric abscess after periapical infection of the mandibular cheek tooth 4 and osteo-myelitis affecting the masseteric fossa of the left mandible of a rabbit. (*A, B*). Oblique radiographic views of the skull. Rt 35° V-Lt D projection (*A*), and Lt 35° V-Rt D projection (*B*). Extensive bone lysis (*A*) affecting the left masseteric fossa (*yellow arrow*) and surrounding the abnormal reserve crown of mandibular cheek tooth 4 (*white arrow*) is present. Elongated and deformed apex of mandibular cheek tooth 4 is also visible (*orange arrow*). The apparent different elongation is owing to opposite obliquities of the 2 projections. (*C, D*). CT scan, 3-dimensional volume rendering of the head at the surface level (*C*), and after subtraction of soft tissues, at the level of the skull surface (*D*). The retromasseteric swelling (*blue arrow*) and the dental and skull abnormalities are displayed as a real model. (*D*) Bone lysis (*yellow arrow*), elongated reserve crown (*white arrow*), and diseased apex (*orange arrow*). The clinical crown of left mandibular cheek tooth 5, and the abnormal clinical crown of cheek tooth 4 just rostral to it, are also visible (*green arrow*). (*E*) Surgical exposure of the extensive and circular bone lysis of the masseteric fossa (*yellow arrow*), of the diseased reserve crown of mandibular cheek tooth 4 (*white arrow*), and of its apex (*orange arrow*) before extraction. Rt, right; Lt, left; V, ventral; d, dorsal; -, to. (*Courtesy of* Vittorio Capello, DVM, Milano, Italy; with permission.)

Patient positioning and anesthesia

Despite the flexibility of viewing modalities, proper positioning of the patient and the patient's head are of critical importance to obtain a good scanning and then interpreted by the radiologist and/or veterinarian.

Modern CT units are capable of scanning the entire head in a few seconds. Although owners are reluctant about anesthesia that is not related to surgery or other procedures, deep sedation or anesthesia are essential for proper positioning for CT and to reduce breathing artifact, especially in smaller mammals with higher respiratory rate.

The patient is positioned commonly in sternal recumbency, with the head elevated slightly and kept horizontal, parallel to the table.[1,6] The endotracheal tube will not create a superimposition as in conventional radiographs. However, care must be taken that the connection with the anesthetic circuit does not prevent proper symmetric positioning of the head. The use of face masks is not recommended during scanning because the rubber material may create artifacts, or simply cover part of the face in the 3-dimensional renderings. Even though the scanning time is short, simple inhalant induction of anesthesia is not an effective option, increasing the chance the patient will revive and move during the scanning procedure. The author's preferred anesthetic protocol for any stable patient is with injectable drugs and oxygen administration via a face mask. The anesthetic effect allows adequate time for positioning, scanning, and verification of the CT images. Before scanning, a scout view is collected in both dorsoventral and lateral projection. Scout projections are standard radiographic images that are used to ensure accurate positioning and symmetry of the patient's head for CT scanning. The dorsoventral scout view is useful for evaluating bilateral symmetry, and the lateral projection is useful to assess the proper angle of the scanning plane. A provisional transverse scan through the tympanic bullae allows a further assessment of symmetric position of the head. The thickness of the slices is selected, as well as the extent of the scan. The face mask is then removed during the short scanning time and replaced once the scanning is completed.

Intravenous contrast medium can be used during CT imaging of rabbits.[16]

Interpretation of computed tomography

Data are usually acquired in the transverse plane (axial views) but can be reformatted by the computer and displayed also in sagittal, coronal, and oblique planes.[5] This capability is called multiplanar reformation. Although the resolution of analog or digital radiography is superior, viewing slices of the patient in sagittal and coronal planes as well as the standard axial plane offers tremendous advantages. Radiologists agree that axial views and additional 2-dimensional views represent the standard interpretation and are the most sensitive for diagnosis. However, dedicated imaging software allows various reconstruction techniques, including 3-dimensional volume rendering techniques and shaded surface displays.[5,6,16] Image volume presented in this fashion is virtually 3-dimensional, because the actual image is obviously 2-dimensional on the computer monitor. Volume rendering can be rotated on the monitor to allow the observer to visualize any surface. Also, additional functions can be performed, such as cropping part of the volume for evaluation of deeper anatomic structures. Both hard and soft tissues can be added virtually or subtracted to different extents and degrees of density, providing detailed relationship between soft and hard tissues. Shaded surface displays presents a contoured surface map of the entire image volume, converting CT data into an image very similar to an image of an anatomic specimen, well within the range of interpretation of a trained clinician. Although it has limited value because deep structures are masked, it is still very important for evaluating abnormalities of the bones of the skull such as deformities, osteomyelitis, and skull fractures. Depending on the specific case, volume and surface renderings may be of critical importance for diagnostic accuracy and to select the best surgical approach, when indicated.[18,19] Software for viewing DICOM images is readily available. Several products with varying operating system requirements and pricing are available; however, freeware is also available. CT images presented in this article have been produced with OsiriX, which is the most popular and user-friendly online freeware currently available to Apple users.

Indication for computed tomography

CT of the skull is a critical diagnostic imaging tool in rabbits for acquired dental disease and its related complications, such as osteomyelitis of the mandible (see **Figs. 3** and **4**)

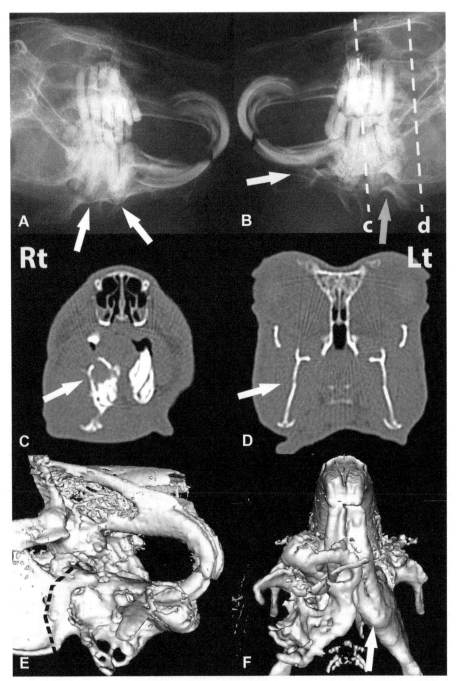

Fig. 4. Comparison between radiography and computed tomography (CT) scan for diagnosis of diffuse osteomyelitis of the incisive portion and of the body of the right mandible, after end-stage dental disease of the mandibular cheek teeth arcade of a rabbit. (*A, B*). Oblique radiographic views of the skull. Rt 15° V-Lt D oblique projection (*A*), Lt 15° V-Rt D oblique projection (*B*). (*A*) Elongation of reserve crowns and apices of left mandibular cheek teeth

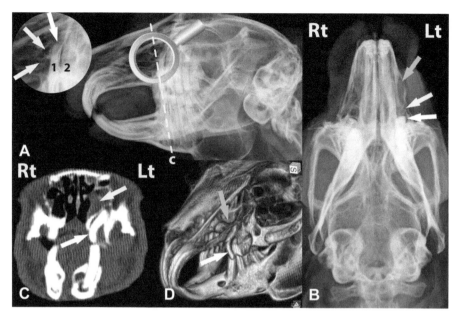

Fig. 5. Comparison between radiography and computed tomography (CT) for diagnosis of a zygomatic abscess after periapical infection of the maxillary cheek tooth 1, and empyema of the maxillary recess in a rabbit. (*A, B*) Radiographic views of the skull. Lt 15° V-Rt D oblique projection (*A*) and ventrodorsal projection (*B*). (*A*) Abnormal coronal and apical elongation of maxillary cheek tooth 1 (*inset, white arrow*), and abnormal radiodensity in the area of the left maxillary recess (*inset, yellow arrows*). (*B*) Abnormal apex of left maxillary cheek tooth 1 (*white arrow*); increased radiodensity of the left maxillary recess (yellow *arrow*); lysis at the perforated area of the maxilla just beneath the facial swelling (green *arrow*). (*C*) CT scan, axial view, of the scanning plane shown in (*A; yellow dotted line*). Abnormal left maxillary cheek tooth 1 (*white arrow*) and empyema of the left maxillary recess (*yellow arrow*). (*D*) CT scan, 3-dimensional volume rendering of the skull at the surface level. Abnormal left maxillary cheek tooth 1 (*white arrow*). After subtraction of soft tissues, the perforated surface of the maxilla may disappear because it is very thin. The green arrow indicates the position of the maxillary recess. (*Courtesy of* Vittorio Capello, DVM, Milano, Italy; with permission.)

with wider interproximal spaces are present. Compression and deformity of the ventral cortical bone of the left mandible is present (*white arrows;* see also *F*), but the overall bone is intact. (*B*) Elongation, deformity, and demineralization of reserve crowns and apices of the right mandibular cheek teeth. The cortical bone of the mandible is lytic and destroyed from the rostral end of the incisive portion (*yellow arrow*) to the incisure for facial vessels between the body and the masseteric fossa of the mandible (*orange arrow*). (*C, D*) CT scan, axial views of the scanning planes shown in (*B; yellow dotted lines*). Extensive lysis of the cortical bone of the incisive portion (*C*) and of the body of the right mandible (*arrow*) is visible; while the masseteric fossa (*arrow*) is intact (*D*). (*E, F*). CT scan, 3-dimensional surface rendering of the skull from the right lateral view (*E*), and from oblique rostroventral view (*F*). The "moth-eaten" enlarged and deformed incisive portion, and body of the right mandible, are displayed as a real model (*E*). The comparison with the destroyed and the intact mandible is emphasized (*F*). The black dotted line in (*E*) indicates the osteotomy line between the rostral diseased bone tissue and the caudal intact masseteric fossa for rostral mandibulectomy. (*Courtesy of* Vittorio Capello, DVM, Milano, Italy; with permission.)

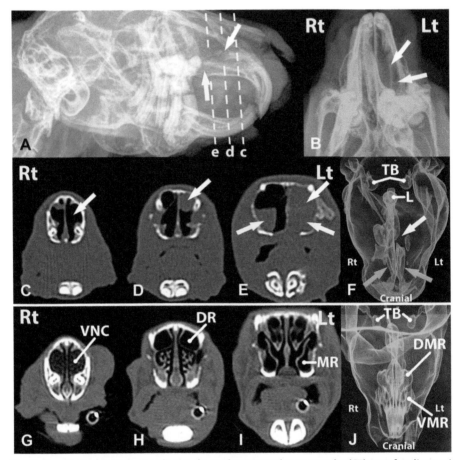

Fig. 6. Comparison between radiography and computed tomography (CT) scan for diagnosis of chronic odontogenic rhinitis with bilateral empyema of the nasal cavities of a rabbit (*A–F*) and the normal nasal cavities as a reference (*G–J*). (*A, B*). Radiographic views of the skull. Rt 15° V-Lt D oblique projection (*A*) and ventrodorsal projection with the mandible shifted to the right side (*B*). Severe acquired dental disease, including osteolysis and deformities of the right mandible after abscesses previously addressed with surgical procedures (*A*) and deformity of the left alveolar bulla. Irregular radiodensities of the nasal cavity in the areas of the ventral nasal concha (*white arrows*), and of the left maxillary recess (*yellow arrows*). (*C–E*). CT scans, axial views, of the scanning planes shown in (*A; yellow dotted lines*). (*C*) Bilateral lysis of the rostral portion of the ventral nasal concha (*arrow*). (*D*) Bilateral lysis of the caudal portion of the ventral nasal concha and empyema of the left dorsal conchal recess (*arrow*). (*E*) Bilateral lysis of turbinates, empyema of the left nasal cavity (*white arrow*), and bilateral empyema of the maxillary recesses (yellow *arrows*). (*F*) CT scan, 3-dimensional volume rendering of the skull applying the "airways" modality. The rostral portion of the nasal cavities is narrowed (*orange arrows*); the empty space of maxillary recesses are reduced, in particular the left (*yellow arrow*). L, larynx; TB, tympanic bullae. (*G–I*). CT scan, axial views, of the normal skull corresponding with the axial views shown in (*C–E*). DR, dorsal nasal concha; MR, maxillary recess; VNC, ventral nasal concha. (*J*) CT scan, 3-dimensional volume rendering of the normal skull applying the "airways" modality. DMR, dorsal portion of the maxillary recess; VMR, ventral portion of the maxillary recess. (*Courtesy of* Vittorio Capello, DVM, Milano, Italy; with permission.)

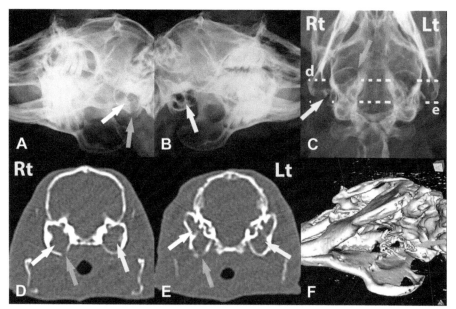

Fig. 7. Comparison between radiography and computed tomography (CT) scan for the diagnosis of bilateral empyema and otitis media of the tympanic bullae of a rabbit. (*A, B*) Radiographic views of the skull. Lt 30° V-Rt D oblique projection (*A*), Rt 30° V-Lt D oblique projection (*B*), and ventrodorsal projection (*C*). (*A*) Abnormal radiodensity within the right tympanic bulla (*white arrow*). The bony wall of the bulla is thinner than normal and lysis is present (*orange arrow*). (*B*) Abnormal radiodensity within the left tympanic bulla (*yellow arrow*). The bone is thinner than normal, but intact. (*C*) Bilateral, abnormal radiodensities within the tympanic bullae. The bony wall is thinner than normal and lytic on the right bulla (*orange arrow*). Periosteal reaction is also present close to the right acoustic meatus (*yellow arrow*). (*D, E*) CT scan, axial views, of the scanning planes shown in (*C; yellow dotted lines*). Bilateral radiodensity of the alveolar bullae indicative of empyema (*white* and *yellow arrows*) including the acoustic meatus (*E, white arrow*) and lysis of the ventral dome of the right bulla (*D, E, orange arrows*). (*F*) CT scan, 3-dimensional surface rendering of the skull with 45° obliquity, displaying the lytic, ventromedial part of the right tympanic bulla (*orange arrow*). (*Courtesy of* Vittorio Capello, DVM, Milano, Italy; with permission.)

and the maxilla[5,6,16,20,21] (**Fig. 5**), empyemas of the bony cavities of the skull (**Figs. 5 and 6**), and the tympanic bullae for diagnosis of otitis media[20,21] (**Fig. 7**). Nasal and paranasal cavities, including meatuses, nasal septum, turbinates, and recesses, can be visualized in detail, making CT complementary to rhinoscopy.[22,23]

Despite smaller patient size, CT is also very important for detailed diagnosis of dental disease in rodent species,[24–28] including space occupying masses such as elodontomas,[29] or pseudoodontomas in prairie dogs, which compress the nasal cavities.[30,31]

Radiography versus computed tomography

CT is generally considered to be superior to standard radiography by default. A recent retrospective study performed on 30 rabbits with dental disease and its related complications compared radiography and CT on 2 different levels: diagnostic consistency and diagnostic accuracy.[18] Observations were statistically consistent for diagnosis between the 2 techniques. Nonetheless, the diagnostic accuracy of CT was superior in 80% of patients with regard to diagnosis and prognosis, and in 56.6% of patients for guiding extraoral dental and surgical treatment. Greater sensitivity and superior accuracy for clinical diagnosis and prognosis was particularly valuable for cases of osteomyelitis after periapical infections, for rhinitis and otitis media. Radiography provided superior accuracy in 16.6% of patients for guiding intraoral dental treatment. Radiography and CT should be ideally performed together in most cases to improve diagnostic quality.

Microcomputed tomography

Micro-CT has recently emerged in private practice for small exotic mammals. Originally designed for laboratory animal imaging,[32] it may represent the new, advanced modality for diagnosis of dental disease in rabbits and rodents. The pet rabbit has been used as a model for a new micro-CT unit of 190 mm diameter, with 5 μm resolution, producing 2-dimensional standard images and 3-dimensional renderings of exceptional quality and with a superior level of detail[33] (**Fig. 8**). The basic principles of CT scanning and operation are the same; however, advantages are represented by a much smaller CT unit, which has been configured with a shield structure so that an additional lead shield chamber is not required to protect the operator from x-ray exposure.

Its compact size and design allows it to be used in a room much smaller than that needed by a traditional CT unit and this particular model can accommodate animals weighing up to 3 kg inside the gantry. A disadvantage of this model is represented by the limited range of species that can fit into the gantry, including large rabbits, precluding its use by small animal veterinarians. Other micro-CT units allow 20 cm of scanning extent, and can accommodate animals up to 15 kg, with lower resolution (**Fig. 9**).

The accurate and detailed images make micro-CT an outstanding diagnostic tool for small exotic patients.

ORAL ENDOSCOPY
Indications

Unlike other diagnostic imaging modalities, endoscopy (meaning *to view inside*) provides direct visualization of internal anatomic structures related to a real or virtual body cavity.[34–36] For this reason, the number of organs that can be evaluated is more limited than with the other diagnostic techniques. The specific name of oral endoscopy is *stomatoscopy*, and it represents an essential tool for diagnosis of dental disease in pet rabbits and rodent species.[1,2,34–39]

The most important advantages of stomatoscopy can be summarized as follows:

- The basic equipment is not very expensive;
- It requires basic skills by the veterinarian;
- The procedures are relatively simple and noninvasive;
- It allows thorough inspection of the narrow oral cavity of herbivorous species and even smaller rodent species;
- It offers a magnified perspective of dental structures;
- It highly reduces the risk of missing subtle lesions, facilitating early diagnosis;
- It facilitates coronal reduction of cheek teeth and other therapeutic procedures;
- It aids endotracheal intubation in selected patients;
- It allows the simultaneous visualization of the clinical case by multiple observers; and
- It allows documentation of images for tracking progress of disease, for medical records, and for both veterinary and client education.

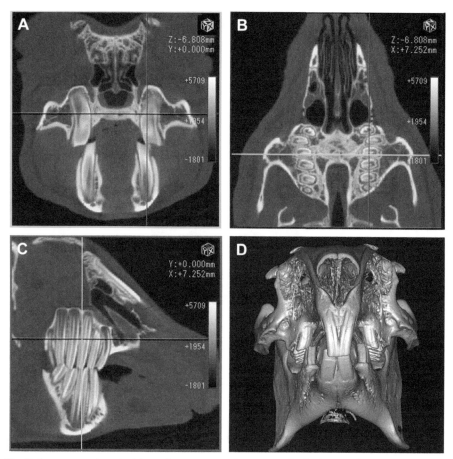

Fig. 8. Images produced with a micro-computed tomography (CT) unit of 190 mm diameter, and 5 μm resolution. This model produces 2-dimensional (2D) standard images and 3-dimensional renderings of exceptional quality and of a superior level of detail compared with standard CT units.[33] (A–C) The 2D multiplanar rendering displays axial (A), coronal (B), and longitudinal (C) views. The area of interest is targeted at the cross-point of the 2 perpendicular lines in each view, shown at the level of the left maxillary cheek tooth 3 in this normal rabbit. Each projection displays the other 2 views with a colored line. (D) These 3-dimensional reconstructions provide images similar to a sharply detailed real animal model. (*Courtesy of* Hiroshi Sasai, DVM; with permission.)

Rhinoscopy and pararhinoscopy (ie, endoscopy of the paranasal recesses) may be adjunct endoscopic procedures in the case of select complications of advanced dental disease such as empyema of the nasal cavity in rabbits.

Equipment

Detailed features of endoscopic instrumentation have been reported.[40] The most commonly used in exotic mammal medicine and surgery are the 2.7-mm (30° view) and the 1.9-mm telescope. Both have dedicated sheaths, either protecting or operating, the latter with several ports and instrument channels. The 1.9-mm semiflexible and the 1.7 flexible miniscopes are available and useful for smaller exotic mammals.

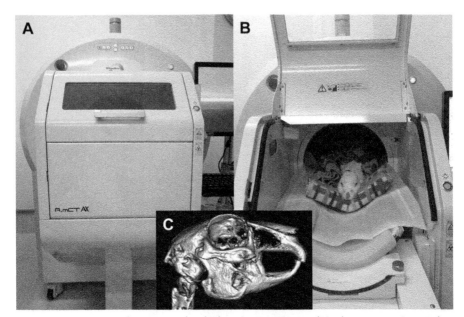

Fig. 9. Micro-computed tomography (CT) unit, R_mCT AX (Rigaku corporation, Tokyo, Japan). The CT unit is mobile and builtin shielding eliminates the requirements for a designated shielded room. Maximum resolution is 0.06 mm, which is superior to conventional CT for small patients. This unit can accommodate animals up to 15 kg. (*A*) External view of the CT unit. (*B*) Inside of the CT unit with a pet rabbit under anesthesia ready for scanning. This model produces excellent 2-dimensional images and high-resolution 3-dimensional renderings (*C*). (*Courtesy of* Yasutsugu Miwa, DVM, Tokyo, Japan; with permission.)

Additional basic endoscopic equipment includes a light source, light cable, endoscopic video camera, monitor, and digital recording device.

As with other endoscopic procedures, stomatoscopy is always performed under general anesthesia. Additional dental instruments for intraoral inspection such as mouth gags and cheek dilators are needed (see Capello V: Intraoral Treatment of Dental Disease in Pet Rabbits; Legendre L: Anatomy and Disorders of the Oral cavity of Guinea Pigs, in this issue).

Endoscopy of the Normal Oral Cavity in the Rabbit, Guinea Pig, and Chinchilla

Rabbit

Entering the mouth, the area on the dorsal aspect of the tongue is the lingual torus (*torus lingualis*). The mucosa of the lingual torus is light pink, thick, and prominent as compared with the rest of the lingual mucosa. Mandibular cheek teeth arcades are visible lateral to the tongue. Normal length of clinical crowns must be assessed. Positioning the endoscope tangential to the occlusal plane allows detailed inspection and assessment of the normal zig-zag pattern. Normal, small enamel points are visible on the lingual aspect of the mandibular cheek teeth (**Fig. 10**A).

The inferior alveolar vessels are visible below the thin oral mucosa distal to mandibular cheek tooth 5. Special attention must be paid to avoid injuring these vessels during coronal reduction of cheek teeth. Clinical crowns of maxillary cheek teeth are normally shorter than those of the mandibular teeth, and maxillary cheek tooth 6 is significantly smaller than the other 5 cheek teeth (**Fig. 10**B). A better view of the maxillary dental arcades may be obtained by turning the endoscope 180°.

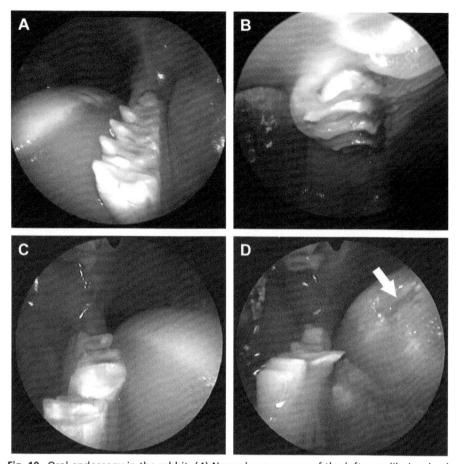

Fig. 10. Oral endoscopy in the rabbit. (*A*) Normal appearance of the left mandibular cheek teeth. Small enamel points visible on the lingual aspect are normal. (*B*) Normal appearance of the right maxillary cheek teeth. The clinical crowns are shorter than those of the mandibular arcade. The tiny clinical crown of cheek tooth 6 is not visible from this view. (*C*) Acquired dental disease and malocclusion of the right mandibular arcade. Abnormal elongation and shortening of clinical crowns, uneven occlusal plane ("step mouth"), and initial lingual bending of the teeth are present. (*D*) Sharp lingual spike of the second premolar tooth (cheek tooth 4) caused by improper wearing and related lesion of the lingual mucosa (*arrow*). (*Courtesy of* Vittorio Capello, DVM, Milano, Italy; with permission.)

Guinea pig

The anatomy, structure, and function of the tongue of guinea pigs are unique. The tongue is divided by a visible groove into a rostral and a caudal portion that move independently. The prominent lingual torus is covered by papillae. Bilateral mucosal folds (frenula) extend laterally from the rostral portion to the mandible.

Food debris on the dental surfaces is a common finding in normal guinea pigs. Before inspection, the oral cavity should be gently flushed and cleaned with cotton swabs.

Cheek teeth of guinea pigs have a 30° sloped occlusal plane from buccal to lingual, dorsal to ventral. The normal oblique angle of the occlusal plane must be carefully assessed, and evaluation should not be affected by improper orientation of the endo-scope (**Fig. 11**A, B).

Chinchilla

Inspection of the oral cavity is easier in chinchillas than in guinea pigs, because there is no angulation of the cheek teeth occlusal plane. The torus of the tongue is not present in chinchillas. The clinical crowns of mandibular cheek teeth are very short, and the occlusal surface is flat but rough because of the presence of dentinal grooves inter-spersed in between enamel ridges. The mandibular first premolar is almost triangle shaped (**Fig. 12**A, B).

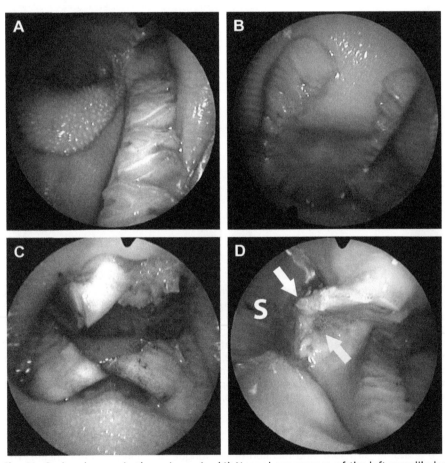

Fig. 11. Oral endoscopy in the guinea pig. (*A*) Normal appearance of the left mandibular cheek teeth. Enamel crests and dentinal grooves are visible over the sloped occlusal plane. (*B*) Normal appearance of the maxillary cheek teeth, with focus on the left arcade. (*C*) Severe coronal elongation and uneven occlusal plane of cheek teeth. Right and left mandibular cheek tooth 1 cross each other in a "bridge-like" malocclusion over the tongue. (*D*) Sharp buccal spike of the first maxillary premolar tooth (*white arrow*) after improper wearing, causing ulcerations of the buccal mucosa (*yellow arrows*). Spikes must be identified thoroughly during inspection by deflecting the buccal mucosa with the aid of a curved spatula (*S*). (*Courtesy of* Vittorio Capello, DVM, Milano, Italy; with permission.)

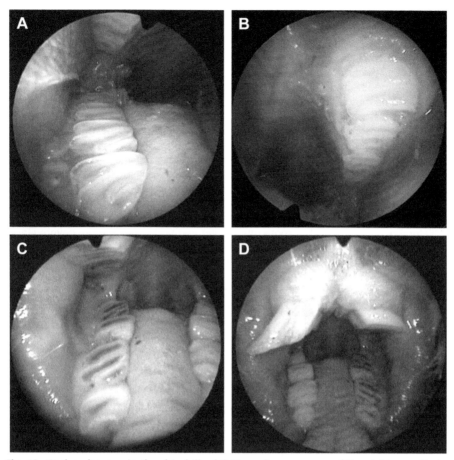

Fig. 12. Oral endoscopy in the chinchilla. (*A*) Normal appearance of the right mandibular cheek teeth. Enamel crests and dentinal grooves are visible over the occlusal plane. (*B*) Normal appearance of the left maxillary cheek teeth. Clinical crowns of cheek teeth are much shorter than in rabbits, and the occlusal plane is not oblique, as in guinea pigs. (*C*) Acquired dental disease of cheek teeth. Coronal elongation, "wave mouth," widened interproximal spaces, and a laterally deviated occlusal plane are present. (*D*) Severe coronal elongation and sharp buccal spikes of the first maxillary premolar teeth caused by improper wearing. Increase of both the alveolar crest and the gingival margin of the maxillary cheek teeth is typical in chinchillas with advanced dental disease. (*Courtesy of* Vittorio Capello, DVM, Milano, Italy; with permission.)

Endoscopic Abnormalities of the Cheek Teeth in the Rabbit, Guinea Pig, and Chinchilla

Many different abnormalities from mild to severe may be recognized in cases of acquired dental disease of cheek teeth. The severity of the pathologic changes can be staged. Early diagnosis is the key to early treatment and resolution of lesions affecting the gingiva, tongue, and oral mucosa. These lesions can be a source of constant discomfort or pain. Prompt treatment also prevents the progression of dental disease.

Rabbit

The earliest stage of acquired dental disease of cheek teeth in rabbits detectable with stomatoscopy is elongation of the clinical crowns. Changes of the occlusal plane are owing to excessive and irregular coronal elongation, with differences in height of up to a few millimeters between 1 cheek tooth and the adjacent tooth. This abnormal occlusal plane is called "wave mouth." When abnormality of the occlusal plane is evident, with marked differences of crown length between 2 adjacent cheek teeth, this abnormal occlusal plane is called "step mouth" (**Fig. 10**C). Usually, in cases of both "wave mouth" and "step mouth," sharp spurs are not present, and clinical signs and symptoms may be mild or absent.

Lingual curvature of clinical crowns of mandibular cheek teeth and buccal curvature of clinical crowns of maxillary cheek teeth lead to the development of points and sharp spikes. Spikes and spurs from mandibular cheek teeth may develop over the tongue, or may be oriented to the side the tongue producing severe damage to the lingual mucosa (**Fig. 10**D). To detect small but sharp spikes, the tongue must be deflected carefully during stomatoscopy. For this reason, these spikes may be very difficult to visualize during examination of the oral cavity in the conscious patient. Symptoms such as excessive salivation can suggest these types of lesions.

Bilateral dental spurs of 1 or more mandibular teeth represent a more severe stage of dental disease than "wave mouth" or "step mouth." The lingual edge may not always be sharp, but overgrown mandibular cheek teeth can impinge on the tongue and affect chewing and swallowing. Discomfort is present and at this stage clinical signs may include teeth grinding, reluctance to chew, changes in food preference, excessive salivation, and signs related to secondary gastrointestinal disorders.

A common sequela of excessive coronal elongation of cheek teeth is fracture, especially of mandibular cheek teeth. The longitudinal fracture of the mandibular first premolar (cheek tooth 1) is relatively common. This often occurs when the rabbit chews improper hard foods such as seeds. Inspection of the oral cavity with a metal cone (especially when improperly inserted between the cheek teeth arcades) may also cause or predispose to this fracture. The most common sequela of fractures is periapical infection and abscess. Fractures often produce no clinical signs and symptoms; therefore, the first clinical sign may be the appearance of a lump representing the developing abscess.

Excessive coronal elongation and malocclusion (including "wave mouth" and "step mouth") also affect maxillary cheek teeth. Coronal elongation is usually accompanied by an increase in the height of both the alveolar crest and the gingival margin. These changes are more apparent in maxillary rather than mandibular cheek teeth malocclusion.

Spurs of maxillary cheek teeth typically form on the buccal aspect of the tooth and may cause ulcerations of the mucosal surface of the cheek. Clinical signs and symptoms are usually less severe than those associated with spurs of mandibular cheek teeth. Nevertheless, in other cases they can lead to odontogenic, nonperiapical abscesses.

Guinea pig

The most common early stage of malocclusion of cheek teeth in guinea pigs is elongation of 1 or both mandibular premolars. Symptoms may be mild or absent, and this stage represents a common finding of early malocclusion in healthy guinea pigs. Bridgelike overgrowth of the mandibular premolars is a common finding and depicts a more advanced form of cheek teeth malocclusion in guinea pigs.

Owing to the peculiar orientation of the cheek teeth and the anatomy of the tongue, abnormal coronal elongation of mandibular cheek teeth is always oriented lingually. However, unlike rabbits, the tongue is almost never traumatized by sharp edges or spurs. Discomfort is a result of entrapment of the tongue by elongated cheek teeth, affecting tongue movements and deglutition (see **Fig. 11**C).

Intermediate stages include malocclusion of the entire mandibular cheek teeth arcade. Coronal elongation and the abnormal occlusal plane must be assessed carefully with the aid of an endoscope. Gingivitis is a common sequela of coronal elongation, impaction of food debris, or hair impaction in long-haired breeds. Severe coronal elongation, malocclusion, and sharp buccal margins develop at maxillary cheek teeth (**Fig. 11**C).

Chinchillas

Coronal elongation and malocclusion of cheek teeth occurs in chinchillas, and is similar to some extent to dental disease in guinea pigs and in rabbits. However, presenting signs and symptoms are usually much less severe when compared with guinea pigs, and may also vary from the typical presentation in rabbits. Mild abnormalities include slight elongation of the clinical crowns, mild alteration of the normal enamel crests and dentinal grooves, and slightly widened interproximal spaces. Pattern of malocclusion similar to "wave mouth" and "step mouth" of rabbits are present in chinchillas (**Fig. 12**C). Like guinea pigs but unlike rabbits, chinchillas seldom develop sharp spurs of mandibular cheek teeth. When present, spurs usually do not traumatize the tongue, but rather impair its movement and entrap it under the elongated crowns. Advanced dental disease exhibits widened interproximal spaces. Food impaction in between the clinical crowns is a common consequence, leading to gingivitis. Unlike rabbits and guinea pigs, cavities are a frequent finding in chinchillas affected by dental disease. Partial or complete fracture of the clinical crowns is a further complication.

Coronal elongation of maxillary cheek teeth and abnormal sharp edges are frequently accompanied by an increase in height of both the alveolar crest and the gingival margin (see **Fig. 12**C). Proliferation of the gingiva makes coronal reduction more difficult and seems to be associated with increased discomfort and a poorer prognosis in chinchillas. Simple burring of elongated crowns may not relieve discomfort and should be considered when formulating a prognosis. In the case of end-stage dental disease, clinical crowns may be worn out and fractured, reserve crowns may no longer replace clinical crowns, and gingiva may heal over reserve crowns.

MRI

MRI is considered a non-invasive imaging modality because it does not use radiation for generating images. Similar to CT, it is a computer-based technique; but in MRI, images are obtained visualizing the movements of hydrogen atoms in the body of the patient in reaction to a very strong magnetic field placed around the patient.[16,20,41] The animal undergoing MRI examination should always be under general anesthesia.

MRI represents the diagnostic imaging procedure of choice for soft tissues. It is most commonly used for the central nervous system, but other soft tissues can be visualized in detail. MRI has superior quality to CT, even exceeding CT with contrast. Different types of sequences (images) can be obtained depending on the tissues to be emphasized. Sequences are produced and visualized in one of the 3 standard views (transverse or axial, dorsal or coronal, lateral or sagittal). Unlike CT, complex manipulation and 3-dimensional volume and surface renderings are not possible, because images are not based on voxels. Acquisition of MRI sequences also depends on several technical factors that are beyond the scope of this article. However, the most important and most practical are the type of sequence, the sequence views, and the overall number of sequences. These factors, together with resolution, have an impact on the time for resonance.

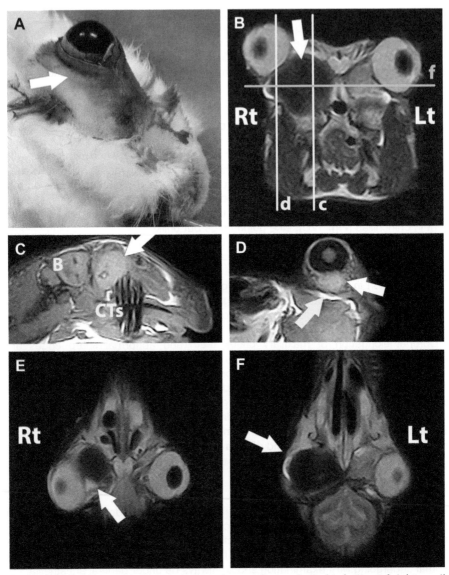

Fig. 13. MRI for diagnosis of a retrobulbar abscess after periapical infection of right maxillary cheek teeth in a rabbit. (*A*) Clinical aspect of the exophthalmos. The *white arrow* indicates the lateral surgical approach to the abscess. (*B*) T2 sequence, axial view, demonstrating a large retrobulbar mass (*white arrow*). Thick pus appears dark in T2 sequences. The yellow lines display the longitudinal views in (*C, D*). The green line displays the coronal view in (*F*). (*C, D*) Longitudinal views, T1 sequences, demonstrating the retrobulbar mass (*white arrow*) over the alveolar bulla (*C*) and the top of the mass (*white arrow*) protruding just over the zygomatic arch (*yellow arrow*) and just below the eye globe (*D*). Thick pus appears white in T1 sequences. (*E, F*) Coronal views, T2 sequences, demonstrating that the caudal approach to the retrobulbar space was not an option because of the dislocation of the optic nerve (*E, white arrow*), and indicating a viable lateral approach to the mass (*F, white arrow*). (*Courtesy of* Vittorio Capello, DVM, Milano, Italy; with permission.)

Two potential disadvantages of MRI are actually resolution (especially for small patients) and prolonged scanning time, when compared with CT. Resolution depends on the magnet of the MRI unit. Low power magnets capable of field strengths of 0.2 to 0.4 T will produce lower resolution images than magnetic fields of 1 T or higher. Higher resolution can also be achieved with prolonged resonance time. The average time for acquisition of diagnostic sequences for a rabbit patient using a low-field MRI unit can range from 20 to 40 minutes, whereas the acquisition time for CT scanning can be less than a minute. Owing to long acquisition time, images may be affected by respiratory and cardiac rate, which are higher in small sized mammals. However, this does not usually represent a concern because they are reduced significantly under anesthesia and when the thorax is not the diagnostic target.

Indications and Applications for Rabbit and Rodent Dental Disease

Thick pus and the capsule, typical of rabbit odontogenic abscesses, have a signal intensity similar to other soft tissues. However, standard fluid pus can be displayed as well. For this reason, MRI of the head for indications other than investigation of the central nervous system represents an interesting and very useful application in pet rabbits and rodents to diagnose the presence and the extent of abscesses[20,21,27] (**Figs. 13** and **14**). In cases of mandibular abscesses, retrobulbar and parabulbar abscesses, and single or multiple empyema affecting 1 or more cavities of the rabbit skull (nasal cavities, maxillary recess, diseased alveolar bulla, and tympanic bulla) MRI provides excellent information, even superior to CT, which is less specific for lower radiodensities.[20,21] Like CT, MRI can provide a high level of diagnostic accuracy, providing

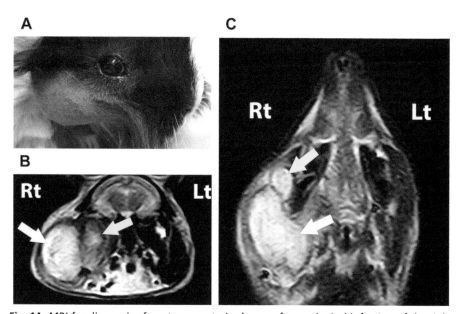

Fig. 14. MRI for diagnosis of a retromasseteric abscess after periapical infection of the right mandibular cheek tooth 4 in a guinea pig. (*A*) Clinical aspect of the facial swelling after fur shaving. (*B, C*) T1 sequences, axial (*B*) and coronal (*C*) views demonstrating a bilobed mass, with a main large lobe (*white arrows*) and a smaller, anteromedial lobe (*yellow arrows*). Owing to the caudal surgical approach to the abscess, the cranial lobe might have easily been missed during surgery without the accurate diagnostic information provided by MRI. (*Courtesy of* Vittorio Capello, DVM, Milano, Italy; with permission.)

a critical guide in preoperative planning. For example, most odontogenic abscesses of guinea pigs are retromasseteric owing to anatomic features of the skull, cheek teeth, and masseter muscle. The exact visualzation of the abscess, superior to the soft tissue window of CT, may optimize the difficult surgical approach.

CT remains superior for diagnosis of dental disease and related bone infection.[16,20,21] For this reason, CT and MRI of the head are best used as complementary tests. In most cases, this is not feasible for practical and financial reasons; therefore, the clinical examination and survey radiographs would guide the clinician to choose the most useful adjunct diagnostic imaging test for the specific case.

SUMMARY

After the clinical examination, several diagnostic imaging techniques are beneficial for diagnosis, prognosis, and treatment of dental disease in rabbits and rodents. Beside standard radiography and stomatoscopy, advanced imaging such as CT and MRI are critical for diagnostic accuracy.

REFERENCES

1. Capello V, Gracis M, Lennox AM, editors. Rabbits and rodents dentistry handbook. Lake Worth (FL): Zoological Education Network; 2005. p. 1–272.
2. Capello V, Lennox AM. Small mammal dentistry. In: Quesenberry KE, Carpenter JW, editors. Ferrets, rabbits and rodents clinical medicine and surgery. 3rd edition. St Louis (MO): Elsevier Saunders; 2012. p. 452–71.
3. Lennox A. Diagnosis and treatment of dental disease in pet rabbits. J Exot Pet Med 2008;17:107–13.
4. Jekl V. The dental examination. In: Harcourt-Brown F, Chitty J, editors. Manual of rabbit surgery, dentistry and imaging, vol. 25, 1st edition. Quedgeley, Gloucester British Small Animal Veterinary Association; 2013. p. 337–48.
5. Capello V, Lennox AM. Clinical radiology of exotic companion mammals. Ames (IA): Wiley Blackwell; 2008.
6. Capello V, Cauduro M. Application of computed tomography for diagnosis of dental disease in the rabbit, guinea pig, and chinchilla. J Ex Pet Med 2008;17:93–101.
7. Jekl V. Principles of radiography. In: Harcourt-Brown F, Chitty J, editors. Manual of rabbit surgery, dentistry and imaging, vol. 3, 1st edition. Quedgeley, Gloucester British Small Animal Veterinary Association; 2013. p. 39–58.
8. Gracis M. Clinical technique: normal dental radiography of rabbits, guinea pigs, and chinchillas. J Ex Pet Med 2008;17:78–86.
9. Boehmer E. Intraoral radiographic technique in lagomorphs and rodents. Exotic DVM 2007;9(3):2–27.
10. Boehmer E, Crossley D. Objective interpretation of dental disease in rabbits, guinea pigs and chinchillas. Tierarzliche Praxis Kleintiere 2009;73:250–60.
11. Silverman S, Tell LA. Radiology of rodents, rabbits and ferrets. An atlas of oral anatomy and positioning. St Louis (MO): Elsevier Saunders; 2005.
12. Reese S, Fehr M. Small mammals. In: Krautwald-Junghanns ME, Pees M, Reese S, et al, editors. Diagnostic imaging of exotic pets. Hannover (Germany): Schlütersche Verlagsgesellschaft GmbH & Co; 2011. p. 143–307.
13. Raftery A. Radiographic interpretation of the skull. In: Harcourt-Brown F, Chitty J, editors. Manual of rabbit surgery, dentistry and imaging, vol. 4, 1st edition. Quedgeley, Gloucester British Small Animal Veterinary Association; 2013. p. 59–68.

14. Fischetti AJ. Diagnostic imaging. In: Quesenberry KE, Carpenter JW, editors. Ferrets, rabbits and rodents clinical medicine and surgery. 3rd edition. St Louis (MO): Elsevier Saunders; 2012. p. 502–10.
15. Boehmer E. Dentistry in rabbits and rodents. Philadelphia: Wiley-Blackwell; 2015.
16. Veraa S, Schoemaker N. CT and MRI scanning and interpretation. In: Harcourt-Brown F, Chitty J, editors. Manual of rabbit surgery, dentistry and imaging, vol. 9, 1st edition. Quedgeley, Gloucester British Small Animal Veterinary Association; 2013. p. 107–14.
17. Van Caelenberg AI, De Rycke LM, Hermans K, et al. Computed tomography and cross-sectional anatomy of the head in healthy rabbits. Am J Vet Res 2010;71(3): 293–303.
18. Capello V, Cauduro A. Comparison of diagnostic consistency and diagnostic accuracy between survey radiography and computed tomography of the skull in 30 rabbits with dental disease. J Exotic Pet Med 2016;25(2):115–27.
19. Van Caelenberg AI, De Rycke LM, Hermans K, et al. Comparison of radiography and CT to identify changes in the skulls of four rabbits with dental disease. J Vet Dentistry 2011;28(3):172–81.
20. Capello V. Application of computed tomography and magnetic resonance in exotic companion mammals. In: Proceedings of the 16th ABVP symposium. St Louis (MO): 2011.
21. Capello V. Novel diagnostics and surgical techniques for treatment of difficult facial abscesses in pet rabbits. In: Proceedings of the North Am Vet Conference. Orlando (FL): 2011. p. 1685–9.
22. Capello V, Lennox AM. Diagnostic imaging of the respiratory system in exotic companion mammals. Vet Clin North Am Exot Anim 2011;14(2):369–89.
23. Capello V. Rhinostomy as surgical treatment of odontogenic rhinitis in three pet rabbits. J Exotic Pet Med 2014;23(2):172–87.
24. Chesney CJ. CT scanning in chinchillas. J Small Anim Pract 1998;39:550.
25. Crossley DA, Jackson A, Yates J, et al. Use of computed tomography to investigate cheek tooth abnormalities in chinchillas (Chinchilla laniger). J Small Anim Pract 1998;39:385–9.
26. Brenner SZG, Hawkins MG, Tell LA, et al. Clinical anatomy, radiography, and computed tomography of the chinchilla skull. Comp Cont Ed Pract Vet 2005; 27:933–44.
27. Capello V, Lennox A. Advanced diagnostic imaging and surgical treatment of an odontogenic retromasseteric abscess in a guinea pig. J Small Anim Pract 2015; 56(2):134–7.
28. Souza MJ, Greenacre CB, Avenell JS, et al. Diagnosing a tooth root abscess in a guinea pig (Cavia porcellus) using micro computed tomography imaging. J Exot Pet Med 2008;15:274–7.
29. Capello V, Lennox AM, Ghisleni G. Elodontoma in Two Guinea Pigs. J Vet Dent 2015;32(2):111–9.
30. Capello V. We are not smaller rabbits, either. Dentistry of other rodent species and ferrets. In: Proceedings of the North Am Vet Conference. Orlando (FL): 2011. p. 1681–4.
31. Pelizzone I, Vitolo GD, D'Acierno M, et al. Lateral approach for excision of maxillary incisor pseudo-odontoma in prairie dogs (Cynomys ludovicianus). In vivo 2016;30:61–8.
32. De Rycke LM, Boone MN, Caelenberg Van, et al. Micro-computed tomography of the head and dentition in cadavers of clinically normal rabbits. Am J Vet Res 2012;73(2):227–32.

33. Sasai H, Iwai H, Fujiita D, et al. The use of micro-computed tomography in the diagnosis of dental and oral diseases in rabbits. BMC Vet Res 2014;10:209.
34. Divers SJ. Exotic mammal diagnostic endoscopy and endosurgery. Vet Clin Exot Anim 2010;13:255–72.
35. Hernandez-Divers SJ. Clinical technique: dental endoscopy of rabbits and rodents. J Ex Pet Med 2008;17:87–92.
36. Divers SJ. Exotic mammal diagnostic and surgical endoscopy. In: Quesenberry KE, Carpenter JW, editors. Ferrets, rabbits and rodents clinical medicine and surgery. 3rd edition. St Louis (MO): Elsevier Saunders; 2012. p. 485–501.
37. Taylor M. Endoscopy as an aid to examination and treatment of the oropharyngeal disease of small herbivorous mammals. Sem Avian Exot Pet Med 1999;8: 139–41.
38. Capello V. Application of rigid oral endoscopy in exotic companion mammals. In: Proceedings of the 16th ABVP Symposium. St Louis (MO): 2011.
39. Melillo A. Endoscopy. In: Harcourt-Brown F, Chitty J, editors. Manual of rabbit surgery, dentistry and imaging, vol. 10, 1st edition. Quedgeley, Gloucester British Small Animal Veterinary Association; 2013. p. 115–22.
40. Divers SJ. Endoscopy equipment and instrumentation for use in exotic animal medicine. Vet Clin Exot Anim 2010;13:171–85.
41. Gavin PR, Bagley RS. Practical small animal MRI. Ames (IA): John Wiley & Sons; 2009.

Intraoral Treatment of Dental Disease in Pet Rabbits

Vittorio Capello, DVM, DECZM (Small Mammal), DABVP-Exotic Companion Mammal[a,b,*]

KEYWORDS

- Incisor teeth • Cheek teeth • Dental instruments • Extraction • Coronal reduction

KEY POINTS

- The intraoral treatment of dental disease in pet rabbits must follow a complete clinical examination, intraoral inspection under general anesthesia, and diagnostic imaging.
- Intraoral inspection and dental procedures require specific instruments and equipment suitable for rabbits.
- Extraction of incisor teeth represents the only definitive and completely effective treatment of severe malocclusion. Rabbits adapt easily to absence of incisors, and the prognosis is good.
- Coronal reduction of incisor teeth must never be performed using trimmers, clippers, or similar instruments because they frequently lead to complications such as fractures, damage of the apical germinative tissue, pulp exposure, endodontic infection, and periapical abscessation; this is a meaningless procedure in cases of severe malocclusion.
- Coronal reduction of clinical crowns of cheek teeth is aimed at restoration of the coronal length and the occlusal planes *as close as possible* to normal anatomy.

INTRODUCTION

The proper planning of dental treatment is feasible after thorough diagnosis using modalities such as intraoral examination (ideally stomatoscopy), radiography, and other advanced imaging. In many cases, treatment immediately follows diagnosis in order to avoid a second anesthetic procedure. Discussion with the owner about long-term prognosis and aftercare is imperative.

Intraoral dental procedures represent an important part of treatment of dental disease in pet rabbits. Treatment includes elimination of dental spurs, restoration of a more normal occlusal plane, extractions, and gingival suture.

Disclosure: The author has nothing to disclose.
[a] Clinica Veterinaria S.Siro, Via Lampugnano, 99, Milano 20151, Italy; [b] Clinica Veterinaria Gran Sasso, Via Donatello, 26, Milano 20134, Italy
* Clinica Veterinaria S.Siro, Via Lampugnano, 99, Milano 20151, Italy.
E-mail address: capellov@tin.it

Vet Clin Exot Anim 19 (2016) 783–798
http://dx.doi.org/10.1016/j.cvex.2016.05.002
1094-9194/16/$ – see front matter © 2016 Elsevier Inc. All rights reserved.

PLANNING DENTAL TREATMENT
Common Presentations

The 3 most common clinical presentations of dental disease in pet rabbits relate to overgrowth of the incisors; reduced food intake, anorexia, or dysphagia; and presence of a facial swelling.[1–3] One, 2, or all 3 of these conditions can be present at the same time. Although dental disease affecting the cheek teeth is more frequent, diseases affecting the incisors are more apparent to the owners. In the most common pattern of malocclusion, diseased incisors enhance the normal curvature of the reserve and clinical crowns. The mandibular incisors tend to elongate labially, and usually do not produce secondary lesions because they are rostral to the upper lip and nose.[1] The maxillary incisors tend to elongate and curve palatally[1,2] and possibly damage the lips and/or the palate (**Fig. 1**). Elongated incisors may fracture at different levels of the clinical crown, or even below the gingival level. In cases of advanced dental disease, growth may be slowed or arrested. Dental disease of the incisors also affects the reserve crown. Abnormal elongation and apical deformity of maxillary primary incisors may lead to partial or complete obstruction of the nasolacrimal duct. Epiphora, dacryocystitis, additional ocular lesions, or facial dermatitis are possible sequelae.[1,4–6]

Rabbits with acquired dental disease of the cheek teeth may present at different stages,[2,7] but symptoms may not be consistent with the degree of disease.[2] The earliest stage is elongation of clinical crowns. Clinical signs are usually not present at this stage, even though some symptoms, such as the rabbit being reluctant to eat hay or other hard food, may be inferred from a detailed history. This condition is caused by the elongated apex impinging on its sensory nerve supply.[7] At a further stage, elongation of the clinical crowns and the abnormal occlusal plane appear as so-called step mouth on the intraoral examination.[1,2,7] Extraoral signs may also appear, such as slight deformity of the ventral profile of the mandibular cortical bone following elongation of reserve crowns.[1,3,7,8] In advanced stages, excessive curvature of clinical crowns of mandibular cheek teeth typically occurs, but is not limited to the lingual direction. In contrast, the maxillary cheek teeth usually curve in the buccal direction, which can result in spur formation and lesions of the lingual or the buccal mucosa.

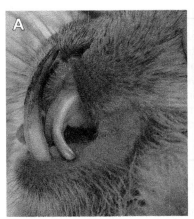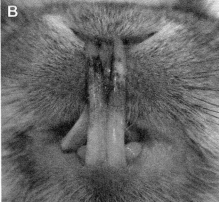

Fig. 1. Common presentation of malocclusion of incisor teeth in a pet rabbit, lateral (*A*), and rostral (*B*) views. The mandibular incisors tend to elongate labially, whereas the maxillary incisors tend to elongate and curve palatally with possible damage to the lips and/or palate. (*Courtesy of Vittorio* Capello, DVM, Milano, Italy; with permission.)

A common complication of coronal elongation of cheek teeth is fracture, especially longitudinal fracture of mandibular premolars.[1] End-stage dental disease of the cheek teeth is frequently associated with resorption of dental tissue and severe changes of cheek teeth arcades.

Instruments and Equipment

The equipment suitable for dentistry of pet rabbits can be divided into 2 groups: instruments for diagnosis and instruments for treatment.[1,2,9]

Instruments for diagnosis

Because of the deep and narrow oral cavity, special mouth gags designed to fit with the clinical crowns of incisors are essential instruments for oral examination. The rabbit and rodent table retractor/restrainer (otherwise named the tabletop mouth gag) is a special platform acting as a combined mouth gag and patient positioner.[1–3] This instrument is useful because it allows the operator to work without the need of an assistant, apart from the anesthetist. It also allows the patient to be placed in an optimal position that facilitates the intraoral examination. The patient is positioned in sternal recumbency. The table restrainer has 2 horizontal bars working as the mouth gag, where the incisor teeth are anchored (**Fig. 2**). The platform can be raised to enhance the operator's view. However, the platform should not be tilted more than 30° to minimize stress on the neck, and to avoid excessive traction on incisor teeth. Various types of gags are used under general anesthesia, but they should be used with extreme caution to prevent excessive stretching of the masticatory muscles and the ligaments of the temporomandibular joint.

The second instrument needed to access the oral cavity is the cheek dilator. Different sizes and shapes are available with longer blades fitting better into the rabbit mouth and being more effective in dilating the cheeks, especially in larger breeds.[1,3] After the mouth gag and cheek dilator have been applied, 2 other instruments are suitable for managing the tongue. Small and smooth-tip anatomic forceps are used to grasp and move the tongue. A flat or concave spatula is also used to deflect and protect the tongue during treatment of cheek teeth.

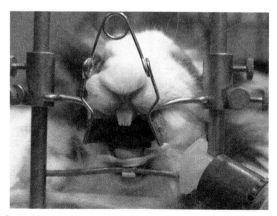

Fig. 2. Close-up of a rabbit positioned on the rabbit and rodent table retractor/restrainer (tabletop mouth gag) with the cheek dilator. Anesthesia is maintained using orotracheal intubation in this rabbit. Depending on the rabbit's size, the orotracheal tube may hinder the procedure. Injectable anesthetic protocols combined with face mask may be an effective alternative option. (*Courtesy of* Vittorio Capello, DVM, Milano, Italy; with permission.)

Proper lighting is critical, and magnification is desirable in rabbits for intraoral inspection. Effective light spots can be connected to magnifying loupes when endoscopy is not an option. Miscellaneous diagnostic instruments include intravenous catheters of 22 to 24 gauge (without the stylet) to assess the patency of the nasolacrimal duct.

TREATMENT

The general guidelines of intraoral dental procedures consist of reduction of abnormal tooth length of clinical crowns, restoration of the occlusal plane to as near normal as possible, and extraction of diseased teeth.[2,10] Complications and secondary diseases, such as periapical infections, osteomyelitis, and odontogenic abscesses, are treated with combined dental procedures and extraoral surgery.

Medical Treatment

Medical therapy alone is not sufficient for the treatment of dental disease. However, it may be important as a temporary palliative or supportive treatment before a dental procedure under general anesthesia, and it is also an important adjunct to surgical procedures. The 3 key points of medical treatment are supportive, antimicrobial, and antiinflammatory/analgesic therapy.[1,2,10] Supportive treatment includes syringeable assist-feeding products for herbivorous species. Fluid therapy may also be necessary in some patients.[1]

The choice of the antimicrobial treatment should be based on both aerobic and anaerobic culture and sensitivity testing when possible, and considering any species-specific contraindications, such as oral administration of penicillins in rabbits.[1,2,11] Analgesia is critical to relieve pain and discomfort as well as to prevent pain-related reduced food intake and anorexia.

Intraoral Treatment

Instruments and equipment

The intraoral dental treatment requires specific instruments. Beside the equipment described earlier for inspection of the oral cavity and protection of soft tissues, other novel instruments are available for extraction and mechanical trimming.[1,2,9] Specialized elevators for rabbit incisor and cheek teeth have been designed by Dr David Crossley. Crossley luxators for rabbit incisor teeth are flat, curved to match the shape of the reserve crowns, and sharp at the concave margin. The 2 ends have different curvatures; 1 for maxillary and 1 for mandibular incisor teeth (**Fig. 3**). This instrument allows the breaking down of periodontal ligaments on the distal (lateral) and mesial (medial) aspect of the incisor teeth. Other luxators have recently been designed to address the labial (rostral) and lingual/palatal (caudal) aspect of incisors. Alternatively, properly contoured 18-gauge needles may be used on these sides.

Crossley luxators for rabbit cheek teeth are designed with 2 sharp working ends angled at about 100° to the handle, and perpendicular to each other (**Fig. 4**). This luxator is used to break the ligament on the 4 aspects of the cheek teeth: one end for the mesial and distal aspect, and the other end for the lingual/palatal and the buccal aspect. Small standard extraction forceps can be used to extract incisors; needle holders and small hemostats can be used as well, depending on the patient's size. Another instrument especially designed for rabbits is the extraction forceps for cheek teeth. The grasping tip is angled at 100° to facilitate its use in the narrow oral cavity (**Fig. 5**).

In the past, Dremel-type (20,000–30,000 rpm) hobby tools have been used for coronal reduction of cheek teeth, but several manufacturers offer precision, higher

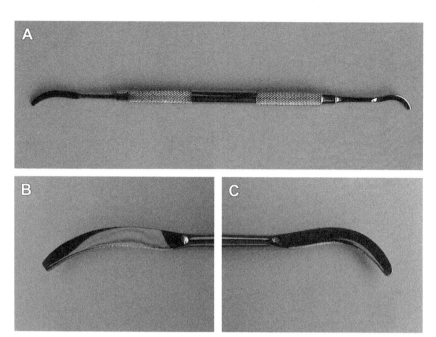

Fig. 3. Crossley luxators for incisor teeth. (*A*) The instrument. (*B*) The end for luxation of mandibular incisor teeth. (*C*) The end for luxation of mandibular incisor teeth. Note the different curvature and the sharp edge of the concave margin. (*Courtesy of* Vittorio Capello, DVM, Milano, Italy; with permission.)

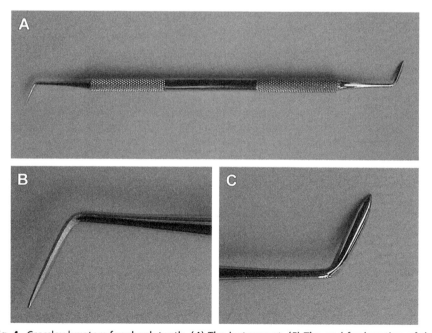

Fig. 4. Crossley luxators for cheek teeth. (*A*) The instrument. (*B*) The end for luxation of the mesial (rostral) and distal (caudal) aspects of cheek teeth. (*C*) The end for luxation of the buccal (lateral) and lingual/palatal (medial) aspects of cheek teeth. The 2 ends are angled at approximately 100° to the handle, and are perpendicular to each other. (*Courtesy of* Vittorio Capello, DVM, Milano, Italy; with permission.)

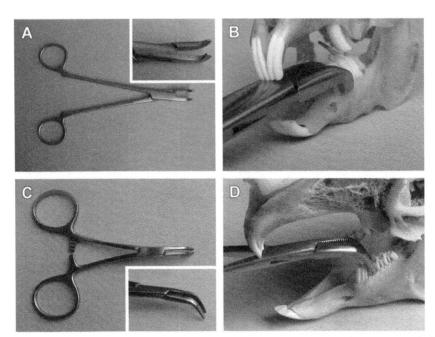

Fig. 5. Extraction forceps for cheek teeth. Standard extraction forceps for cheek teeth (*A*) and related size in relationship to a skull of a 1.5-kg dwarf rabbit (*B*). Smaller extraction forceps (*C*) and related size in relationship to a skull of a 1.5-kg dwarf rabbit (*D*). (*Courtesy of* Vittorio Capello, DVM, Milano, Italy; with permission.)

speed handpieces. A dental unit is adequate and recommended for dental treatment of pet rabbits. A straight dental handpiece is needed because the standard angled dental handpiece used for dog and cat dentistry cannot access the mouth of rabbits, and its use is limited to coronal reduction of incisor teeth.

Many different types, shapes, and sizes of burrs are available. Sheats protecting the metal bur can be mounted on straight handpieces. Old diamond rasps and cutters for rabbit cheek teeth are still available on the market, but their use must be discouraged because forces applied by these instruments can fracture cheek teeth and may cause severe damage to adjacent soft tissues.

Treatment of Incisor Teeth

Extraction
Extraction of the incisor teeth is the only definitive and completely effective treatment of severe malocclusion, both with and without associated acquired dental disease.[1,2,10,12,13] Maloccluded incisor teeth are not functional, and rabbits adapt easily to the absence of incisors. They are able to eat normally using their lips and tongue for food prehension. Also, repeated coronal reductions are not recommended because of frequent anesthesia, complications such as pulp overgrowth and exposure,[14] or abnormal reserve crowns affecting the function of nasolacrimal ducts. Financial reasons may also be a concern.

In most cases, extraction of the entire set of 6 incisor teeth is necessary, even if, in selected cases in which a single mandibular incisor tooth is fractured or infected, extraction of that single mandibular incisor tooth may be indicated. For those patients, the maxillary incisor on the same quadrant may be able to keep a normal occlusal plane because of lateral chewing movements.

Diagnostic radiographs are taken before extraction of incisor teeth, in particular to assess the reserve crowns.[2,15] The use of mouth gags is possible after extraction of incisor teeth, but it is a bit more difficult, and mouth opening may be suboptimal. For this reason, intraoral dental procedures on cheek teeth should be performed before extraction of the incisor teeth.

Extraction of mandibular incisors before maxillary incisors is not a specific guideline, but it is the author's preference and the recommendation is to begin by extracting the mandibular incisor teeth (**Fig. 6**).

The anesthetized patient is placed in dorsal recumbency. The gingiva is scrubbed with 0.1% chlorhexidine solution. For optional adjunct local anesthesia, local block of the mental nerve is performed.[16,17] The gingival attachment is incised circumferentially around the 4 aspects of the clinical crown with the tip of a number 11 scalpel blade. The longer edge of the Crossley luxator is inserted in the periodontal space on the mesial side of the tooth, until resistance is felt. The luxator is held in position for a few seconds to stretch and damage the periodontal ligament. The tip of the

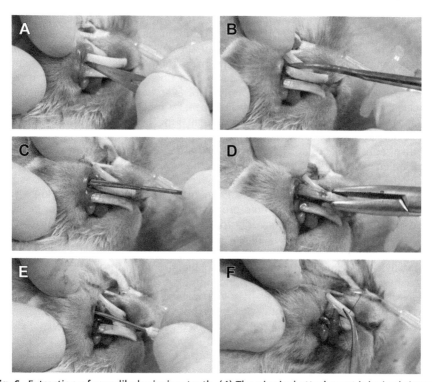

Fig. 6. Extraction of mandibular incisor teeth. (*A*) The gingival attachment is incised circumferentially around the 4 aspects of the clinical crown with the tip of a number 11 scalpel blade. (*B*) The mandibular edge of the Crossley luxator is inserted in the periodontal space on the distal side of the tooth. (*C*) A flattened and curved contoured 18-gauge needle is used to break down the periodontal ligament on the labial aspect. (*D*) The tooth is grasped with the extraction forceps (a needle holder in this case) as close to the gingival margin as possible. It is extracted using steady, slowly increasing force, following the curvature of the root and with slight torsional movements. (*E*) After extraction, damage of the geminal tissue is performed by inserting a needle into the alveolus to curette the alveolar walls, which helps to prevent possible tooth regrowth. (*F*) Suture of the gingiva using 4-0 absorbable suture material (poliglecaprone, Monocryl). (*Courtesy of* Vittorio Capello, DVM, Milano, Italy; with permission.)

luxator is gradually moved toward the apex of the tooth. The free hand is used to stabilize the mandible. The same procedure is then performed on the distal aspect of the tooth. With the same technique, either a dedicated luxator for the lingual and labial sides of the tooth or a contoured, 18-gauge hypodermic needle is used to break down the periodontal ligament on those aspects. The tooth should be loose and very mobile at this point. The tooth is grasped with the extraction forceps as close to the gingival margin as possible. It is extracted using steady, slowly increasing force, following the curvature of the root and with slight torsional movements. When the tooth is loosened and ready to be extracted, the tooth is repeatedly inserted back in the socket before extraction to damage the germinal tissues at the bottom of the alveolus. If the periodontal ligament has been completely and correctly severed and the tooth is not severely deformed, it can be extracted without the use of significant force. Bleeding is usually minimal and can easily be controlled with sterile cotton swabs. After extraction, the tooth is examined to ensure that the entire tooth and its pulp tissues have been removed. In addition to repeated insertion of the tooth before extraction, further damage of the geminal tissue is performed by inserting a needle into the alveolus to curette the alveolar walls after extraction, which helps to prevent possible tooth regrowth. The alveolar cavity is thoroughly flushed with saline solution to remove any debris. If periapical infection is present, dilute 2% povidone iodine or 0.1% chlorhexidine solution is used for flushing. The alveolus is closed by suturing the gingiva with simple interrupted sutures or a purse-string suture pattern using 3-0 or smaller absorbable suture material. However, when infection is present the alveolus is left open, allowing the gingiva to heal by second intention.

Before extraction of the maxillary incisor teeth (**Fig. 7**), the gingiva is scrubbed with 0.1% chlorhexidine solution. For optional adjunct local anesthesia, local block of the rostral infraorbital nerve is performed.[16,17] The upper harelip is lifted with the free hand, which is used to hold and stabilize the patient's head. Either a dedicated luxator for the labial and palatal sides of the tooth or a contoured, 18-gauge hypodermic needle is used to sever the periodontal ligament on the labial and palatal sides of the maxillary incisor teeth, similar to the procedure described for mandibular incisors. When working on the palatal aspect, special attention should be paid to prevent damage to the small secondary incisor teeth. The periodontal ligament is severed on the mesial and distal aspects of the primary incisor teeth using the Crossley luxator. The periodontal ligament is particularly strong on the mesial aspect, and the tooth will be significantly loose after the ligament is cut. When the tooth is loosened, the clinical crown is grasped with suitable extraction forceps or a pair of needle holders. To avoid dental and bony fractures, the tooth is pulled gently, following the natural curvature of the reserve crown, and applying a slight distal (lateral) rotation during extraction. After extraction, the tooth is examined to ensure that the entire tooth and its pulp tissues have been removed. The procedure is repeated on the primary incisor tooth of the contralateral quadrant, and bleeding is controlled with sterile cotton swabs. A thin, 22-gauge, contoured hypodermic needle is used to loosen the secondary incisor teeth. When the small peg tooth is completely luxated, it is extracted with small extraction forceps or thin hemostats, taking care to avoid crushing the tooth. After extractions, the alveoli are curetted with a needle to remove any remaining pulp tissues, and rinsed with saline or 0.1% chlorhexidine solution. The gingiva is closed with simple interrupted sutures or a purse-string suture pattern with 3-0 or 4-0 absorbable suture material to promote gingival healing. However, the extraction site is not sutured when infection is present. When using a purse-string pattern, the suture material is fixed at a minimum of 6 points through the gingiva before tightening it.

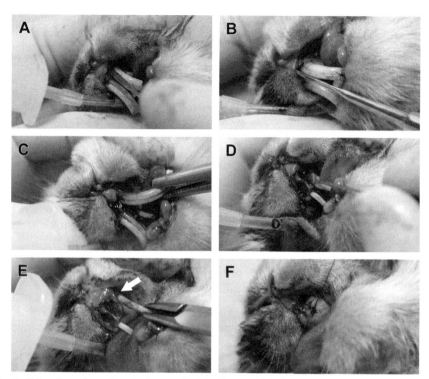

Fig. 7. Extraction of maxillary incisor teeth. (*A*) A flattened and curved contoured 18-gauge needle is used to break down the periodontal ligament on the labial aspect of the primary incisor tooth. (*B*) The maxillary edge of the Crossley luxator is inserted in the periodontal space on the mesial aspect of the tooth. (*C*) When the tooth is loosened, the clinical crown is grasped with suitable extraction forceps (a large hemostat, in this case). The tooth is pulled gently, following the natural curvature of the reserve crown, and applying a slight distal (lateral) rotation during extraction. (*D*) A flattened and curved contoured 21-gauge needle is used to perform luxation of the rostral aspect of the secondary (peg) incisor tooth. (*E*) The peg tooth is extracted using a small needle holder. Note the red germinative tissue at the apex (*arrow*), showing complete extraction. (*F*) Purse-string suture of the gingiva using 4-0 absorbable suture material (poliglecaprone, Monocryl). (*Courtesy of* Vittorio Capello, DVM, Milano, Italy; with permission.)

At the end of the dental procedure, a postoperative lateral radiographic view is taken to confirm complete extraction of all 6 incisor teeth.

Incomplete removal of teeth or failure to destroy pulp tissues can result in partial or complete regrowth.[1,15] In the first case, a bud of reserve crown may regrow, not followed by eruption of a clinical crown. This latter case is rare,[18] and can be addressed should it occur.

Possible complications are represented by fracture of the incisive bone and retention of fragments in the case of preexisting tooth ankylosis, and dehiscence of the gingival suture. Extraction of the retained reserve crown may require an extraoral approach.[15] Dehiscence typically heals by second intention and does not require specific treatment.[1]

Coronal reduction
Coronal reduction is limited to selected cases in which malocclusion is minimal, has been diagnosed early, and proper occlusion of both incisor and cheek teeth can be restored.[1,2,10]

Trimmers, clippers, or similar instruments must not be used because they do not allow the restoration of a normal incisal edge, and frequently lead to complications such as fractures, damage of the apical germinative tissue, pulp exposure, endodontic infection, and periapical abscessation.[1]

Reduction of coronal length and reshaping of the occlusal plane must be performed on anesthetized patients with a fissure-cut bur on a high-speed angled dental handpiece, or with a diamond disc on a low-speed straight handpiece. In case of pulp exposure, partial pulpectomy and pulp capping have been described.[1,14]

Treatment of Cheek Teeth

Coronal reduction

Coronal reduction of clinical crowns of cheek teeth is intended to restore the coronal length and the occlusal planes as close as possible to normal anatomy.[2,7,19] It should be performed with a low-speed straight handpiece and longer grinding-type burs that can be safely introduced into the small oral cavity of the rabbit. Small rasps and molar cutters should not be used.[1]

Standard orotracheal intubation may be routinely performed during anesthesia for intraoral procedures. However, depending on the rabbit's size, effective application of mouth gag and cheek dilators, and the difficulty of the procedure, the orotracheal tube may significantly hamper the movements and the procedure. Although intubation is a mainstay of anesthesia, intraoral procedures should never be suboptimal because of the endotracheal tube. Injectable anesthetic protocols combined with face mask, and nasal or nasotracheal intubation, may be effective alternative options.

Depending on severity of acquired dental disease, coronal reduction may be more or less effective. With regard to prognosis for treatment of malocclusion, several considerations should be kept in mind and discussed with the owner[19]:

1. Coronal reduction is a palliative treatment by default, because acquired dental disease is progressive.[20] Apart from very early stages at which minimal correction would help normal chewing preventing further changes, coronal reduction does not stop or address the underlying bone and/or dental disease.
2. The goal of proper coronal reduction is burring of spurs, restoration of the proper length of clinical crowns, and restoration of an even occlusal plane. Even is mostly synonymous with flat, and does not correspond with anatomically normal. Clinicians are aware that it is impossible to restore the normal zigzag occlusal plane, and slightly bent in a dorsoventral and rostrocaudal direction.
3. Coronal reduction does not address abnormal elongation of reserve crowns. Despite this obvious limitation, it does help to relieve pain. Elongation of apices of cheek teeth leads to pressure, deformity, and even perforation of the periapical cortical bone, which may be painful. When clinical crowns are elongated, coronal reduction helps to reduce apical pressure during chewing movements.
4. Coronal reduction does not address abnormal curvature of reserve and clinical crowns. Depending on the severity of this trait of dental disease, formation of new spurs occurs more or less frequently. The owners should be informed that repeated intraoral treatments may be necessary for the patient's life. However, the slowing or cessation of eruption caused by advancing dental disease and repeated treatments usually occurs.

Despite this being a palliative procedure compared with the normal anatomy of cheek teeth, coronal reduction is usually very effective, and it dramatically improves the patient's clinical condition.

With regard to the dental procedure, several points and tips should be considered:

1. The simple burring of spurs does not represent a proper and complete dental treatment. This procedure relieves some pain and allows healing of mucosal wounds, but the discomfort elicited by the excessive elongation of clinical crowns and the abnormal occlusal plane is not improved. This omission leads to partial remission of symptoms, and to frequent relapse.

2. Coronal reduction must never be performed beyond restoration of normal length in order to reduce time until the next dental treatment; for example, burring all cheek teeth to the gingival level. Excessive coronal reduction results in improper occlusion with risk of increased discomfort and/or exposure of the pulp. Also, excessive coronal reduction may result in exposure of the pulp cavity,[20] eliciting pain and predisposing to endodontic disease.

3. However, abnormal elongation of clinical crowns of mandibular cheek teeth is accompanied by stretching or hyperplasia of the gingiva in some patients. This stretching or hyperplasia may allow the clinical crowns (the portion of the tooth beyond the gingival margin) of cheek teeth (in particular the mandibular) to appear normal at intraoral inspection, whereas the reserve crown is elongated, both the portion inside the alveolus and the short portion buried under the gingival margin but not within the socket. In order to detect this misleading abnormality, clinicians must carefully compare the visual findings at intraoral inspection with the radiographic findings in the lateral projection of the skull (**Fig. 8**). Because the radiograph does not show any evidence of gingival tissue, the whole length of the cheek teeth (from the occlusal plane through the apex) can be properly evaluated. In this case, the clinical crown will have to be burred shorter than the gingival margin. The clinical crown will appear shorter than normal, but the whole length of the tooth will be correct.

4. Some patients have severe step mouth (uneven length of adjacent cheek teeth), in which a clinical crown might be longer than normal, and others might be shorter than normal. The abnormally short clinical crowns should not be used as a landmark for restoration of an even occlusal plane. Doing so can result in excessive reduction of length. If 1 or more cheek teeth are shorter than normal, the final result will still be a form of step mouth, because the elongated (or the normal) clinical crowns will be longer than those that are abnormally short.

5. Special attention must be paid to coronal reduction of elongated mandibular CT4 and CT5, because the lower alveolar vein lies just under the mucosa of the pharyngeal commissure, in close proximity. Accidental injury of this vein may cause significant intraoral hemorrhage.

In general, when early diagnosis and treatment are performed before severe changes of the cheek teeth have occurred, coronal reduction combined with proper nutrition is often effective in preventing ongoing dental disease.[20]

The dental procedure consists of the application of a rotating bur to the dental occlusal surface. The tooth is moistened with saline before coronal reduction to reduce the amount of tooth dust and prevent thermal injury to dental pulp.[1,2,10,19–21]

Proper coronal reduction of cheek teeth can be verified with a post-treatment radiograph in lateral projection, which is compared with the same projection taken before the intraoral dental treatment.

Extraction

Indications for extraction of cheek teeth are significantly different from indications for extraction of incisor teeth.[19] Although incisor teeth can be extracted with a good anatomic and functional prognosis, cheek teeth play a primary role for normal crushing

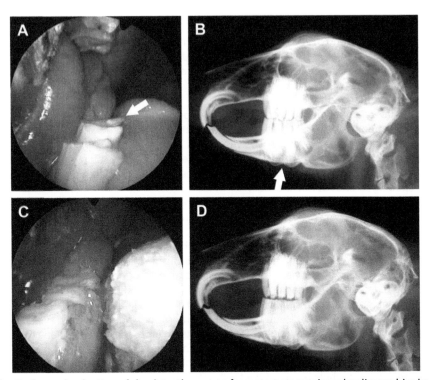

Fig. 8. Coronal reduction of cheek teeth, as seen from stomatoscopic and radiographic view-points. (*A*) Elongation and malocclusion of clinical crowns of the right mandibular cheek teeth arcade. Clinical crowns of CT1, CT3, and CT4 are bent lingually. Step mouth is present, as well as a lingual spike on CT4 (*arrow*). Dental disease of mandibular cheek teeth arcades was bilateral, associated with mild elongation and malocclusion of the clinical crowns of maxillary cheek teeth arcades. (*B*) Radiography in the same patient, laterolateral view. Overall elongation of reserve crowns of cheek teeth is present, with deformity of the ventral cortical bone of the mandible (*arrow*). The occlusal plane of cheek teeth is abnormal, and the normal zigzag radio-transparent line is lost. (*C*) Right mandibular cheek teeth arcade in the same patient, after cor-onal reduction. The occlusal plane is now even. Note the apparently short clinical crowns, caused by stretching or hyperplasia of the gingiva. (*D*) Control radiograph postoperatively following coronal reduction. Even though it is impossible to restore the normal occlusal plane, a small gap is present between the cheek teeth arcades, and the occlusal plane is more regular. Also, the control radiograph shows that coronal reduction was adequate, considering the gingival elongation masking part of the clinical crown of the cheek teeth. (*Courtesy of* Vittorio Capello, DVM, Milano, Italy; with permission.)

of food, and the goal of therapy should be retention of as many cheek teeth as prac-tically possible.[15,19] Dental indications for carnivorous mammals typically include the extraction of a tooth that is significantly damaged and this may not apply to rabbit dentistry. Because of the peculiar palisade pattern of rabbit cheek teeth, extraction of even a single tooth may cause instability of adjacent teeth.

Indications for extraction of cheek teeth include:

- When a cheek tooth is loose
- When a tooth is associated with periapical infection (typically it is also loose)
- When a cheek tooth is fractured; sometimes complete extraction of the reserve crown is not b possible, as in the case of some longitudinal fractures

- For selected teeth (ie, maxillary premolars) to reduce the need for frequent and repeated coronal reduction
- In selected cases, special extractions might be required, as in the case of diseased maxillary molars to create access to the alveolar bulla for treatment of empyema or a retrobulbar abscess

The 2 sharp working ends of the Crossley luxator for cheek teeth are used to sever the periodontal ligaments on all 4 aspects of the cheek teeth[1,2,10,19,21] (**Fig. 9**). Luxation and extraction are easier depending on the degree to which a diseased tooth is loose. Because of the small size, the short clinical crown, and the long reserve crown of cheek teeth, small extraction forceps with tips angled at about 100° to the handle are critical to perform a proper extraction.

When a cheek tooth is extracted, it is not necessary to extract the opposing tooth because:

- With the exception of the maxillary CT1 and CT6, the occlusal plane of every cheek tooth matches with 2 portions of the occlusal plane of opposing teeth, in a domino fashion
- Overgrowth of opposing teeth can be controlled with repeated coronal reductions

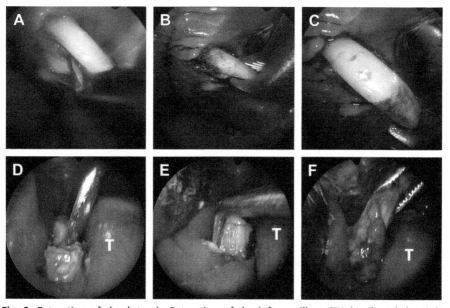

Fig. 9. Extraction of cheek teeth. Extraction of the left maxillary CT1 (*A–C*) and the right mandibular CT1 (*D–F*). (*A*) The perpendicular end of the Crossley luxator for cheek teeth is inserted on the distal aspect of the diseased tooth. (*B*) After luxation on the 4 aspects and when the tooth is loosened, the clinical crown is grasped with the extraction forceps (standard size, in this case) and (*C*) extracted following the abnormal curvature of the diseased reserve crown. (*D*) The perpendicular end is inserted on the distal aspect of the diseased tooth, affected by periapical infection. (*E*) The other end of the Crossley luxator works the buccal aspect of the tooth. Pus is visible on the distal aspect, after luxation of that side. (*F*) The clinical crown is grasped with the extraction forceps (small size, in this case) and extracted. The elongated and deformed reserve crown and apex are clearly visible. T, tongue. (*Courtesy of* Vittorio Capello, DVM, Milano, Italy; with permission.)

- Acquired dental disease may eventually result in slowing or arrested elongation of opposing teeth
- Contact between the dental occlusal plane and gingiva may provide sufficient and effective wearing

Combined intraoral and extraoral extraction

For information on surgical treatment of periapical infections, debridement of odontogenic abscesses and osteomyelitis, and related extraoral extraction of cheek teeth (or their fragments), please see Vittorio Capello: Surgical Treatment of Facial Abscesses and Facial Surgery in Pet Rabbits, in this issue.

When the reserve crown of cheek teeth is fractured (even with multiple fragments), or when ankylosis of the reserve crown is present, complete extraction from the intraoral approach is not possible. In these cases, complete extraction of the remainder of the reserve crown may require a combined intraoral/extraoral approach. Extraction of the clinical crown and part of the reserve crown is performed intraorally; extraction of the remaining reserve crown is performed through the extraoral approach.[1,2,15]

Suture of the gingiva

Suture of the gingiva may or may not be performed after extraction of cheek teeth[19] (**Fig. 10**). Because of small patient size and the narrow opening of the oral cavity, it

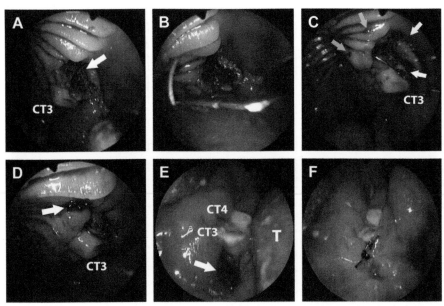

Fig. 10. Suture of the gingiva after extraction of maxillary (*A–D*) and mandibular (*E, F*) cheek teeth. (*A*) Large defect after extraction of both left maxillary premolar teeth (*arrow*). (*B*) The curved needle of a 5-0 absorbable suture material (poliglecaprone, Monocryl) is inserted through the palatal mucosa to create a horizontal mattress suture between the palatal mucosa and the gingiva. (*C*) The suture passes through the palatal mucosa (*green arrow*), laterally through the gingiva (*yellow arrow*), again through the gingiva on the same buccal side (*white arrow*), and back again through the palatal mucosa (*orange arrow*). (*D*) The suture is tightened (*arrow*), closing the defect. (*E*) Large defect after extraction of both right mandibular premolar teeth (*arrow*) (*F*) Suture of the gingiva in a mattress fashion using a 5-0 absorbable suture material (poliglecaprone, Monocryl). (*Courtesy of* Vittorio Capello, DVM, Milano, Italy; with permission.)

is a challenging procedure that requires proper lighting, magnification, and instruments. A small and long needle holder, and fine-tipped scissors are particularly useful. Special suture material with a curved needle is available from dental suppliers, otherwise an ordinary curved needle can be bent appropriately to allow suture of margins inside the small space.

As a general guideline, gingival suture should be performed anytime it is feasible and the defect is large, and when periapical infection is not present. In case of infection, the gingiva is allowed to heal by second intention. Gingival suture after extraction of 1 or 2 proximal mandibular cheek teeth may be performed in cases of combined extraoral access for debridement of osteomyelitis and marsupialization. If feasible, suture of the gingiva is designed to prevent drainage of food debris through the osteomyelitic site, or the formation of an oral/extraoral permanent fistula.

Suture is deliberately not performed after extraction of several maxillary molar teeth when the goal is to maintain patency with the alveolar bulla.

Complications

Complications during intraoral procedures are rare. Flat or curved spatulas are designed to reflect the tongue and soft tissues, and to protect them during coronal reduction. Hemorrhage from the lower alveolar vein should be prevented when the most distal (caudal) cheek teeth are manipulated.[19] In some patients affected by advanced dental disease of maxillary cheek teeth with severe elongation and deformity of reserve crowns, luxation might accidentally damage the descending palatine artery or the maxillary artery. Hemorrhage of these important vessels may be challenging to control and requires the use of gelatin sponge hemostatic material and/or pressure.

SUMMARY

The intraoral treatment of dental disease in pet rabbits follows a complete clinical examination, intraoral inspection under general anesthesia, and diagnostic imaging. The most common intraoral procedures are extraction of incisor teeth, coronal reduction, and extraction of cheek teeth. These dental procedures require specific instruments and equipment.

REFERENCES

1. Capello V, Gracis M, Lennox AM. Rabbits and rodents dentistry handbook. Lake Worth (FL): Zoological Education Network; 2005.
2. Capello V, Lennox AM. Small mammal dentistry. In: Quesenberry KE, Carpenter JW, editors. Ferrets, rabbits and rodents clinical medicine and surgery. 3rd edition. St Louis (MO): Elsevier Saunders; 2012. p. 452–71.
3. Jekl V. The dental examination. In: Harcourt-Brown F, Chitty J, editors. Manual of rabbit surgery, dentistry and imaging, vol. 25, 1st edition. Quedgeley (United Kingdom): British Small Animal Veterinary Association; 2013. p. 337–48.
4. Burling K, Murphy CJ, da Silva Curiel J, et al. Anatomy of the rabbit nasolacrimal duct and its clinical implications. Prog Vet Comp Ophthalmol 1991;1:33–40.
5. Harcourt-Brown FM. Dacryocystitis in rabbits. Exotic DVM 2002;4:47–9.
6. van der Woerdt A. Ophthalmologic diseases in small pet mammals. In: Quesenberry KE, Carpenter JW, editors. Ferrets, rabbits and rodents: clinical medicine and surgery. 2nd edition. St Louis (MO): Elsevier Saunders; 2004. p. 421–8.
7. Harcourt-Brown F. Normal rabbit dentition and pathogenesis of dental disease. In: Harcourt-Brown F, Chitty J, editors. Manual of rabbit surgery, dentistry and

imaging. 1st edition. Quedgeley (United Kingdom): British Small Animal Veterinary Association; 2013. p. 319–36.

8. Capello V, Lennox AM. Clinical radiology of exotic companion mammals. Ames (IA): Wiley-Blackwell; 2008.

9. Capello V. The dental suite: equipment needed for handling small exotic mammals. J Exot Pet Med 2006;15(2):106–15.

10. Lennox A. Diagnosis and treatment of dental disease in pet rabbits. J Exot Pet Med 2008;17:107–13.

11. Rosenthal KL. Therapeutic contraindications in exotic pets. Sem Avian Exot Pet Med 2004;13:44–8.

12. Brown SA. Surgical removal of incisors in the rabbit. J Small Exot Anim Med 1992; 1:150–3.

13. Capello V. Extraction of incisor teeth in pet rabbits. Exotic DVM 2004;6(4):32–7.

14. Crossley DA. The risk of pulp exposure when trimming rabbit incisor teeth. In Proceedings 10th Ann Cong Europ Vet Dent. Berlin, Germany, October 25-26, 2001. p. 21–22.

15. Easson W. Tooth extraction. In: Harcourt-Brown F, Chitty J, editors. Manual of rabbit surgery, dentistry and imaging, vol. 27, 1st edition. Quedgeley (United Kingdom): British Small Animal Veterinary Association; 2013. p. 370–81.

16. Lichtenberger M, Ko J. Anesthesia and analgesia for small mammals and birds. Vet Clin North Am Exot Anim Pract 2007;10:293–315.

17. Lennox AM. Small exotic mammal dentistry-anesthetic considerations. J Exot Pet Med 2008;17:102–6.

18. Steenkamp G, Crossley DA. Incisor tooth regrowth in a rabbit following complete extraction. Vet Rec 1999;145:585–6.

19. Capello V. Beyond burring of cheek teeth: intraoral treatment of dental disease in pet rabbits. Proceedings of the North American Veterinary Conference. Orlando (FL): 2011. p. 1674–1676.

20. Harcourt-Brown F. Treatment of dental problems: principles and options. In: Harcourt-Brown F, Chitty J, editors. Manual of rabbit surgery, dentistry and imaging, vol. 26, 1st edition. Quedgeley (United Kingdom): British Small Animal Veterinary Association; 2013. p. 349–69.

21. Capello V. Endoscopic assessment and treatment of cheek teeth malocclusion in pet rabbits. Exotic DVM 2004;6(2):21–7.

Surgical Treatment of Facial Abscesses and Facial Surgery in Pet Rabbits

Vittorio Capello, DVM, DECZM (Small Mammal), DABVP-Exotic Companion Mammal[a,b,*]

KEYWORDS

- Abscess • Osteomyelitis • Empyema • Retrobulbar • Marsupialization
- Mandibulectomy

KEY POINTS

- Understanding of dental and anatomic features of the jaws and the skull is critical for interpretation of diagnostic imaging and for the surgical treatment of odontogenic facial abscesses and their complications.
- Thorough diagnostic imaging (including radiography, oral endoscopy, computed tomography, and magnetic resonance) is of paramount importance for diagnostic accuracy, prognosis, and for planning surgical treatment.
- Medical therapy alone is unrewarding, but important as an adjunct to the surgical therapy.
- Aggressive surgical treatment is necessary to remove the abscess capsule, extract the diseased teeth involved, and address the focal osteomyelitis.
- Further complications, such as retromasseteric and retrobulbar abscesses, extensive osteomyelitis of the mandible, and empyemas of the skull, should be addressed with specific surgical techniques and approaches.

INTRODUCTION

The most common complications of acquired dental disease in pet rabbits are periapical infections, osteomyelitis of the jaw, and facial abscesses.[1–4] They comprise a considerable portion of acquired and progressive dental disease syndrome (ADD). Facial abscesses appear as large masses, usually located at the ventrolateral aspect of the mandible or the lateral aspect of the maxilla.[1,2,4] Some rabbits may have an obvious unilateral exophthalmos.[4,5]

The abscess does not represent the primary disease, therefore thorough diagnosis (including standard or advanced diagnostic imaging) should be pursued to make a

Disclosure: The author has nothing to disclose.
[a] Clinica Veterinaria S. Siro, Via Lampugnano, 99, Milano 20151, Italy; [b] Clinica Veterinaria Gran Sasso, Via Donatello, 26, Milano 20134, Italy
* Clinica Veterinaria S. Siro, Via Lampugnano, 99, Milano 20151, Italy.
E-mail address: capellov@tin.it

proper prognosis, identify surgical candidates, and plan the most effective treatment using the most appropriate surgical approach.[5] Medical therapy alone is unrewarding, although it is an important adjunct to the dental and surgical treatment, which is usually a combined intraoral and extraoral approach. Numerous variations of surgical techniques have been reported, but the extraoral treatment is intended to address all 3 pathologic components: to remove the entire abscess including the capsule, extract the tooth fragments involved, and debride the osteomyelitic bone.[2]

Further complications, such as retromasseteric and retrobulbar abscesses, extensive osteomyelitis of the mandible, and empyemas of the skull, may require more invasive and challenging surgical techniques.[5]

ANATOMY AND SURGICAL ANATOMY

Detailed knowledge of the normal, topographic, and surgical anatomy of the teeth and skull with a focus on the mandible and maxilla is important for understanding classification of the abscesses and empyemas and their pathophysiology. It is also critical for interpretation of diagnostic imaging techniques, and to perform surgical techniques.

Mandible

The topographic anatomy outlines 3 portions of the rabbit mandible.[5,6]

1. The incisive part, in which the 2 mandibles are joined rostrally by the mandibular symphysis. This portion includes the reserve crown and apex of the incisor teeth.
2. The body of the mandible, which includes the reserve crowns and apices of the premolar and molar teeth.
3. The masseteric fossa and the branch of the mandible, with the condylar process. The area of the masseteric fossa is very thin, because it accommodates the masticatory muscles in a double groove both laterally and medially. The masseter muscle, positioned laterally, is composed of 2 main layers (the superficial and the deep part) and is of particular surgical interest.

Maxilla and Skull

The alveolar bulla is a unique bony structure specific to rabbits, which includes the reserve crowns and apices of the 4 distal (caudal) maxillary cheek teeth (the third premolar, and the 3 molar teeth, CT3–CT6).[1,5–7] Reserve crowns of the first 2 premolars (CT1 and CT2) are located more cranially and outside the alveolar bulla. The dome of the alveolar bulla is adjacent to the cranioventral aspect of the orbital fossa, and caudolaterally adjacent to the lacrimal bone.

The lacrimal bone separates the cranial aspect of the alveolar bulla from the nasolacrimal duct, and craniomedially from the maxillary recess.[8]

Rabbits have 3 main lacrimal glands (lacrimal gland proper, accessory lacrimal gland, and the gland of the nictitating membrane) of which 2 are divided into multiple lobes.[6,7,9,10] The lacrimal gland proper is located in the caudodorsal area of the orbit. The accessory lacrimal gland is much larger and divided in 3 lobes: the orbital, the retro-orbital, and the infraorbital. The gland associated with the nictitating membrane is commonly referred to as the harderian gland and is divided into the superficial gland and the deep gland.

The nasolacrimal duct runs from the orbital fossa to the nasal cavity. It curves medially, passes through the infratrochlear incisure and the foramen of the lacrimal bone, and enters the bony nasolacrimal canal medial to the maxillary bone, being adjacent to the maxillary recess.[8,11,12]

The conchae, also called nasal turbinates, are highly convoluted cartilaginous membranes covered by mucosa filling the nasal cavities. They outline empty spaces (meatuses) and blind cavities (recesses).[8] The paranasal cavities of rabbits are represented by the paired dorsal conchal, the sphenoidal, and the large double-chambered maxillary recesses.[8,13]

The tympanic bulla is well developed in rabbits. Unlike the alveolar bulla, it is a normally cavitary bone located caudally and laterally at the base of the skull.[6,14] The tympanic bulla communicates laterally with the ear canal entering the alveolar bulla through the external acoustic meatus (but separated by the tympanic membrane), and medially with the pharynx through the eustachian tubes.

CLINICAL PRESENTATION

Facial abscesses appear as large masses, usually located at the ventrolateral aspect of the mandible or the lateral aspect of the maxilla (**Fig. 1**).[1,2,4] Some rabbits show an obvious unilateral exophthalmos.[4,5] Abscesses are typically firm, cool, and nonpainful on palpation.[4] Early small masses are usually missed by the owners because of their location and the presence of fur, especially in long-haired rabbits. However, they may increase to considerable size. Occasionally, part of the overlying skin is necrotic, and a fistula or rupture may occur.

PATHOPHYSIOLOGY AND CLINICAL CONSIDERATIONS

Periapical infections represent the most common complications of acquired dental disease in pet rabbits.[1–4] They comprise a considerable portion of the ADD. Because of the specific anatomy of rabbit teeth, and the relationship between the reserve crown and the adjacent alveolar bones, periapical infections often quickly involve surrounding bone and adjacent soft tissues, producing abscesses and osteomyelitis.[2]

Facial abscesses can be single or multiple, or multilobed within a single entity. They are typically surrounded by a thick and well-developed capsule, and contain white, creamy pus.[1]

Part of the pathophysiology and clinical implications of periapical infections and abscessations in rabbits are not yet completely understood, especially compared with the same disease in non-herbivorous species. Rabbits are a prey species, therefore naturally prone to hide the symptoms of a disease, which may explain why clinicians frequently see advanced stages of acquired dental disease already complicated by periapical infection, abscessation of soft tissues, and osteomyelitis before early symptoms are detected by the owners.[2] However, this is not sufficient to explain the various clinical conditions displayed by different individuals.

The pain component seems to be extremely variable among patients, and it is not clear which component of this complex disease produces the most pain. Patients without concurrent severe intraoral dental disease and related complications, such as coronal spikes creating lesions to the tongue and other soft tissues, do not seem to be painful even at an advanced stage.[2] Those patients lacking intraoral lesions and evident malocclusion are usually able to eat normally. Pain can be elicited on palpation at the bony infection site, but is usually absent on palpation of the mass. With regard to further complications, such as extensive osteomyelitis or exophthalmos, the range of symptoms is even broader. Most patients with end-stage dental disease complicated by chronic, extensive osteomyelitis produce very large and multiple facial abscesses that can rapidly progress to weight loss and emaciation if aggressive treatment is not pursued. However, other animals with single or multiple foci of osteomyelitis and/or empyemas may live for several years in fair overall health.

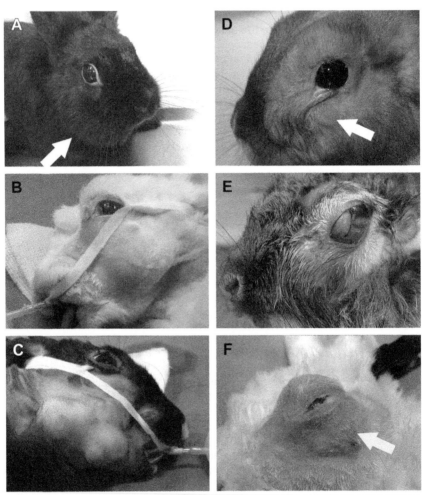

Fig. 1. Clinical presentation of odontogenic facial abscesses. (*A*) Mandibular swelling following periapical infection of the right CT1 (*arrow*). These masses are typically not as evident before shaving. Palpation is critical to evaluate size and position. (*B*) Swelling of the zygomatic area caused by periapical infection of the maxillary CT1 (*arrow*). Epiphora is present. (*C*) Retromasseteric abscess following periapical infection of mandibular CT4. (*D*) Exophthalmos caused by a retrobulbar abscess. Ocular complications such as conjunctivitis, keratitis, and prolapse of the third eyelid are present. (*E*) Multiple mandibular abscesses in a rabbit with extensive osteomyelitis of the mandible following advanced dental disease. (*F*) Parabulbar abscess affecting the accessory lacrimal gland (*arrow*). Exophthalmos is present, but the swelling is more lateral to the orbit compared with the deep retrobulbar abscesses. (*Courtesy of* Vittorio Capello, DVM, Milano, Italy; with permission.)

Three more aspects having important clinical and surgical impact are related to hyperthermia, local pathologic features, and anatomic features.[2] Periapical infections and osteomyelitis represent a true septic inflammatory process; however, they do not elicit hyperthermia. Also, the local infection tends to be encapsulated (while it progressively destroys the surrounding bone), and this likely plays a critical role in the antimicrobial treatment alone being ineffective.

Advanced ADD (coupled with specific anatomic features of the rabbit skull) may also elicit the formation of empyemas.[5] An empyema is defined as a collection or gathering of pus within a naturally existing anatomic cavity. It is different from an abscess because the latter is a collection of pus in a newly formed cavity surrounded by a capsule. The rabbit skull has at least 3 preformed anatomic cavities that may be involved following ADD and bacterial complications: the nasal cavity with its meatuses, the maxillary recess, and the tympanic bulla.[5,6] A fourth bony cavity of the skull can also be affected by empyema: the alveolar bulla. Although this preformed cavity is not normally empty, because it includes the reserve crowns of maxillary CT3 to CT6, in the case of dental disease or tooth extraction, it can be enlarged and/or partially empty, acting as a pathologic cavity (without a capsule) and therefore be affected by an empyema. Empyemas of the skull may or may not be concurrent with odontogenic abscesses, in cases of advanced ADD. Similarly, 1 or more empyemas can be subsequently or even concurrently present in the same patient, leading to the rabbit skull empyema syndrome.[5]

The anatomic features and the small size of the skull and teeth of rabbits make the dental and/or the surgical treatment difficult in general.[2] In select advanced or complicated cases, it can be very challenging. The presence of the orbit and the eye globe makes surgical access especially difficult when treating certain maxillary abscesses.

PROGNOSIS

The many complications leading to facial abscesses, empyemas, and possible further involvement of facial structures make discussion of prognosis in general virtually limitless and impossible. Prognosis should therefore be tailored to the specific patient and case.

The first critical element for a proper prognosis is diagnostic accuracy.[15] The diagnosis must be correct and as detailed as possible, specifically with regard to dental and bony involvement. Therefore, diagnostic imaging, both standard (radiography, oral endoscopy) and advanced (computed tomography, magnetic resonance) is of paramount importance.[6]

Several practical, even nonmedical, factors should be considered when formulating the prognosis. They include the management during the postoperative period, the owner's understanding and compliance (in particular with regard to advanced and chronic disease), and cost.[4]

Because of enhanced diagnostic imaging, improved surgical techniques, and overall treatment advances, prognosis is more favorable even for complex cases, than it was just a few years ago. Rabbits can show surprising improvements after facial surgery, and even chronic cases can be managed for years with a good quality of life.

MEDICAL TREATMENT VERSUS SURGICAL TREATMENT: THE ROLE OF OSTEOMYELITIS

Because periapical infection, osteomyelitis, and abscesses are bacterial infections, antimicrobial therapy is indicated.[2,4] The best therapeutic choices come from culture/sensitivity, keeping in mind that the core of the abscess is usually sterile and that a portion of the capsule should be submitted for sensitivity; that anaerobic organisms are frequently involved, therefore different culture techniques should be pursued; and taking into consideration the potential toxicity of many common antibiotics in rabbits.[1,2,4,16]

Bacteria isolated from complications of ADD in rabbits have been extensively published, as well as their sensitivity to antibiotics. According to one study, both anaerobic gram-negative[17] and aerobic gram-positive pathogenic bacteria have been identified,[17] including *Fusobacterium nucleatum*,[17,18] *Prevotella* spp, *Pseudomonas* spp, *Streptococcus* spp, and *Actinomyces israelii*.[17] Common rabbit pathogens such as *Pasteurella multocida* were not isolated.[17] Sensitivity testing indicated that 100% of pathogens were susceptible to clindamycin and chloramphenicol, 96% to penicillin, 86% to tetracycline, and 54% to metronidazole and ciprofloxacin.[17]

A more recent, large-scale, retrospective study performed on 81 rabbits[19] reported that the most common bacterial aerobic isolates were *Pseudomonas* spp, *Pasteurella* spp, *Streptococcus* spp, and *Staphylococcus* spp; and the most common bacterial anaerobic isolates were *Fusobacterium* spp, *Peptostreptococcus* spp, and *Bacteroides* spp. Antimicrobial susceptibilities varied depending on the bacterial isolate, with *Pseudomonas* spp most susceptible to amikacin and gentamicin; *Pasteurella* spp susceptible to trimethoprim-sulfamethoxazole, aminopenicillins, amikacin, and gentamicin; *Streptococcus* spp susceptible to most antibiotics evaluated; and *Staphylococcus* spp susceptible to amikacin, gentamicin, chloramphenicol, trimethoprim-sulfamethoxazole, and aminopenicillins.

Nevertheless, with the exception of some anecdotal reports, no clinical trials have shown that medical therapy alone is effective. This finding is easy to understand if the 3 distinguishing traits of periapical infections and abscesses of rabbits are considered: the presence of a capsule, the osteomyelitis, and the diseased tissue (soft, dental, and bony) acting as a sequestrum.[2,4] Treatment of all 3 pathologic conditions must be pursued and addressed in order to obtain long-term therapeutic success and prevent frequent reoccurrence. The combined dental and surgical treatment is designed to remove the entire capsule and the affected tooth/teeth, and to thoroughly debride the osteomyelitic bone.[1,2,4,20,21] This outcome ultimately facilitates the efficacy of antibiotic therapy.

In addition to antibiotic therapy, the key points of medical treatment should include supportive (fluids and nutrition with assisted feeding formulas for herbivores) and analgesic therapy when indicated.[1,4] Both should be tailored for every patient, because many of them have a normal appetite even in presence of an abscess, and may show little to no evidence of pain. Medical and supportive treatment is critical for debilitated patients before surgical intervention, and in general when gastrointestinal complications are present following reduced food intake. Rabbits typically resume eating well soon after a dental or extraoral surgical treatment, and show noticeable improvement even after an aggressive surgery, compared with the clinical conditions before the surgical treatment of the abscess.

PRINCIPLES OF SURGICAL TREATMENT

The surgical treatment of facial abscesses has been extensively reported in the literature. The goal of most surgical procedures, except wound packing, is to remove the entire abscess including the capsule, extract the tooth fragments involved, and debride the osteomyelitic bone.[1,2,4,20,21] Various surgical options have been reported beyond the simple (and usually ineffective) incision of the abscess followed by flushing of the purulent content. Minimal surgical debridement, without removing the capsule, has been reported as an effective treatment option in rabbits with dental abscesses.[22] This technique involves the incision of the abscess, minimal debridement and cleaning of the abscess cavity, and packing the cavity with strips of sterile gauze 3 to 5 mm in diameter and impregnated with antibiotics, most commonly ampicillin or clindamycin. The gauze is changed weekly until granulation tissue fills the cavity and the abscess is resolved. Rabbits are concurrently treated with systemic antibiotics such as trimethoprim and metronidazole, enrofloxacin and metronidazole, or azithromycin.

Placement of antibiotic-impregnated polymethyl methacrylate (AIPMMA) beads may be necessary in conjunction with gauze packing in cases with early osteomyelitis and bone defects. This procedure may be an option in rabbits with minimal osteomyelitis. However, efficacy in rabbits with extensive bony involvement is not known.

Excision of the abscess may be followed by either primary closure after packing of the surgical site with AIPMMA beads,[1,3,23–27] or marsupialization.[1,2,21] Additional local treatment of the open site has been reported in many different ways, including packing with calcium hydroxide,[1,28] honey,[3,29,30] sugar[31] solution, Intrasite Gel (Smith & Nephew, London, United Kingdom),[3] or bioactive ceramics.[20]

Marsupialization of the soft tissues around the area of the affected bone has been the author's treatment of choice for more than 15 years because this procedure is associated with a high percentage of successful outcomes and long-term postoperative follow-up, particularly in cases of deep or severe osteomyelitis, which are common. Ideally, the surgical technique should allow postoperative flushing and debridement of the surgical site, application of antiseptics or other products to promote healing, and constant direct monitoring of healing. This method is based on the same basic principles of orthopedics as when a grade III open fracture and an osteomyelitic site are present.[2] The fracture repair is usually performed with an external fixation technique and the infected site left partially exposed. Marsupialization of the surgical site allows these same surgical principles in cases of osteomyelitis of the skull.

Possible hospitalization for management of the wound during the first days, a longer postoperative period, frequent rechecks, temporarily unattractive cosmetic appearance, and significant owner commitment should be discussed with the owner before surgery.[2,4]

ABSCESSES AND OSTEOMYELITIS OF THE MANDIBLE
Periapical Infection of Mandibular Premolar Teeth and Focal Osteomyelitis of the Body of the Mandible

Following induction of general anesthesia, the patient is maintained via orotracheal intubation and positioned in dorsal or lateral recumbency, depending on the location of the abscess.[1,2,5,21] Adjunct local anesthesia can be achieved by performing local nerve blocks of the mental and the inferior alveolar nerves.[32,33] The surgical site is shaved, aseptically prepared, and draped. Transparent or semitransparent drapes are preferred because they facilitate visualization of the orientation of the head. A skin incision is made over the mass, preserving the capsule and taking care not to enter the underlying abscess. The subcutaneous tissue and muscle layers are bluntly dissected to expose the capsule of the abscess. The junction between the capsule and the underlying cortical bone is dissected with a scalpel blade or sharp scissors. The wall of the abscess is removed, including thin bone when cortical reaction is present. A small portion of the capsule is submitted for culture and sensitivity testing, because the purulent material inside is often sterile. The purulent exudate is removed using cotton-tipped applicators, and the bone cavity is thoroughly flushed using saline or 0.1% chlorhexidine solution. The infected or necrotic cortical bone is debrided using a bone curette. If present, fragments of the diseased teeth are meticulously worked with small dental elevators or contoured needles, to free the attachment to the bone, and extracted. In some cases, the tooth fragment is ankylotic to a small piece of necrotic alveolar bone. The bone cavity is again flushed as described earlier. Marsupialization of the soft tissues around the surgical site is performed using 3-0 or smaller nonabsorbable suture material (**Fig. 2**).

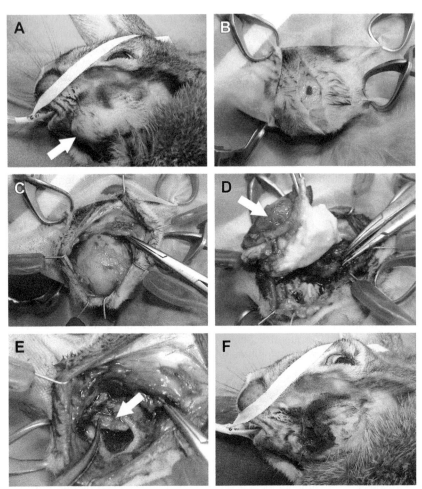

Fig. 2. Surgical treatment of a mandibular abscess with focal osteomyelitis of the body of the mandible. (*A*) The anesthetized patient is placed in lateral recumbency. (*B*) The area is surgically prepared with a plastic, semitransparent, nonadhesive drape. A skin incision is performed over the abscess, preserving the capsule. (*C*) The subcutaneous tissue and muscle layers are bluntly dissected and retracted to expose the capsule of the abscess. (*D*) The abscess is dissected free from the underlying bone. The thick purulent exudate is removed and a small portion of the capsule (*arrow*) is submitted for culture and sensitivity testing. (*E*) The bone cavity is thoroughly flushed with saline and debrided using a bone curette. The diseased tooth is worked with small dental elevators or contoured needles, and extracted (*arrow*). (*F*) Marsupialization and cosmetic appearance at the end of the surgical procedure. The surgical site has been filled with iodopovidone cream. (*Courtesy of* Vittorio Capello, DVM, Milano, Italy; with permission.)

Periapical Infection of Mandibular Incisor Teeth and Osteomyelitis of the Incisive Portion of the Mandible

The involvement of the incisive portion of the mandible is less common because both inspection and extraction of incisor teeth are easier than for premolar teeth.[1,5] The surgical technique is similar to the previous description; however, the approach is slightly more cranial. Because of anatomic proximity, periapical infection of a mandibular incisor tooth may be associated with periapical infection of the ipsilateral premolar, making the approach combined.

Extensive osteomyelitis involving the incisive portion (unilaterally or bilaterally) may create large and challenging ventral abscesses firmly attached to underlying bone. They require deep and thorough debridement (**Fig. 3**).

Periapical Infection of Distal Molar Teeth and Osteomyelitis of the Masseteric Fossa

The most distal (caudal) mandibular cheek teeth (CT4 and CT5) can be affected by abnormal elongation of the reserve crown and periapical infection. CT5 is rarely

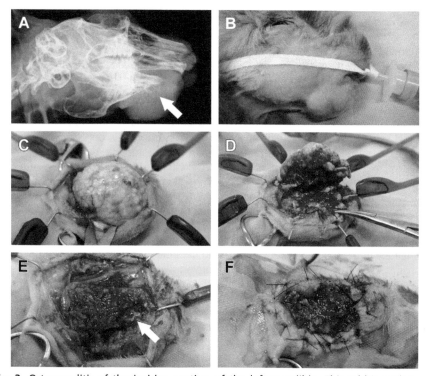

Fig. 3. Osteomyelitis of the incisive portion of the left mandible. This rabbit underwent extraction of the incisor teeth 6 months earlier because of malocclusion and periapical infection of the left mandibular incisor. (*A*) Right ventral to left dorsal 30° oblique projection of the head showing infection and periosteal reaction of the incisive part of the left mandible (*arrow*). The other oblique projection did not confirm involvement of the right incisive portion. (*B*) Clinical appearance of the abscess, which is well attached and non-mobile. (*C*) With the rabbit placed in dorsal recumbency, exposure of the abscess is performed after incision of the skin and blunt dissection of the overlying soft tissues. Note that this abscess does not have an overall capsule; it appears to be an aggregate of small abscesses. The bases of the abscesses are dissected free from the incisive part of the mandible. (*D*) When dissection is complete, removal exposes the underlying moth-eaten appearance of the osteomyelitic bone, including many pockets filled with pus. (*E*) The affected bone must be thoroughly debrided and flushed to the point of bleeding, for healing by second intention. Note the discolored portion of the bone, on the left side (*arrow*). (*F*) The overlying part of the skin is removed, and skin margins are simply apposed over the bone. (*Courtesy of* Vittorio Capello, DVM, Milano, Italy; with permission.)

primarily involved, but is frequently involved in conjunction with CT4.[1,4,5,34] Because of the normal curvature of their reserve crown, the apices of those teeth lie just cranial to the borderline between the body of the mandible and the masseteric fossa.[1] In the case of ADD of those teeth, caudal elongation of the reserve crown and perforation of the cortical bone occurs at the cranial aspect of the masseteric fossa. The periapical infection and the abscess develop beneath the masseter muscle, leading to a retro-masseteric abscess.

The surgical treatment of a retromasseteric abscess is more challenging than a standard mandibular abscess involving the 2 more cranial portions of the mandible. The basic principles are similar, but in this case the abscess capsule lies beneath the double-layered masseter muscle, and the underlying thin bone is often lytic and perforated. Deep and thorough debridement of the diseased bone is not always feasible, and the risk of intraoperative complications (ie, fracture of the mandible during the debridement of the osteomyelitic bone) is higher. However, possible fracture of the mandible during debridement of this area may not be associated with poor prognosis because the masseter muscle can provide enough stabilization to allow the fracture to heal during the postsurgical period. Computed tomography is highly recommended before this surgery to evaluate the position of the diseased reserve crown and the extent of the lysis, and to rule out possible fracture of the branch of the mandible. Intraoral extraction of CT4 and CT5 should be attempted before the extraoral surgical procedure. However, complete extraction is unrewarding in most cases because the clinical or the reserve crown can fracture.

The skin incision over the swelling is performed in an oblique dorsoventral and craniocaudal direction. After gentle retraction of the skin, the superficial zygomatic muscle is exposed. Blunt dissection and retraction allow exposure of the aponeurosis covering the superficial part of the masseter muscle. The aponeurosis is then dissected and retracted to expose the body of the superficial masseter. The superficial and the deep parts are then dissected and retracted as well, until the white capsule of the abscess is exposed. The retromasseteric capsule is usually thinner than in other abscesses. The capsule is opened and removed along with the abundant pus. The diseased tooth or its remainder is extracted, but thorough debridement of the surrounding bone may not be feasible because it may be very thin and lytic. The author has performed 2 different variations of this surgical approach. In the past, thorough cleaning and flushing of the infected area followed by suturing of the muscle layers has been unrewarding. Relapse of infection may carry a poor prognosis, because the masseter muscle can be affected by necrosis and gangrene. Although the function of the masseter muscle is affected after complete incision and marsupialization, chewing does not seem to be affected. Food is masticated primarily in a horizontal or lateral plane by only 1 side of the cheek teeth at a time; therefore, the rabbit is able to chew with the contralateral muscle/teeth functional unit. The author currently performs and recommends this technique (**Fig. 4**).

Extensive Osteomyelitis of the Mandible

Rabbits affected by advanced to end-stage dental disease may be presented with extensive osteomyelitis of the mandible.[2–5,34] Typically, 2 different stages of this condition can be encountered: (1) extensive osteomyelitis of the mandible involving the incisive portion and the body of the mandible, without involvement of the masseteric fossa; or (2) extensive osteomyelitis of the mandible involving the incisive portion, the body of the mandible, and the masseteric fossa.

In those cases in which most of the supporting bone is lytic and moth-eaten, usually with additional multilobed abscesses, thorough debridement is not sufficient to stop

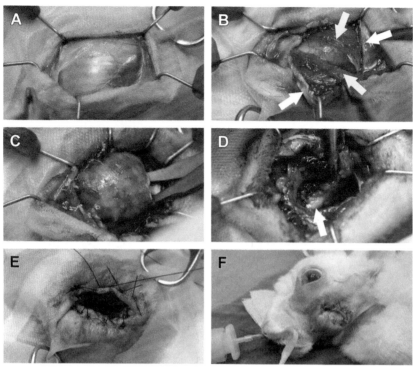

Fig. 4. Surgical treatment of a retromasseteric abscess, in the same case as shown in **Fig. 1**C. (A) Following incision and blunt dissection of the superficial zygomatic muscle, the aponeurosis of the masseter muscle is exposed using the Lone Star Retractor. (B) The aponeurosis and the superficial part of the masseter muscle are dissected and retracted (*white arrows*). The deep part of the muscle is dissected (*yellow arrows*) revealing the underlying capsule of the retromasseteric abscess. (C) The capsule of the abscess is dissected and removed, and the cavity cleaned and repeatedly flushed. (D) The affected tooth is extracted using an extraoral approach. Note the forceps grasping the elongated and L-shaped apex, and the clinical crown (*arrow*). (E) Marsupialization of the dissected layers is performed with nonabsorbable suture. (F) Cosmetic appearance at the end of the surgical procedure. The surgical site has been filled with HEALx Soother Plus cream. (*Courtesy of* Vittorio Capello, DVM, Milano, Italy; with permission.)

the infection. The involved portions of the mandible should be removed en-bloc. In the case of an intact, caudal masseteric portion of the mandible, unilateral rostral (partial) mandibulectomy can be a feasible treatment option (**Fig. 5**). In the second case, the surgical options can be subtotal unilateral mandibulectomy with transverse resection of the branch of the mandible, or total mandibulectomy. Computed tomography is mandatory to make a proper prognosis and a surgical plan. Mandibulectomy has also been reported in case of mandibular neoplasia.[35]

The steps of this challenging surgical procedure can be summarized as follows:

- The anesthetized rabbit is placed in lateral recumbency. During surgery, the dorsal recumbency also helps to expose the ventral and the medial aspects of the mandible.
- The area is shaved and surgically prepared as routine.
- A skin incision parallel to the long axis of the body of the mandible is performed.

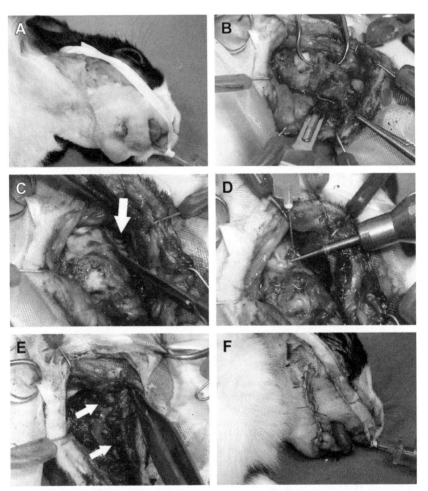

Fig. 5. Rostral right subtotal mandibulectomy. (*A*) The patient is placed in lateral recumbency for most of the surgical procedure, and converted to dorsal recumbency when necessary. Note the multiple abscesses following extensive osteomyelitis of the body and the incisive part of the mandible. (*B*) The deformed and moth-eaten osteomyelitic portion is widely exposed after dissection of overlying and surrounding soft tissues. The mandibular symphysis is separated using a scalpel blade. (*C*) Buccotomy is performed, dissecting the oral mucosa from the surrounding bone. Mandibular cheek teeth are visible (*arrow*). (*D*) The caudal aspect of the body of the mandible is dissected just cranial to the masseteric fossa with a ball-tipped bur mounted on a straight handpiece. After osteotomy of the mandible, the medial muscles are detached for the medial surface, and the diseased portion is removed. (*E*) The suture of the buccotomy is performed with absorbable 4-0 suture (*arrows*). The author prefers a simple interrupted pattern to reduce the risk of dehiscence. The overlying muscles and the skin are sutured as routine. (*F*) Cosmetic appearance at the end of the surgical procedure. (*Courtesy of Vittorio Capello, DVM, Milano, Italy; with permission.*)

- Overlying abscesses and infected tissue are dissected and removed.
- Exposure of the osteomyelitic bone of the body and the incisive part of the mandible, including exposure of the facial artery and vein, is made after blunt dissection of surrounding tissue, also on the ventral aspect of the mandible.

- The facial artery and vein are ligated.
- Separation of the mandibular symphysis is performed using a scalpel blade or a periosteal elevator. Attention must be paid to preventing fracture of the contra-lateral incisive portion of the mandible.
- Lateral buccotomy is performed by dissection of the buccal mucosa from the diseased portion of the mandible, to expose caudally all cheek teeth.
- Transverse osteotomy of the body of the mandible, just cranial to the border of the masseteric fossa, is performed with a small bur.
- The digastric muscle is gently dissected from the medial aspect of the mandible. At this stage, the diseased part of the mandible is free from surrounding tissues and is removed.
- The suture of the buccal mucosa is performed from the extraoral side in a simple interrupted pattern using a 3-0 absorbable suture (eg, polydioxanone).
- The overlying muscles are sutured over the defect.
- The skin incision is sutured as routine. Marsupialization or healing by second intention is not an option with this technique.

Techniques for subtotal and total mandibulectomy are even more challenging than for the rostral subtotal mandibulectomy, because detachment of the masticatory muscles medial to the masseteric fossa and ligation of the mandibular artery are required.

POSTOPERATIVE CARE

Marsupialization allows postoperative flushing and treatment, and facilitates healing by second intention, reducing the risk of recurrence. Despite exposure of part of the deep bone, marsupialization is well tolerated by rabbits, and typically they do not need an Elizabethan collar or assisted feeding, usually being able to eat on the day after surgery.[2,4] Antibiotics and analgesics are administered as routine. Occasionally, anorexic rabbits must be encouraged to eat. Commercially available assisted-feeding products for herbivores are excellent for this purpose. Adjunct fluid therapy is necessary in some patients.

The local postoperative treatment consists of flushing the surgical site twice daily with further gentle debridement, applying antiseptics or other products to promote healing (**Fig. 6**).[1,2,4] The author prefers the use of healing-promoting cream containing quaternary ammonium suspended in aloe vera distillate and monoglyceride of fatty acid (HEALx Soother Plus, Lake Worth, FL). This wound care can be performed with gentle restraint and without the use of sedation or anesthesia. Most owners, following adequate instructions from the veterinarian, are able to perform part of the local treatment at home.

When a layer of granulation tissue begins to cover the exposed bone, the marsupialization suture is removed from the marsupialization site (typically 4–7 days postoperatively). At 3 weeks after surgery, the bone cavity fills with new connective tissue and other deep soft tissues are usually healed. Approximately 4 weeks after surgery, the overlying skin is completely healed (**Fig. 7**). Slow healing by secondary intention is also critical in cases of simultaneous extraction of 1 or 2 cheek teeth, in which suturing the gingiva may be difficult to impossible. In these cases, the alveolus may become impacted with food if the extraoral access is completed with a suture. Marsupialization allows flushing of the intraoral-extraoral fistula through the cutaneous opening, until the fistula closes after healing of the gingiva and extraoral soft tissues, and the apposition of new bone.

Intensive postoperative care of the wound should be performed with special care after marsupialization of the masseter muscle. Temporary exposure of the masseteric fossa leads to formation of a fistula that eventually heals by second intention[5] (**Fig. 8**).

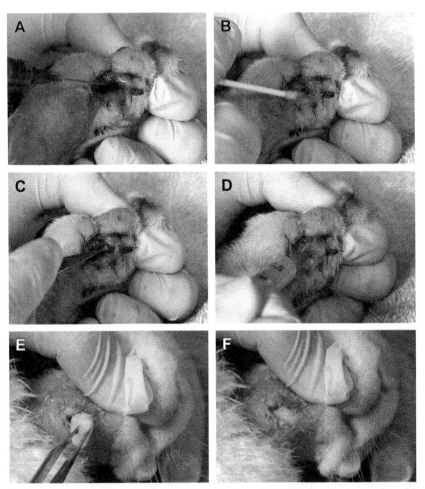

Fig. 6. Postoperative treatment after marsupialization of mandibular abscesses. The rabbit is manually restrained in dorsal (*A–D*) or lateral (*E, F*) recumbency without the use of sedation. (*A*) The surgical site and the bone cavity are flushed with saline or with 2% iodopovidone solution. (*B*) Debris and fibrin are removed using a cotton-tipped applicator. (*C*) Further gentle debridement is performed to stimulate bleeding of bone and soft tissues. (*D*) The area is flushed with saline, and healing-promoting cream is applied locally. (*E, F*) When an intraoral-extraoral fistula is present, a cotton ball wet with saline solution and impregnated with healing-promoting cream may be inserted to fill the bone cavity and prevent food debris from delaying the healing process. The cotton ball is replaced twice daily until the fistula closes. (*Courtesy of* Vittorio Capello, DVM, Milano, Italy; with permission.)

Edema of surrounding tissues is expected to some extent during the first days after rostral mandibulectomy. Complications include edema of tongue or dehiscence of the buccotomy suture.[5] The author has experienced several cases in which rabbits were able to eat soft food on their own within a few days after surgery.[5]

FOLLOW-UP

Periapical abscesses and osteomyelitis are associated with a high rate of reoccurrence. Short-term follow-up shows healing of the surgical site and the surrounding soft tissues (see **Figs. 7** and **8**; **Fig. 9**). Medium-term follow-up (8–12 weeks after surgery) includes radiographic evaluation to show remodeling and apposition of new bone in previous sites of osteomyelitis.[1]

ABSCESSES OF THE MAXILLA AND EMPYEMAS OF THE SKULL
Odontogenic Non-periapical Abscesses

Most odontogenic abscesses are periapical.[3,5] However, exceptions can be encountered. Coronal spikes of cheek teeth creating a wound on the buccal mucosa can develop into facial abscesses. Because of the typical pathophysiology of dental spikes, those abscesses are more likely to originate from maxillary cheek teeth. Extraction of the affected tooth is usually intraoral, and then complete surgical excision is performed as routine.

Periapical Infection of Maxillary Mesial (Rostral) Premolar Teeth (CT1 and CT2)

This abscess, typically presenting with a swelling of the rostral maxillary area and epiphora, is commonly named maxillary abscess or zygomatic abscess.[1,5] Pathophysiology and combined intraoral dental/extraoral surgical treatment are similar to the corresponding abscess of mandibular premolars (**Figs. 10** and **11**). Adjunct local anesthesia can be achieved by performing a local nerve block of the rostral infraorbital

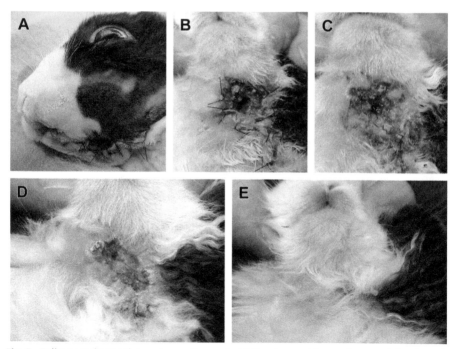

Fig. 7. Follow-up during the postoperative period following excision and marsupialization of a mandibular abscess. This patient was treated with local application of HEALx Soother Plus cream. (*A*) Marsupialization at the end of the surgical procedure. (*B*) Seven days after surgery, granulation tissue is present within the bone cavity and around the marsupialization site. (*C*) Ten days after surgery and suture removal, the stoma is reducing in size. (*D*) Eighteen days after surgery the surgical site is almost completely healed. (*E*) Four weeks after surgery, healing and fur regrowth are complete. (*Courtesy of* Vittorio Capello, DVM, Milano, Italy; with permission.)

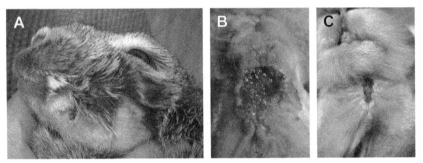

Fig. 8. Follow-up of surgical procedures shown in **Fig. 2** (*A*) and **Fig. 3** (*B*, *C*). (*A*) Follow-up 25 days after surgery. (*B*) Follow-up 17 days after surgical debridement shows formation of bleeding granulation tissue over the diseased bone. (*C*) Healing is almost complete 4 weeks after surgery. (*Courtesy of* Vittorio Capello, DVM, Milano, Italy; with permission.)

nerve.[32,33] Because of the different anatomy compared with the mandible, focal osteomyelitis may not be present. However, in advanced cases, it may also be complicated by dacryocystitis or by involvement of the maxillary recess.[3,5] Exophthalmos is usually absent.

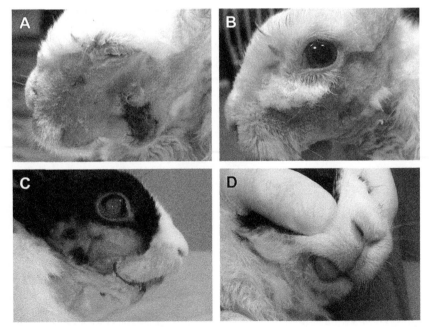

Fig. 9. Follow-up during the postoperative period of surgical procedures shown in **Fig. 4** (*A*, *B*) and **Fig. 5** (*C*, *D*). (*A*) Follow-up after 6 days and (*B*) 23 days. Further improvement progressed to complete healing and fur regrowth. (*C*) Follow-up after 10 days and removal of the skin suture. (*D*) Follow-up 35 days after rostral mandibulectomy. Mild protrusion of the tongue on the right side is caused by the lack of mandibular support, and did not affect the rabbit's eating and drinking capabilities. (*Courtesy of* Vittorio Capello, DVM, Milano, Italy; with permission.)

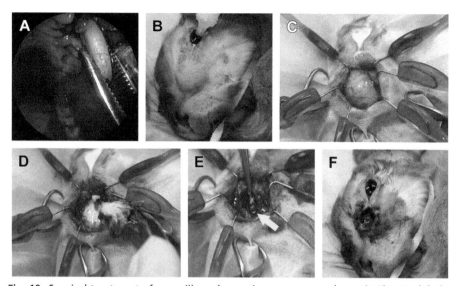

Fig. 10. Surgical treatment of a maxillary abscess, in same case as shown in **Fig. 1**D. (*A*) The diseased left CT1 has been completely extracted via an intraoral approach. (*B*) The rabbit is placed in lateral recumbency. The cornea is protected with ophthalmic lubricant before draping. (*C*) The abscess is exposed after incision of the skin, blunt dissection, and retraction of the surrounding soft tissues. (*D*) The capsule is dissected and removed, and the abscess is cleaned of pus. (*E*) The diseased area over the abnormal perforated surface of the maxillary bone is debrided. The fistula created by the periapical infection (*arrow*) is checked and cleaned using a Williger bone curette. (*F*) Marsupialization and cosmetic appearance at the end of the surgical procedure. (*Courtesy of* Vittorio Capello, DVM, Milano, Italy; with permission.)

Bacterial Dacryocystitis

Bacterial infection of the nasolacrimal duct is usually odontogenic because secondary involvement (subocclusion or obstruction) follows overgrowth of reserve crown and apical deformity of the ipsilateral primary incisor tooth (more commonly), or of the rostral premolar teeth (less commonly).[1,5] It may or may not be associated with a periapical infection of those teeth, but even in the latter case it may develop into a facial abscess. Presentation is similar to the maxillary or zygomatic abscesses mentioned earlier.

Surgical treatment is designed for debridement and marsupialization, but abscess of the distal portion of the nasolacrimal duct involving the naris or the upper lip might require cosmetic surgery (see **Figs. 11** and **16**).

Periapical infection of molar teeth

Bacterial involvement of several periocular structures (maxillary teeth, alveolar bulla, lacrimal glands), single or combined, can lead to the clinical sign of exophthalmos.[1,2,4,5] Those causes have all been generally reported as retrobulbar abscess. Even if this pathologic condition is common in pet rabbits as a complication of dental disease, a proper classification is useful not only because exophthalmos may show slightly different traits but because several different surgical approaches can be pursued, depending on the type of abscess. Advanced cases presenting late in the course of the disease result in loss of the eye globe and necessitate enucleation. This procedure allows dorsal surgical access to the alveolar bulla but also risks

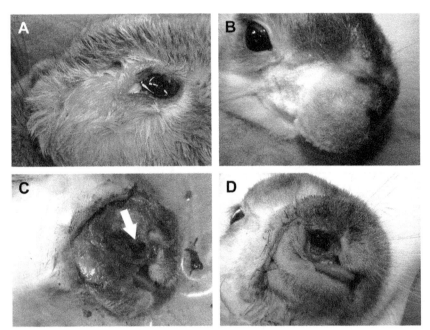

Fig. 11. (*A*) Odontogenic dacryocystitis and abscessation of the nasolacrimal duct. (*B*) Abscess involving the distal tract of nasolacrimal duct and the surrounding upper lip. This rabbit previously underwent extraction of incisor teeth. (*C*) Intraoperative stage after surgical excision, and core of the abscess (*arrow*). (*D*) A combined suture and marsupialization technique was performed to improve the cosmetic appearance at the end of the surgical procedure. (*Courtesy of* Vittorio Capello, DVM, Milano, Italy; with permission.)

exposure of the optic nerve and the optic foramen, and in addition is not ideal for cosmetic reasons. Detailed diagnosis and appropriate surgical access can allow resolution, saving the affected eye.

Deformity and Empyema of the Alveolar Bulla

The alveolar bulla is a virtual cavity, because it is a preformed bony structure including the reserve crowns of maxillary CT3 to CT6.[2,4,5,7] In cases of elongation of reserve crowns, widened interproximal space, and apical deformity, the dome of the alveolar bulla can enlarge. In other cases, a small cavity can form within the alveolar bulla, in particular when a single cheek tooth has been previously extracted. It may partially fill with food debris and an empyema may follow. The result of this pathologic change is mild to intermediate exophthalmos, but a retrobulbar abscess is not present at this stage. Dedicated oblique projections, or advanced diagnostic imaging (computed tomography, MRI) are needed for differential diagnosis (**Fig. 12**). At least 3 different options can be considered to prevent formation of a retrobulbar abscess:

1. Flush the empyema intraorally. This option may not be practical, because repeated anesthesia is necessary and the empyema may not be resolved.
2. Extract all the cheek teeth and allow the inner surface of the alveolar bulla to heal by second intention.
3. Perform a lateral maxillotomy to access the alveolar bulla and fill the defect with AIPMMA beads.

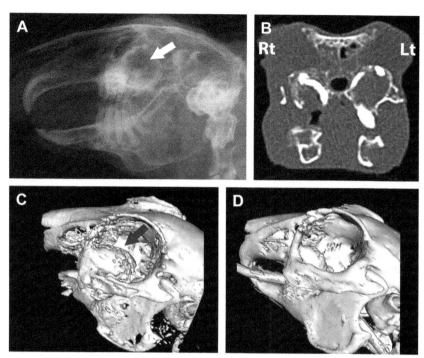

Fig. 12. Deformity and empyema of the alveolar bulla. (*A*) Radiography of the head, slight oblique view in the rostrocaudal direction, showing deformity of the alveolar bulla (*arrow*). This rabbit previously underwent extraction of the maxillary CT4. Note the gap between CT3 and CT5. This deformity, uncomplicated by a retrobulbar abscess, may or may not elicit mild exophthalmos. (*B*) Computed tomography of the head, axial view, in a different rabbit with advanced dental disease. Bilateral deformity and empyema of the alveolar bullae are visible, more evident on the left side. (*C*) Three-dimensional surface rendering of the same patient as in (*B*), emphasizing the enlargement and deformity of the left alveolar bulla (*arrow*). (*D*) Appearance of the normal alveolar bulla, for comparison. (*Courtesy of* Vittorio Capello, DVM, Milano, Italy; with permission.)

The steps of this surgical procedure can be summarized as follows:

- With the patient in lateral recumbency, shaved, and surgically prepared as routine, a skin incision is made followed by blunt dissection of the underlying soft tissues to expose the cranial third of the zygomatic arch.
- The insertion of the masseter muscle is dissected free from the cranial part of the zygomatic arch.
- Partial ostectomy of the cranial portion of the zygomatic arch is performed using a bur, the goal being to expose the lateral aspect of the maxillary bone and the alveolar bulla.
- The lateral osteotomy of the alveolar bulla is performed with the tip of a small bur.
- The cavitary alveolar bulla is flushed and cleaned. Small AIPMMA beads can then be introduced to fill the defect.
- The suture of the overlying muscular and cutaneous tissues is performed as routine. Marsupialization of this surgical site is not a practical option because the small linear opening is prone to closure.

However, in the author's experience, conservative treatment and monitoring of the deformity and/or empyema of the alveolar bulla can be an alternative option to the surgical approach, being prepared to address the retrobulbar abscess should the empyema progress to a further stage.

Retrobulbar Abscess

A retrobulbar abscess originates from periapical infection and perforation of the dome of the alveolar bulla.[2,4,5,34] The abscess can be as large as the eye globe, and the position is exactly at the bottom of the orbital fossa, therefore ventromedial to the eye globe. Pressure usually elicits an obvious and severe exophthalmos that can rapidly evolve to panophthalmitis, with possible damage to the optic nerve. Radiography including several oblique views is diagnostic regarding the involvement of teeth and the alveolar bulla, but provides little information about the size and position of the abscess. Computed tomography and/or MRI are important for diagnosis and surgical planning. Computed tomography allows detection of the cheek teeth involved and more details about the alveolar bulla, whereas MRI provides the precise size and position of the retrobulbar abscess, including the optic nerve. Ideally they should be performed in combination; however, when only 1 is an option, MRI is more specific.

A combined intraoral and extraoral surgical approach is needed for a salvage procedure of the eye. Extraction of the affected cheek teeth (sometimes involving the entire maxillary arcade) is mandatory. Following extraction, the access to the retrobulbar abscess may[36,37] or may not be feasible, because the top of the alveolar bulla may not be reached through the intraoral approach. When the retrobulbar abscess is very large and dislocation of the eye globe is very dorsal, a lateral approach slightly dorsal to the lateral margin of the orbital fossa can be attempted (**Fig. 13**), as described later for the lateral parabulbar abscess. Depending on periorbital edema, immediate reposition of the eye globe may or may not be possible. Even in the latter case, postoperative antiinflammatory treatment can be effective to improve the exophthalmos.

Parabulbar Abscesses

Periapical infection with subsequent involvement of the accessory lacrimal gland leads to a lateral (or infraorbital) parabulbar abscess.[5] Because exophthalmos is evident and severe, these abscesses have usually been reported as retrobulbar. However, the difference is critical because the abscess is not located at the bottom of the orbital fossa, and surgical access can be successfully achieved with a ventrolateral approach to the exophthalmic eye globe. Repositioning of the eye globe is accomplished after removal of the pus, debridement, and thorough flushing. Marsupialization of this surgical site is not a practical option because the small linear opening is prone to closure. However, part of the incision may be left open, allowing flushing for a few days postoperatively (**Fig. 14**; see **Fig. 16**).

Periapical infection with subsequent involvement of the main lacrimal gland leads to a caudal parabulbar abscess. Surgical debridement is straightforward, with a caudal approach to the eye globe.

Empyema of the Maxillary Recess

An empyema of the alveolar bulla (or a periapical infection of premolar teeth, with or without concurrent involvement of the nasolacrimal duct) can spread to the adjacent maxillary recess.[5,7,8] Depending on individual patients and further development, clinical signs can be more consistent with an ipsilateral rhinitis, or with a swelling of the infraorbital area. The empyema of the maxillary recess may require a double or triple combined surgical access: intraoral extraction of diseased cheek teeth, an extraoral

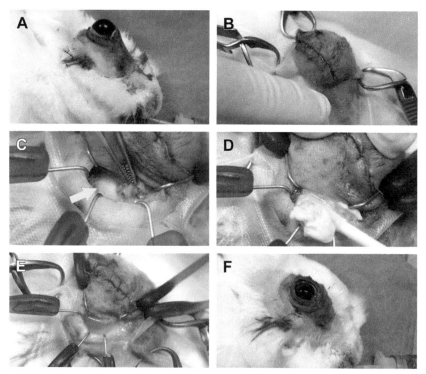

Fig. 13. Lateral approach to a retrobulbar abscess. (*A*) Exophthalmos, conjunctivitis, and episcleritis following a large retrobulbar abscess. (*B*) The cornea is protected beneath the surgical drape with a temporary suture of the eyelid. The surgeon's finger palpates the lateral dome of the abscess. (*C*) A skin incision has been performed just below the exophthalmic eye globe and just above the zygomatic arch. The normal intact accessory lacrimal gland (*arrow*) is exposed after blunt dissection and retraction. (*D*) Beneath the gland, incision of the abscess is performed, and a large amount of pus is removed using cotton-tipped applicators. The abscess cavity is thoroughly flushed. (*E*) After the abscess cavity is emptied, the exophthalmos is reduced. (*F*) Marsupialization of this surgical access is not a practical option because the small linear opening is prone to closure, so the skin incision is partially closed. In this case, the eye was repositioned at the end of the surgery. (*Courtesy of* Vittorio Capello, DVM, Milano, Italy; with permission.)

approach through the perforated area of the maxilla (pararhinotomy) (**Figs. 15** and **16**), and/or a dorsal approach via a rhinostomy. The pararhinotomy and rhinotomy techniques have been reported in the literature.[8]

Empyema of the Nasal Cavity and Odontogenic Septic Rhinitis

Chronic septic rhinitis secondary to severe or end-stage dental disease can be a sequela of empyema of the alveolar bulla and/or empyema of the maxillary recess.[5,8] Long-term medical treatment is usually unrewarding, but it can provide temporary and palliative improvement. The rhinotomy approach followed by temporary or permanent rhinostomy has been reported in the literature.[8,38,39]

Empyema of the Tympanic Bulla/Otitis Media

Empyemas of the alveolar bulla, maxillary recess, and/or nasal cavities can spread the infection to the tympanic bulla through the pharynx and the eustachian tubes.[5,14,34]

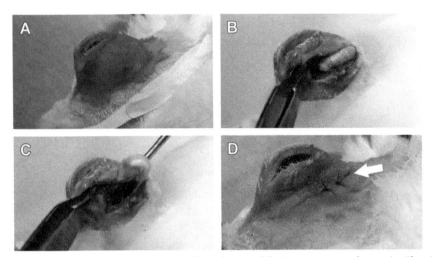

Fig. 14. Lateral approach to a parabulbar abscess. (*A*) Same case as shown in **Fig. 1F**, scrubbed with 5% diluted iodopovidone solution. (*B*) After the skin incision, the abscessed accessory lacrimal gland is entered. In this case, a thick capsule was not present. (*C*) The pus is removed using cotton-tipped applicators and a Williger bone curette. (*D*) The eye globe is repositioned, and the suture is closed leaving a small part open (*arrow*) for postoperative flushing. (*Courtesy of* Vittorio Capello, DVM, Milano, Italy; with permission.)

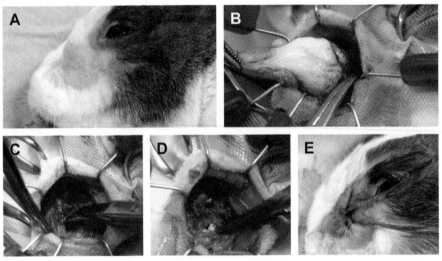

Fig. 15. Surgical excision of a maxillary abscess and pararhinotomy for treatment of the empyema of the maxillary recess. (*A*) In this rabbit showing an ordinary maxillary abscess, computed tomography showed the underlying empyema of the maxillary recess. (*B*) The abscess is exposed and excised as routine. (*C*) A small fenestration, which represents a pararhinotomy, is created over the abnormal diseased portion of the perforated surface of the maxillary bone. The thin bone can be entered using the tip of sharp scissors. (*D*) The maxillary recess is emptied by flushing, or using a Williger bone curette. (*E*) Marsupialization of the surgical site allows postoperative flushing of the recess until healing of the overlying soft tissues. (*Courtesy of* Vittorio Capello, DVM, Milano, Italy; with permission.)

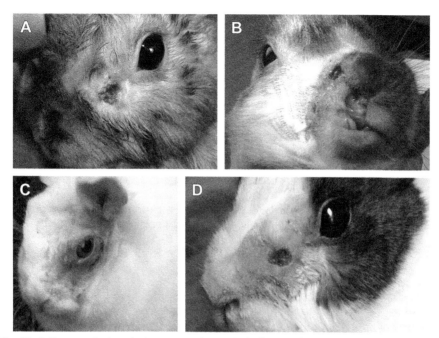

Fig. 16. Follow-up during the postoperative period of surgical procedures shown in **Fig. 10** (*A*), **Fig. 11** (*B*), **Fig. 14** (*C*) and **Fig. 15** (*D*). Further improvement progressed to complete healing and fur regrowth. (*Courtesy of* Vittorio Capello, DVM, Milano, Italy; with permission.)

Empyema of the tympanic bulla may or may not be clinically evident as otitis media with neurologic signs and symptoms, and these patients may or may not be affected by concurrent otitis externa. The surgical approaches and techniques for treatment of the tympanic bulla have been extensively reported.[40–44]

SUMMARY

Facial abscesses associated with periapical infections and osteomyelitis of the jaw are frequent in pet rabbits affected by acquired dental disease. Retromasseteric and retrobulbar abscesses, extensive osteomyelitis of the mandible, and empyemas of the skull represent possible further complications. Definitive therapy requires surgical treatment via numerous extraoral and facial approaches, depending on the exact diagnosis, position, and anatomic structures involved.

REFERENCES

1. Capello V, Gracis M, Lennox AM. Rabbit and rodent dentistry handbook. Lake Worth (FL): Zoological Education Network; 2005.

2. Capello V. Clinical technique: treatment of periapical infections in pet rabbits and rodents. J Exot Pet Med 2008;17:124–31.

3. Harcourt-Brown F, Chitty J. Facial abscesses. In: Harcourt-Brown F, Chitty J, editors. Manual of rabbit surgery, dentistry and imaging. 1st edition. Quedgeley (Gloucester): British Small Animal Veterinary Association; 2013. p. 395–422, 29.

4. Capello V, Lennox AM. Small mammal dentistry. In: Quesenberry KE, Carpenter JW, editors. Ferrets, rabbits and rodents clinical medicine and surgery. 3rd edition. St Louis (MO): Elsevier Saunders; 2012. p. 452–71.

5. Capello V. Novel diagnostics and surgical techniques for treatment of difficult facial abscesses in pet rabbits. Proceedings of the North Am Vet Conference. Orlando (FL): 2011. p. 1685–89.

6. Popesko P, Rjtovà V, Horàk J. A colour atlas of anatomy of small laboratory animals. Vol. I: rabbit, guinea pig. Vol. II: rat, mouse, hamster. London: Wolfe Publishing; 1992.

7. Capello V. Surgical treatment of prolapse of the deep lacrimal gland in a pet rabbit. J Exot Pet Med 2016;25(1):44–51.

8. Capello V. Rhinostomy as surgical treatment of odontogenic rhinitis in three pet rabbits. J Exot Pet Med 2014;23(2):172–87.

9. Janssens G, Simoens P, Muylle S, et al. Bilateral prolapse of the deep gland of the third eyelid in a rabbit: Diagnosis and treatment. Lab Anim Sci 1999;49(1):105–9.

10. Harcourt-Brown FM. Ophthalmic diseases. In: Harcourt-Brown FM, editor. Textbook of rabbit medicine. Oxford (United Kingdom): Butterworth-Heinemann; 2002. p. 292–306.

11. Burling K, Murphy CJ, Da Silva Curiel J, et al. Anatomy of the rabbit nasolacrimal duct and its clinical implications. Prog Vet Comp Ophthalmol 1991;1:33–40.

12. van der Woerdt A. Ophthalmologic diseases in small pet mammals. In: Quesenberry KE, Carpenter JW, editors. Ferrets, rabbits and rodents: clinical medicine and surgery. 2nd edition. St Louis (MO): Saunders, imprint of Elsevier; 2004. p. 421–8.

13. Casteleyn C, Cornillie P, Hermens A, et al. Topography of the rabbit paranasal sinuses as a prerequisite to model human sinusitis. Rhinology 2010;48:300–4.

14. Capello V, Mancinelli E, Lennox A. Anatomy of the ear. In: Kling M, editor. Ear surgery of pet rabbits. Milano (Italy): ebooksdynamic.vet; 2015. p. 1–6.

15. Capello V, Cauduro A. Comparison of diagnostic consistency and diagnostic accuracy between survey radiography and computed tomography of the skull in 30 rabbits with dental disease. J Exot Pet Med 2016;25(2):115–27.

16. Rosenthal KL. Therapeutic contraindications in exotic pets. Sem Avian Exot Pet Med 2004;13:44–8.

17. Tyrrel KL, Citron DM, Jenkins JR, et al. Periodontal bacteria in rabbit mandibular and maxillary abscesses. J Clin Microbiol 2002;40:1044–7.

18. Ward GS, Crumrine MH, Mattloch JR. Inflammatory exostosis and abscessation associated with *Fusobacterium nucleatum* in a rabbit. Lab Anim Sci 1981;31:280–1.

19. Gardhouse S, Sanchez-Migallon Guzman D et al. Microbiology and antimicrobial susceptibilities of odontogenic abscesses in domestic rabbits. Proceedings of the ExoticsCon. San Antonio (TX): 2015. p. 357.

20. Aiken SA. Small mammal dentistry (part II). In: Quesenberry KE, Carpenter JW, editors. Ferrets, rabbits and rodents: clinical medicine and surgery. 2nd ed. St Louis (MO): Saunders, Imprint of Elsevier; 2004. p. 379–82.

21. Capello V. Extraction of cheek teeth and surgical treatment of periodontal abscessations in pet rabbits with acquired dental disease. Exotic DVM 2004;6:31–8.

22. Taylor WM, Beaufrère H, Mans C, et al. Long-term outcome of treatment of dental abscesses with a wound packing technique in pet rabbits: 13 cases (1998-2007). J Am Vet Med Assoc 2010;237:1444–9.

23. Bennet RA. Management of abscesses of the head in rabbits. Proceedings. North Am Vet Conf. Orlando, FL, 1999. p. 822–23. .

24. Divers SJ. Mandibular abscess treatment using antibiotic-impregnated beads. Exotic DVM 2000;2:15–8.
25. Ethell MT, Bennet RA, Brown MP, et al. In vitro elution of gentamicin, amikacin, and ceftiofur from polymethylmethacrylate and hydroxyapatite cement. Vet Surg 2000;29:375–82.
26. Hernandez-Divers SJ. Molar disease and abscesses in rabbits. Exot DVM 2001; 3:65–9.
27. Weisman DL, Olmstead ML, Kowalski JJ. In vitro evaluation of antibiotic elution from polymethylmethacrylate (PMMA) and mechanical assessment of antibiotic-PMMA composites. Vet Surg 2000;29:245–51.
28. Remeeus PG, Verbeek M. The use of calcium hydroxide in the treatment of abscesses in the cheek of the rabbit resulting from a dental periapical disorder. J Vet Dent 1995;12:19–22.
29. Harcourt-Brown FM. Honey to treat rabbit abscesses. Exotic DVM 2002;3:13–4.
30. Mathews KA, Binnington AG. Wound management using honey. Comp Cont Ed 2002;24:53–60.
31. Mathews KA, Binnington AG. Wound management using sugar. Comp Cont Ed 2002;24:41–50.
32. Lichtenberger M, Ko J. Anesthesia and analgesia for small mammals and birds. Vet Clin North Am Exot Anim Pract 2007;10:293–315.
33. Lennox AM. Small exotic mammal dentistry-anesthetic considerations. J Exot Pet Med 2008;17:102–6.
34. Capello V. Management of difficult periapical infections in rabbits. Proceedings Annu Conf Assoc Exot Mam Vet. Providence, RI, 2007. p. 91–7.
35. Miwa Y. Mandibulectomy for treatment of oral tumors (cementoma and chondrosarcoma) in two rabbits. Exotic DVM 2006;8:18–22.
36. Martinez-Jimenez D, Hernandez-Divers SJ, Dietrich U, et al. Endosurgical treatment of a retrobulbar abscess in a rabbit. J Am Vet Med Assoc 2007;230:868–72.
37. Ward ML. Diagnosis and management of a retrobulbar abscess of periapical origin in a domestic rabbit. Vet Clin North Am Exot Anim Pract 2006;9:657–65.
38. Lennox AM. Respiratory disease and pasteurellosis. In: Quesenberry KE, Carpenter JW, editors. Ferrets, rabbits and rodents clinical medicine and surgery. 3rd edition. St Louis (MO): Elsevier Saunders; 2012. p. 205–16.
39. Lennox A. Rhinotomy and rhinostomy for surgical treatment of chronic rhinitis in two rabbits. J Exot Pet Med 2013;22(4):383–92.
40. Capello V. Surgical treatment of otitis externa and media in pet rabbits. Exotic DVM 2004;6(3):21–6.
41. Chow EP, Bennett RA, Dustin L. Ventral bulla osteotomy for treatment of otitis media in a rabbit. J Exot Pet Med 2009;18(4):299–305.
42. Chow EP. Surgical management of rabbit ear disease. J Exot Pet Med 2011;20(3): 182–7.
43. Capello V, Lennox AM. Diagnosis and surgical treatment of otitis externa, otitis media, and empyema of the tympanic bulla in the pet rabbit. Proc AEMV Conf. Oakland, CA, 2012. p. 110–11.
44. Eatwell K, Mancinelli E, Hedley J, et al. Partial ear canal ablation and lateral bulla osteotomy in rabbits. J Small Anim Pract 2013;54:325–30.

Anatomy and Disorders of the Oral Cavity of Guinea Pigs

Loic Legendre, DVM, FAVD, Diplomate AVDC, EVDC

KEYWORDS

- Guinea pig • Oral cavity • Dentistry • Malocclusion • Dental abscesses

KEY POINTS

- Guinea pigs are -*chomorpha* rodents; their incisors and cheek teeth grow continuously (elodont) and are long crowned (hypsodont).
- The cheek teeth of guinea pigs are different than those of other -*chomorpha* rodents, having curved reserve crowns and oblique occlusal planes.
- Clinical signs and symptoms of oral disorders are not pathognomonic; they include vague symptoms such as reduced food intake, weight loss, and difficulty eating.
- The inspection of the oral cavity, with or without anesthesia, is not completely diagnostic for dental disease; additional diagnostic imaging is essential for diagnosis, prognosis, and treatment.
- The most common dental disease is coronal elongation of cheek teeth which is usually due to inappropriate nutrition. Secondary malocclusion of incisor teeth typically accompanies cheek teeth disease as well as other complications.

INTRODUCTION

Acquired dental disease represents the most common oral disorder of guinea pigs, as in other small mammals with continuously growing teeth, such as the rabbit, chinchilla, and other cavy-like rodents. Several anatomic features characteristic of this species, such as curved cheek teeth and an associated oblique occlusal plane, make diagnosis and treatment more challenging than in rabbits. Most patients are presented with nonspecific clinical signs and symptoms, such as reduced activity, weight loss, reduced food intake, and difficult chewing and/or swallowing. The physical examination must be followed by radiologic diagnosis with standard radiography and/or computed tomography (CT), and thorough inspection under general anesthesia. Several complications may follow early and intermediate stages of malocclusion,

The author has nothing to disclose.
West Coast Veterinary Dental Services Ltd, 1350 Kootenay Street, Vancouver, British Columbia V5K 4R1, Canada
E-mail address: ledentiste58@gmail.com

Vet Clin Exot Anim 19 (2016) 825–842
http://dx.doi.org/10.1016/j.cvex.2016.04.006

including periodontal disease, subluxation of the temporomandibular joint, periapical infection, and abscessation.

The dental treatment is aimed to restore the proper length and shape of both the incisor and the cheek teeth, associated with medical and supportive treatment. Abscesses should be surgically addressed by complete excision.

ANATOMY AND PHYSIOLOGY OF DENTITION

The guinea pig belongs to the order *Rodentia*, which includes more than 2000 species of placental mammals.[1–3] The anatomic feature typical of members of this order is that they possess large, continuously growing incisor teeth that are used for gnawing.[2,4–6] Rodents are monophyodont[2,5] (having a single set of teeth, of which none are replaced at a later stage of growth)[5] and *simplicidentata*, possessing a single pair of maxillary incisor teeth for each arcade (ie, unlike lagomorphs, which have a single maxillary incisor tooth for each quadrant).[2,5–7] Guinea pigs belong to the suborder *Caviomorpha* (or *Hystrychomorpha*).[2] The species in this group are more or less strict herbivores and (unlike other suborders of rodents) have a full set of continuously growing teeth.[2,5,8] This group includes selected other species kept as pets, such as the chinchilla, degu, and Patagonian cavy.[2]

Classifications of suborders of rodents depend on the position and function of the superficial and deep portion of the masseter muscle.[2] They have an enlarged deep masseter muscle and a prominent, anteriorly displaced, infraorbital zygomaticomandibularis section of the masseter.[9] Unlike rabbits, guinea pigs lack the masseteric fossa of the mandible. The masseter muscle covers the lateral surface of the body of the mandible and the angular process.[10]

The dental formula is 2(I 1/1, C 0/0, P 1/1, M 3/3) for a total of 20 teeth (**Fig. 1**). The premolars and molars are anatomically similar and are commonly described as cheek teeth.[2] Guinea pig teeth are aradicular (open-rooted, with germinal cells producing dental tissue at their apical end), elodont (continuously growing and erupting), and hypsodont (long crowned).[2,5,6] The clinical crown (the portion above the gingiva) is short, whereas the reserve crown (the portion below the gingiva and within the alveolous) is long. Guinea pigs are anisognathic with the mandible wider than the maxilla.[2] The cheek teeth of guinea pigs are different than cheek teeth of other hystrocomorph rodent species because their reserve crown is curved, having a buccal convexity for mandibular cheek teeth, and a palatal convexity for maxillary cheek teeth.[2,5] The result is their occlusal plane is an approximate 30° angle from dorsobuccal to ventrolingual.[2]

Guinea pigs are grazers and use their incisor teeth to cut grass and hay. The incisors are covered by white enamel, which is thicker on the labial surface, thinning out on mesial and distal aspects toward the lingual surface, where it is absent. This enamel distribution is most likely responsible for their chisel-shaped occlusal plane. The maxillary incisors grow 1.9 mm per week, whereas the mandibular incisors grow 2.4 mm per week.[6,11]

The temporomandibular joint allows both side-to-side and rostrocaudal movements. This combined movement has a propalineal (lateral and rostrocaudal, ie, diagonal) chewing action.[2]

PATHOPHYSIOLOGY OF DENTAL DISEASE

Most dental problems are related to inappropriate nutrition. When elodont teeth do not wear sufficiently to match the rate of eruption, the clinical crowns will elongate.[12–14] Elongated clinical crowns result in the mouth being forced open, and the increased slope of the occlusal plane increases the leverage effect. When the strength of the

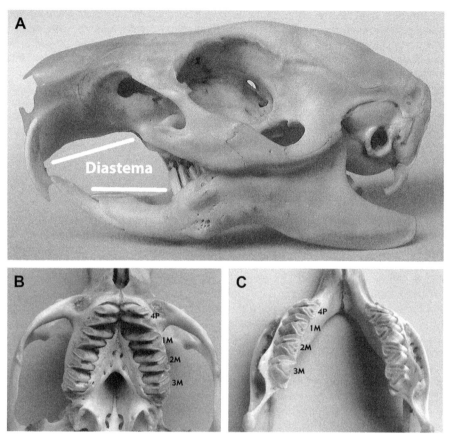

Fig. 1. Dentition of the guinea pig (*Cavia porcellus*) shown on a bony specimen. (*A*) Lateral view of the skull. (*B*) Ventrodorsal view of the maxilla and (*C*) dorsoventral view of the mandible displaying the cheek teeth. The standard system numbering the premolars as P4 is used in this figure. (*Courtesy of* Vittorio Capello, DVM, Milano, Italy; with permission.)

masticatory muscles prevents further elongation of the clinical crowns, the reserve crowns and the apices start to elongate. Apical elongation deforms the cortical bone and can end in perforation. When the strength weakens, coronal elongation of cheek teeth (especially when not symmetric) not only forces the mouth open but also may force the mandible in a lateral position, causing further (usually unilateral) subluxation of the temporomandibular joint. This complication represents a frequent finding in advanced cases and makes a prognosis more guarded. Elongated teeth also get misaligned and loosened, leading to or exacerbating periodontal disease. Severe periodontal disease may also lead to tooth root abscesses. Malocclusion following primary prognathism of the mandible has not been reported in the guinea pig. Unlike rabbits, coronal elongation and malocclusion of incisor teeth (mostly mandibular incisors) are usually secondary to dental disease of cheek teeth.[2,13]

Nutritional deficiencies may represent a predisposing factor for acquired dental disease. An adequate supply of ascorbic acid (vitamin C) is necessary for the production of collagen and dentin and for the maintenance of capillary strength. Hypovitaminosis C (scurvy) can cause irregular dentin formation as well as clinically evident hemarthrosis and severe arthropathy, followed by degenerative joint disease and pathologic fractures.[15,16] Secondary nutritional hyperparathyroidism with fibrous osteodystrophy has been reported in 3 guinea pigs.[17] All 3 had been placed on a low calcium diet to prevent urolithiasis. Diets with a low calcium to phosphorus ratio resulted in calcification of soft tissues, joint stiffness, reduced growth rates, and even pathologic fractures. The 3 patients exhibited lethargy, difficulty eating, and reluctance to move. None of them recovered despite supportive care. Radiographs showed thin cortical bone, and oral examination revealed loose teeth.

Both excess and deficiency of selenium affect collagen formation, resulting in a weakening of the periodontal ligament.[3] Hypovitaminosis A decreases dentin production and tooth eruption.

DIAGNOSIS OF DENTAL DISEASE

Clinical signs and symptoms of dental disease in guinea pigs are numerous and can range from reduced food intake, weight loss, dehydration, ptyalism and drooling, unkempt fur, facial swelling, nasal and/or ocular discharge, production of small fecal pellets, severe debilitation, to death.[2,6,11] Early symptoms of oral discomfort include difficult prehension of food, dropping of food particles, labored chewing, and dysphagia while the guinea pig is still interested in food.[7] Because the signs and symptoms are not pathognomonic, a thorough history should be obtained to help with the diagnosis. The owner should be questioned about nutrition, habits, previous medical and surgical history, and previous dental treatments, if any. The actual components of the diet and the amounts (including any supplements) should be recorded.

The oral and dental examination should include direct visualization with an otoscope (preferably with a speculum) and palpation. However, only an incomplete examination can be performed with the patient awake. Deep sedation or general anesthesia is necessary for indirect, complete inspection via stomatoscopy, and for radiographic diagnostic imaging such as standard radiography of the head and teeth,[2] CT,[7] or even micro-CT, if available. The use of MRI has been reported in the guinea pig.[10]

Dedicated dental equipment is required for diagnosis and treatment of dental disease in guinea pigs as well as good illumination and magnification.[2,7,18] The basic set of instruments for diagnosis includes a mouth gag, cheek dilators, and a spatula (**Fig. 2**). Specific "open-blade" cheek dilators have been designed to prevent slipping from the double-folded cheek opening of guinea pigs. A special patient positioner (the "rabbit and rodent table retractor/restrainer," commonly named "tabletop mouth gag") is combined with a mouth gag and allows optimal positioning of the patient in sternal recumbency (**Fig. 3**). Several investigators are strong proponents of using endoscopy to improve the intraoral examination and to support the dental treatment.[2,7,19–21] The author finds that with appropriate light and magnification devices (**Fig. 4**) one can complete a thorough dental examination.

Extraoral views of the entire skull are by far the most commonly used method to perform dental radiography. A complete study includes one or both laterolateral projections, dorsoventral or ventrodorsal, rostrocaudal, and lateral oblique projections.[2,22] The most informative views are the lateral (**Fig. 5**) and the oblique. The dorsoventral view is less helpful because of the superimposition of teeth and other anatomic parts of the skull. The anteroposterior view is somewhat more difficult to obtain, but it is good for evaluation of the occlusal angle and of the temporomandibular joint.

Boehmer and Crossley[23] devised a quantitative way of evaluating the normal radiographic anatomy versus the abnormal findings using laterolateral and ventrodorsal

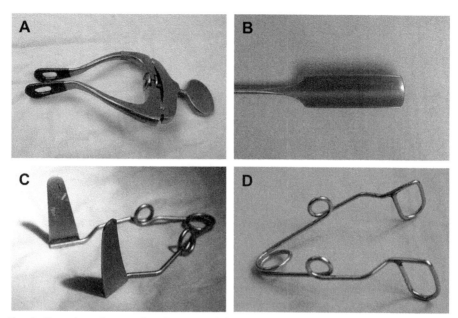

Fig. 2. Dental equipment for diagnosis. (*A*) Standard mouth gag. (*B*) Curved (concave/convex) tongue spatula. (*C*) Small cheek dilators with tapered wings. (*D*) Small "open blade" cheek dilators. ([*B, D*] *Courtesy of* Vittorio Capello, DVM, Milano, Italy; with permission.)

views.[3] The use of lines may facilitate diagnosis; however, they should only be applied to optimal projections in order to be reliable. Moreover, standard radiographic projections remain of limited use when dealing with individual teeth as opposed to general elongation because of the superimposition of quadrants.[24] The use of small intraoral films has been reported as alternative or complementary radiographic technique, to prevent superimposition of anatomic structures.[2,3,22,25] In recent years, the use of

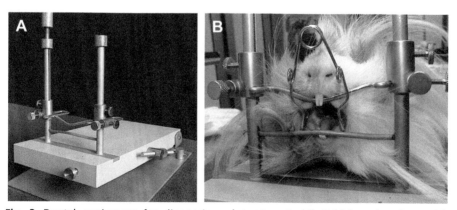

Fig. 3. Dental equipment for diagnosis and treatment. (*A*) Rabbit and rodent table retractor/restrainer. (*B*) Guinea pig positioned in sternal recumbency, with open blade cheek dilators. The anesthetic face mask has been temporarily removed for demonstration purposes. (*Courtesy of* Vittorio Capello, DVM, Milano, Italy; with permission.)

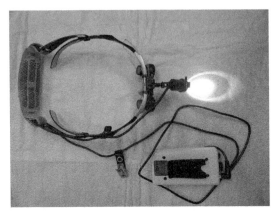

Fig. 4. LED (light-emitting diode) light and magnification loupes mounted on a headband enhance the intraoral examination.

CT and micro-CT has been evaluated for the diagnosis of dental disease in small mammals. They have been found to be more diagnostic because they bypass the intrinsic limit of standard radiography where anatomic structures are superimposed on a single 2-dimensional plane.[26] Micro-CT has yet to gain popularity or practicality due to its small viewing field. However, it does provide higher resolution for small mammals and birds.

Other diagnostic testing should include hematology, biochemistry, bacterial culture, and sensitivity when dealing with periapical infections and abscess, and histopathology when indicated.[2]

DENTAL DISEASE
Incisor Teeth

Fractures of the incisors are occasionally encountered in the guinea pig following trauma or chewing at the cage bars.[2] The most common dental disease of incisor teeth is coronal elongation, particularly of the mandibular incisors (**Fig. 6**).[2,6,7,13] However, the typical pattern of malocclusion is different than in rabbits and other rodent

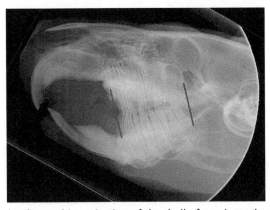

Fig. 5. Laterolateral radiographic projection of the skull of a guinea pig with normal dentition. The alignment of maxillary and mandibular dental arcades is normal (*red lines*).

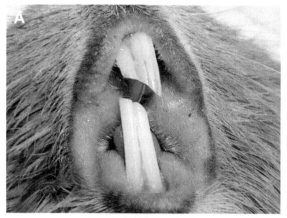
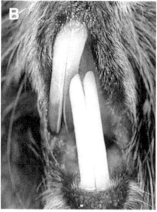
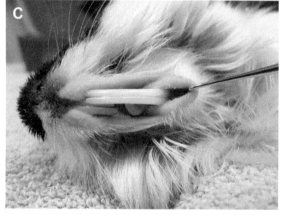

Fig. 6. Common presentations of coronal elongation and malocclusion of incisor teeth with oblique occlusal plane (*A*) and lateral deviation of mandibular incisors (*B, C*). Labial elongation and rostral cross-bite are also present in (*C*). Malocclusion of incisor teeth is usually associated with dental disease of cheek teeth.

species: the mandibular incisors do not usually elongate labially, and the maxillary incisors do not curl palatally.[2,7,13] Lateral deviation with an oblique occlusal plane is frequent, and this usually corresponds to asymmetrical elongation and malocclusion of clinical crowns of cheek teeth, often exacerbated by subluxation of a temporomandibular joint contralateral to the deviation of the mandibular incisors.

An elodontoma of a mandibular incisor tooth has been reported.[27]

Cheek Teeth

The most common dental disease of cheek teeth is coronal elongation.[2,6,7,13] Following anatomic orientation of the cheek teeth and their sloped occlusal plane, mandibular clinical crowns always elongate lingually, whereas the maxillary clinical crowns elongate in the buccal direction. Because of anatomically shorter clinical crowns, overgrowth may not be so evident, especially at the early stage. Spur formation on the mandibular crowns is not common, whereas it is relatively frequent on the buccal edge of maxillary cheek teeth, causing ulcerations of the buccal mucosa. Entrapment of the tongue is a particular type of overgrowth and malocclusion. Usually bilateral and affecting the clinical crowns of mandibular premolars, the overgrown spurs completely cover the tongue in a "bridge-like" fashion, hampering tongue movements and preventing normal deglutition (**Fig. 7**).

Wider interproximal spaces, impaction of food debris, apical elongation (**Fig. 8**), and periodontitis are a common sequela of coronal elongation and malocclusion of cheek teeth. Long-haired guinea pigs (ie, Peruvian) are prone to impaction of hair within the gingival sulcus, even if this is likely secondary to self-licking and self-barbering for skin or behavioral problems.[2] Fur impaction of the mouth creates discomfort and labored chewing and may lead to coronal elongation and malocclusion.

An elodontoma of the right maxillary premolar tooth, which extends into the ipsilateral nasal cavity, has been reported.[27] Elodontoma is a hamartoma of continuously developing odontogenic tissue and the alveolar bone at the periapical bud of elodont teeth.[28] Fully differentiated dental components do not form toothlike structures.[27] Radiography and histopathology are essential for the diagnosis. However, prognosis is guarded to poor because of the locally invasive and expansile nature of this lesion.

Complications of Dental Disease

A frequent complication following coronal elongation and malocclusion of cheek teeth is stretching of the masticatory muscles. In more severe cases, this condition can be associated with unilateral subluxation of the temporomandibular joint following chronic deviation of the mandible.

Although more common in other rodent species such as chinchillas and degus, apical elongation of maxillary cheek teeth may lead to external pressure on the nasolacrimal duct leading to epiphora, dacryocystitis, and other ocular signs or complications. Excessive elongation of rostral maxillary apices may also create compression of the nasal cavities with secondary respiratory problems.

Acquired dental disease results in elongation, malalignment, and loosening of teeth. Once the teeth are loose, impaction of food material occurs in the periodontal space and may be followed by severe periodontal disease, which can lead to infection and abscess formation (**Fig. 9**). Abscessation is also a possible complication of fractured teeth or periapical infection but occurs less commonly than in rabbits. Like most rodents, guinea pigs present with appreciable facial swellings and produce large amounts of caseous purulent material, making the diagnosis of an abscess fairly straightforward. However, differential diagnosis with cervical lymphoadenopathy is of paramount importance in the guinea pig. Because of the anatomy of the cheek teeth

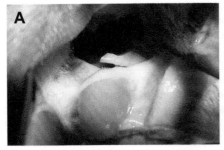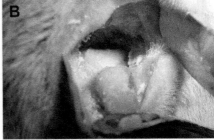

Fig. 7. Coronal elongation of mandibular premolars in a "bridge-like" fashion over the tongue shown before (*A*) and after (*B*) coronal reduction. This condition hampers tongue movements and deglutition.

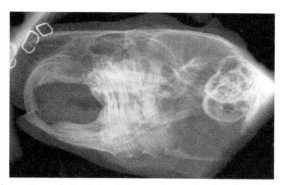

Fig. 8. Coronal elongation of cheek teeth in a guinea pig with dental disease. The oblique projection emphasizes the apical elongation of mandibular and contralateral maxillary cheek teeth.

and of the masseteric muscle with its insertion onto the zygomatic arch, most odontogenic abscesses of the mandible are retromasseteric in the guinea pig.[10]

TREATMENT OF DENTAL DISEASE
Medical Treatment

Prognosis for treatment of dental disease in guinea pigs is fair to good, unless the patient is presented in poor general condition,[13] or if severe complications such as abscesses or subluxation of the mandible are present.

Therapy for dental disease is always combined: dental (intraoral, and in selected cases also extraoral); medical; and supportive. Also, the dental treatment should be coupled with improvement of husbandry and nutrition. The diet should be modified by increasing crude fiber and eliminating soft, carbohydrate-rich treats.

The 3 key points for successful medical treatment are general supportive therapy both before and after dental treatment (assist feeding products for herbivores and fluids), the administration of analgesic drugs, and the use of antibiotics when indicated.[2,13]

Intraoral Treatment of Cheek Teeth

In addition to mouth gags and cheek dilators, the most important instruments for intraoral treatment include burs for coronal reduction (**Fig. 10**), luxators for incisor

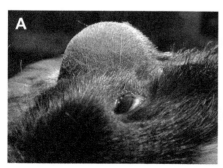
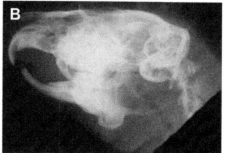

Fig. 9. Periapical infection and odontogenic abscesses present with a large facial swelling, shown after sedation and fur shaving (*A*). Radiography is essential to identify the diseased tooth involved. This oblique projection (*B*) shows severe apical elongation of the fourth mandibular cheek tooth and evident deformity of the cortical bone.

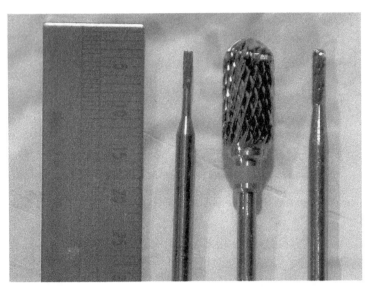

Fig. 10. Burs for coronal reduction.

and cheek teeth, and extraction forceps (**Fig. 11**). Extraoral treatment of dental-related abscesses requires a basic surgical set of small instruments. A light and versatile retractor such as the Lone Star retractor (Lone Star Medical Products, Inc, Stafford, TX, USA) is beneficial during surgery of small patients such as the guinea pig (**Fig. 12**).

Coronal reduction

Treatment of elongation and malocclusion of cheek teeth is aimed at restoring the length of clinical crowns and the proper oblique occlusal plane as close as possible to the normal anatomy.[2,13]

Dental treatment may actually follow diagnostic procedures while the patient is still under general anesthesia. The patient should be placed in the sternal recumbency position and the mouth held open using a mouth gag and cheek dilators. First, the mouth is cleaned of food debris with the aid of cotton tip applicators. In early cases of symmetric elongation of cheek teeth, it may be difficult to evaluate the extent of the coronal elongation just by looking at the clinical crowns. As the crown elongates, the gingival migrates coronally resulting in the visible clinical crown appearing shorter or even normal in length, whereas the suprabony portion of the reserve crown is definitely elongated. Therefore, radiology is also essential for proper evaluation of cheek teeth elongation, because it does not display soft tissues that can mask the actual, abnormal coronal elongation.

Special attention should also be paid to spurs that may be present at the buccal edge of maxillary cheek teeth. The use of a concave/convex spatula is particularly useful to move the buccal mucosa while looking for hidden dental spurs.

Coronal reduction is then performed, restoring the normal coronal length and the anatomic sloped occlusal plane. Because the gingiva has also moved coronally, trimming of the clinical crown may have to be performed very close the gingival level, in order to achieve anatomic and functional reduction. In cases of marked coronal elongation, with or without gingival migration, the complete coronal reduction performed during a single treatment may not be appropriate, or one may not be able to reduce the crowns sufficiently. The coronal reduction below the gingival level would be painful

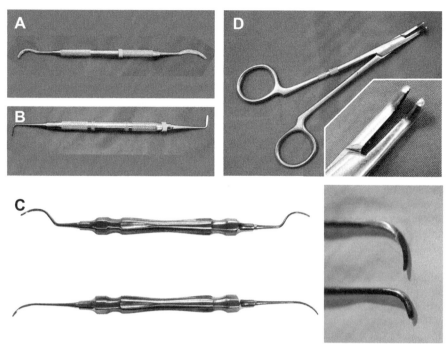

Fig. 11. Dental equipment for treatment. (*A*) Crossley luxator for the mesial and distal aspect of rabbit incisor teeth. Note the narrower curvature of the end for the maxillary incisors, and the wider curvature of the end for the mandibular incisor teeth. (*B*) Crossley luxator for cheek teeth. The Crossley luxator has 2 blades bent approximately at 90° with the handle. One blade (*right end*) is parallel to the long axis of the handle fitting for the lingual and buccal aspect of the cheek teeth; the other blade is perpendicular to the long axis of the handle fitting for the mesial and distal aspect. (*C*) Luxators for the labial and lingual/palatal aspect of rabbit maxillary (*top*) and mandibular (*bottom*) incisor teeth, with close-up of their ends (*right inset*). (*D*) Extraction forceps for cheek teeth, with close-up of the short flat ends suitable to grasp the cheek teeth (*inset*).

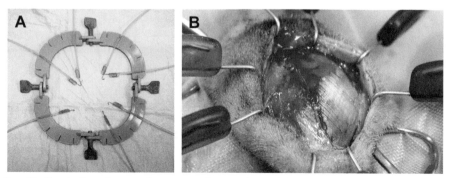

Fig. 12. Surgical equipment for extraoral procedures. (*A*) Lone Star retractor (Lone Star Medical Products, Inc). (*B*) Lone Star retractor in place during surgical excision of a retromasseteric odontogenic abscess. ([*B*] *Courtesy of* Vittorio Capello, DVM, Milano, Italy; with permission.)

and likely result in an anorexic patient. The patient may adjust better to a gradual coronal reduction, which allows the gingival to recede physiologically. In those cases, a second dental procedure is recommended 3 to 4 weeks later, while the patient is supported with assisted feeding if difficulty in eating should continue.

For coronal reduction, burs should be mounted on a straight, low-speed (30,000–40,000 rpm) hand piece. Two types of burs are available: cutters and grinders (see **Fig. 10**). Cutters are more abrasive and thus more rapid, but they function only when rotating in a clockwise direction, making them more difficult to handle when working on a tooth edge where they are prone to slide off. They can also produce vibrations harmful to the periodontal ligament health,[29] and they may also be more dangerous to the soft tissues. Grinders are less abrasive and take more time to perform reduction; however, they allow more precise control and are gentler when touching soft tissues, preventing tears or severe damage. For these reasons, grinders are preferred by the author. Alternatively, proper spatulas to protect the tongue (the author uses coffee stir sticks; **Fig. 13**), and soft tissue protectors mounted on a straight hand piece are available. Frequent cleaning of the oral cavity using cotton tip applicators moistened with saline is recommended to evaluate the coronal reduction and to allow the teeth to cool down. When the dental procedure is complete, a final clean is performed. Coronal elongation as well as passive movements of the lower jaw is evaluated with the mouth closed. At this stage, coronal reduction of incisor teeth with their normal chisel-shaped occlusal plane is performed if needed.

After coronal reduction, dental wear should equate physiologic growth, and reoccurrence of coronal elongation should not ideally happen. However, this rarely happens in cases of severe elongation of cheek teeth. Even if adequate dental treatment is followed by correction of the diet and the patient is supported with feeding formula for herbivores during the recovery phase, coronal elongation may reoccur.

Because coronal elongation forces the mouth open and stretches the masticatory muscles, guinea pigs may frequently experience difficulty in closing and moving the lower jaw because of loose muscles during the first days following coronal reduction of cheek teeth, possibly exacerbated in the case of subluxation of the temporomandibular joint. With the mouth slightly open, the cheek teeth do not properly grind and wear, undergoing repeated abnormal coronal elongations. By increasing the congruency of cheek teeth, the wear would increase as well, delaying the need for further

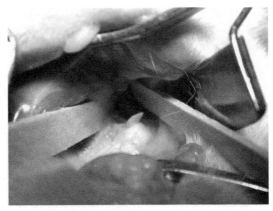

Fig. 13. Plain stir sticks (used here in a rabbit) are very useful to protect soft tissues during coronal reduction of cheek teeth.

dental procedures of coronal reduction. The "chin sling" was designed to accomplish exactly this purpose.[30] This specific device is made of neoprene and provides the support necessary to keep the cheek teeth in constant touch necessary for adequate wear (**Fig. 14**). In order to be effective, the sling needs to be worn at least 6 hours a day. Undesired side effects and owners' complaints have been about head shaking and alopecia on the back of the head where the sling band rubs against the skin and fur. However, in the author's experience, this device proved to be effective in increasing the time span between dental treatments.

In the case of incomplete return to normal chewing function, the patient should be rechecked after 6 to 8 weeks. Follow-ups allow evaluation of whether the dental treatment has been successful and to plan how often the patient should undergo further dental procedures.

Extraction

Extraction of cheek teeth can be performed with the intraoral or the extraoral approach. The latter may include either extraction or apical amputation (apicectomy).

The intraoral approach is challenging because of the small size of the oral cavity and the anatomic curvature of the reserve crowns. The diseased tooth is luxated by cutting the periodontal ligament on the 4 aspects and then extracted intraorally.[31] When the cheek tooth is loose, the clinical crown is grasped with an extraction forceps. Specialized extractors, which have very short ends almost perpendicular to the long arms, are necessary for this procedure (**Fig. 11**). The tooth should be twisted and pushed apically before extraction. Twisting is aimed to break the remaining fibers of the periodontal ligament around the apical part of the reserve crown. Pushing is aimed to damage the apical germinal tissue to prevent regrowth. After extraction, the alveolus is flushed; the gingiva is elevated on either side, and the defect is sutured with 5-0 monofilament absorbable material. Although suturing is difficult in this species, it is crucial to close the gingiva to prevent food impaction of the alveolus, which can cause

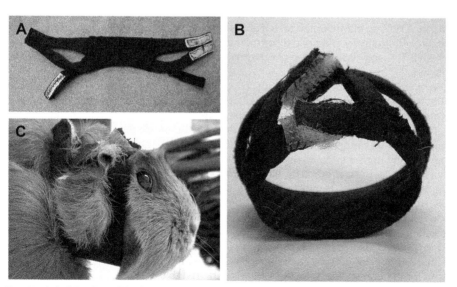

Fig. 14. (*A*) Chin sling. (*B*) Chin sling shown in the position as it would be placed onto the guinea pig and affixed with Velcro. (*C*) Guinea pigs wearing the chin sling, supporting the mandible.

infection. This challenging procedure is made easier by using fine needle holders and a 13-mm, half curve, reverse cutting needle.

The extraoral approach is primarily indicated for mandibular teeth. The extraoral access to the rostral maxillary cheek teeth requires a rhinotomy procedure and should not be performed without adequate experience. The exact position of the diseased tooth can be determined radiographically and is followed by an incision is made on the ventrolateral border of the mandible. The cortical bone is exposed, and a window is created over the apical aspect of the tooth with a small rotating burr. The reserve crown is carefully luxated and extracted through the opening. After the suture of the skin incision, the gingiva is sutured intraorally as described above. The cheek tooth can be seated firmly within the alveolus even in the face of periapical disease. To prevent the risk of an iatrogenic fracture of the mandible during extraction, apicectomy can be an alternative option. The apical aspect of the tooth, including the germinal tissue and a small portion of the reserve crown, is amputated and removed. The remaining portion of the reserve crown and the clinical crown remain in situ, and the incision is closed routinely. The remainder of the tooth will move coronally until it will eventually be shed.

Extraction of the opposing cheek tooth to prevent an uneven occlusal plane or "step mouth" has proven to not be necessary. Because of the propalineal motion of the mandible, a cheek tooth wears against more cheek teeth of the opposite arcade; therefore, physiologic wear would occur.

Treatment of Incisor Teeth

Coronal reduction of abnormally elongated incisor teeth is usually performed in conjunction with dental treatment of cheek teeth.[2,6,7,13] If malocclusion is not severe, or it is secondary to abnormal conditions of the cheek teeth and mandible, which can be corrected, coronal reduction is curative. This dental procedure should never be performed with toenail clippers, wire cutters/nippers, or other such instruments. These types of instruments when used to perform "trimming" can cause oblique fractures that are painful, can result in pulp exposure, and ultimately result in periapical abscessation. A cutting bur mounted on a high-speed angled hand piece is used for this procedure. Alternatively, diamond discs mounted on low-speed hand pieces are available as well. The soft tissues are protected by placing a tongue depressor caudal to the incisors.

In other cases where occlusion can no longer be restored and maintained, treatment options are either repeated coronal reduction or extraction. As in rabbits, the latter is preferred because repeated treatment may eventually lead to complications.

The standard technique is not different than the technique reported in rabbits. Standard Crossley luxators for the mesial and distal aspect of rabbit incisor teeth (**Fig. 11**A) may or may not be suitable depending on the patient's size. In the latter case, contoured needles are a practical alternative. Also, curved luxators for the labial and lingual/palatal aspect of incisor teeth are especially useful (**Fig. 11**C).

Luxation of the incisor teeth should begin on the mesial aspect where the periodontal ligament is stronger. The luxator is introduced in the periodontal space until resistance is encountered. Pressure is applied along the tooth axis for a minimum of 15 to 30 seconds to allow breakage of the ligamental fibers. The luxator is then introduced into the periodontal space on the distal aspect. The appropriate luxator is then used for the convex labial aspect of the tooth, and the procedure is repeated on the concave lingual/palatal aspect. When the incisor tooth is loose, the tooth should be pushed apically and twisted before extraction, similar to the procedure on cheek teeth. If the apical end of the reserve crown is empty after tooth extraction, the apical germinal tissue is still in place and the tooth may regrow, even if it may not erupt. The gingiva is sutured over the alveolus with 5-0 monofilament absorbable material to prevent food debris from entering the alveolus. After extraction of an incisor tooth, and depending on severity of malocclusion, extraction of the opposing incisor may not be needed. In selected patients, effective occlusion can be maintained by a single incisor meeting and wearing with the 2 opposing teeth (**Fig. 15**).

Periapical Infection and Abscessation

An odontogenic abscess presents with an evident clinical sign: a noticeable swelling, which is usually painful on palpation. The associated skin may be erythemic and alopecic or it may be necrotic and already ruptured, resulting in a fistula. Abscesses are usually large and deep, and they are often multilobed[14] with several pockets. The purulent material may range from very thick, to caseous, to fluid. As extensively discussed for odontogenic abscesses in rabbits, aggressive treatment with complete excision including the capsule and extraction of the affected tooth or teeth is the treatment of choice.[2,7,10,13,32] After the extraoral surgical procedure, the gingiva is sutured intraorally as described above; this is aimed to prevent food material from entering the alveolus and causing ongoing infection.

Various adjunct treatments have been reported after excision. The most common is marsupialization of the skin to the underlying connective tissue. The surgical site may then be packed with an antibiotic or an antiseptic. Established or potential toxicity of common antibiotics in the guinea pig should be considered[13] when choosing an

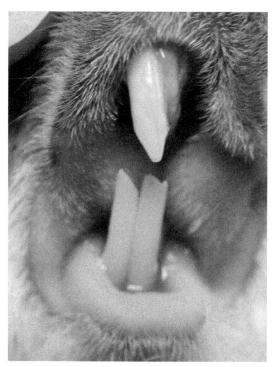

Fig. 15. Follow-up in a guinea pig after extraction of the left maxillary incisor tooth. The single, right incisor is sufficient to wear both mandibular incisors and to keep a functional occlusion.

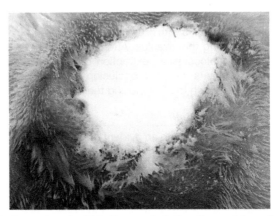

Fig. 16. Antibiotic slurry placed within the surgical site after excision of an abscess.

antibiotic because some can cause enterotoxemia when administered systemically.[33] Methylmethacrylate beads impregnated with drugs such as gentamycin, tobramycin, amikacin, vancomycin, cetiofur, and metronidazole have been used to treat abscesses after the excision. They present several disadvantages, such as cost and size, and the skin must be sutured to hold them in place. Removal requires that the site be reopened, and they are typically impregnated with macrolides that are quite toxic to guinea pigs. Some antibiotics are available in a powder form, which can be moistened to form a slurry or paste, which can be packed within the surgical site. Once the slurry dries, it will stay in place by conforming to the cavity (**Fig. 16**). Antibiotics that have successfully been used in the slurry are ampicillin, clindamycin, tetracycline, doxycycline, and minocycline. Doxycycline hyclate mixed with a plastic carrier has also been successfully used to sterilize abscesses. The area is thoroughly flushed with saline after 2 weeks to remove any residual medication. If the surgical site is covered by healthy granulation tissue, the area is either left to heal by secondary intention or sutured. If the surgical site still appears septic, the slurry is replaced for another 2 weeks. The author typically replaces the antibiotic every 2 weeks until healing has

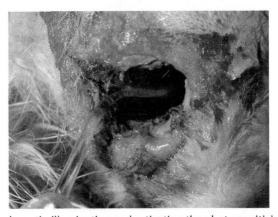

Fig. 17. Periowave laser tip illuminating and activating the photosensitizing solution. Treatment of the surgical site via the laser is achieved in 1 minute.

occurred. In selected cases, the marsupialized area may take up to 8 weeks to heal. Antiseptic products such as calcium hydroxide have also been used.[33,34] Some investigators have described an undesired dry necrosis on the tissues treated[2]; however, this has not occurred in the author's experience.

A laser system designed for treatment of infected periodontal pockets in humans has also been shown to be a promising therapeutic modality (**Fig. 17**). A photosensitizing solution is placed into the cavity, which is then illuminated by the laser that activates the solution, destroying bacteria and their toxins. The treatment session takes approximately 1 minute and is completely painless.

REFERENCES

1. Wiggs RB, Lobprise HB. Dental disease in rodents. J Vet Dent 1990;7:6–81.
2. Capello V, Gracis M. In: Lennox AM, editor. Rabbit and rodent dentistry handbook. Philadelphia: Wiley-Blackwell; 2005. p. 1–272.
3. Bohmer E. Dentistry in rabbits and rodents. Philadelphia: Wiley-Blackwell; 2015.
4. Croft DA, Niemi K, Franco A. Incisor morphology reflect diet in caviomorph rodents. J Mammal 2011;92:871–9.
5. Crossley DA. Clinical aspects of rodent dental anatomy. J Vet Dent 1991;8:131–4.
6. Legendre LF. Oral disorders of exotic rodents. Vet Clin North Am 2003;6:601–28.
7. Capello V, Lennox AM. Small mammal dentistry. In: Quesenberry KE, Carpenter JW, editors. Ferrets, rabbits and rodents: clinical medicine and surgery. 3rd edition. Philadelphia: Elsevier/Saunders; 2012. p. 452–71.
8. Crossley DA. Rabbit and rodent oral anatomy and physiology. In: Proceedings of the North American veterinary conference. Orlando, Gainesville (FL): Eastern States Veterinary Association; 2000. p. 990–2.
9. Cox PG, Rayfield EJ, Fagan MJ, et al. Functional evolution of the feeding system in rodents. PLoS One 2012;7:1–11.
10. Capello V, Lennox AM. Advanced diagnostic imaging and surgical treatment of an odontogenic retromasseteric abscess in a guinea pig. J Small Anim Pract 2015;56(2):134–7.
11. Osofsky A, Verstraete FJM. Dentistry in pet rodents. Compendium on Continuin Education for the Practicing Veterinarian 2006;28(1):61–74.
12. Crossley AD. Dental disease in chinchillas. Manchester (United Kingdom): Department of Dental Medicine and Surgery; University of Manchester; 2003.
13. Capello V. Diagnosis and treatment of dental disease in pet rodents. J Exot Pet Med 2008;17(2):114–23.
14. Reiter AM. Pathophysiology of dental disease in the rabbit, guinea pig, and chinchilla. J Exot Pet Med 2008;17(2):70–7.
15. Redrobe S. Imaging techniques in small mammals. Semin Avian Exot Pet Med 2001;10:187–97.
16. Kalnins V, Petrov N, Greenman V. Malleting injuries of teeth in scorbutic and normal guinea pigs. Oral Surg 1971;31:400–8.
17. Hawkins MG. Secondary nutritional hyperparathyroidism with fibrous osteodystrophy in 3 guinea pigs. Proceedings of 31st Annual AAV Conference and Expo. San Diego (CA): 2010. p. 121.
18. Capello V. The dental suite: equipment needed for handling small exotic mammals. J Exot Pet Med 2006;15(2):106–15.
19. Taylor WM. Endoscopy as an aid to the examination and treatment of oropharyngeal disease in small herbivorous mammals. Semin Avian Exot Pet Med 1999; 8(3):139–41.

20. Jekl V, Knotek Z. Evaluation of a laryngoscope and a rigid endoscope for the examination of the oral cavity of small mammals. Vet Rec 2007;160(1):9–13.

21. Hernandez-Divers SJ. Dental endoscopy of rabbits and rodents. J Exot Pet Med 2008;17(2):87–92.

22. Gracis M. Clinical technique: normal dental radiography of rabbits, guinea pigs, and chinchillas. J Exot Pet Med 2008;17(2):78–86.

23. Boehmer E, Crossley D. Objective interpretation of dental disease in rabbits, guinea pigs and chinchillas. Tierarzliche Praxis Kleintiere 2009;73:250–60.

24. Van Thielen B, Jacqmot O, Siguenza F, et al. Explorative investigation of cone beam CT for maxillofacial imaging in rabbits, rodents and small carnivores. Proceedings 21st ECVD. Lisbon: 2012. p. 54–7.

25. Boehmer E. Intraoral radiographic technique in lagomorphs and rodents. Exotic DVM 2007;9(3):2–27.

26. Souza MJ, Greenacre CB, Avenell JS, et al. Diagnosing a tooth root abscess in a Guinea pig (*Cavia porcellus*) using micro computed tomography imaging. J Exot Pet Med 2006;15:274–7.

27. Capello V, Lennox A. Elodontoma in two guinea pigs. J Vet Dent 2015;32(2): 111–9.

28. Boy SC, Steenkamp G. Odontoma-like tumours of squirrel elodont incisors–elodontomas. J Comp Pathol 2006;135(1):56–61.

29. Gabriel S. Technical aspects of abrasive dental tools. Proceedings of the 18th European Congress on Vet Dent. Zurich: 2009.

30. Legendre LFJ. Malocclusions in guinea pigs, chinchillas and rabbits. Can Vet J 2002;43:385–90.

31. Legendre LFJ. Rodent and lagomorph tooth extractions. J Vet Dent 2012;29: 204–9.

32. Legendre LFJ. Treatment of oral abscesses in rodents and lagomorphs. J Vet Dent 2011;28:30–3.

33. Legendre LFJ. What antibiotics-impregnated materials are available for treating abscesses. Proceedings of NAVC. 2013.

34. Remeus PGK, Verbeek M. The use of calcium hydroxide in the treatment of abscesses in the cheek of the rabbit resulting from dental periapical disorder. J Vet Dent 1995;12:19–22.

Anatomy and Disorders of the Oral Cavity of Chinchillas and Degus

Christoph Mans, Dr med vet, DACZM[a],*,
Vladimir Jekl, MVDr, PhD, DECZM (Small Mammal)[b]

KEYWORDS

- Dental disease • Dentistry • Periodontal • Caries • Resorption • Teeth
- *Chinchilla lanigera* • *Octodon degus*

KEY POINTS

- In chinchillas, apical elongation of the mandibular cheek teeth can be palpated on the ventral aspects of the mandibles; apical elongation can be palpated in the preorbital fossa.
- Apical elongation of maxillary cheek teeth in degus commonly leads to partial obstruction of nasal meatuses with subsequent dyspnea.
- Periodontal disease, caries, and tooth resorption are common findings in chinchillas; an intraoral examination should be performed carefully to avoid missing these lesions.
- Diagnostic imaging is essential in the diagnosis of dental disease, and should be performed in all cases of suspected dental disease in chinchillas and degus.
- Endoscopy-guided examinations are recommended for chinchillas and degus to minimize the risk of missing intraoral pathology and iatrogenic trauma during the intraoral treatment.

INTRODUCTION

Dental disease is commonly diagnosed in pet chinchillas and degus as it is in other small herbivorous mammals with elodont (continuously growing) incisors and cheek teeth. However, subclinical dental disease has been detected in 35% of clinically healthy chinchillas and in 60% of degus examined; therefore, subclinical dental abnormalities should not be always assumed to be responsible for clinical signs and symptoms, such as anorexia.[1,2] Animals of all ages can be affected by dental disease, but older animals are more likely to be diagnosed with acquired dental disease.[1] Most animals with dental disease present with weight loss, reduced food intake or anorexia,

The authors have nothing to disclose.
[a] Department of Surgical Sciences, School of Veterinary Medicine, University of Wisconsin-Madison, 2015 Linden Drive, Madison, WI 53706, USA; [b] Avian and Exotic Animal Clinic, Faculty of Veterinary Medicine, University of Veterinary and Pharmaceutical Sciences Brno, Palackého tr. 1946/1, Brno 61242, Czech Republic
* Corresponding author.
E-mail addresses: christoph.mans@wisc.edu; jeklv@vfu.cz

Vet Clin Exot Anim 19 (2016) 843–869
http://dx.doi.org/10.1016/j.cvex.2016.04.007
1094-9194/16/$ – see front matter © 2016 Elsevier Inc. All rights reserved.

drooling, or poor fur quality. Degus are also commonly presented with dyspnea. In the scientific literature, dental disease in chinchillas and degus has been primarily referred to as elongation and malocclusion of the cheek teeth. However, periodontal disease, caries, and tooth resorption are common diseases in chinchillas, although they are frequently missed during routine intraoral examination, even if the examination is performed under general anesthesia. For this reason, a thorough diagnostic evaluation, including an endoscopy-guided intraoral examination and diagnostic imaging of the skull, is necessary to detect oral disorders and to perform the appropriate therapy.

ANATOMY AND PHYSIOLOGY OF THE ORAL CAVITY

All teeth in chinchillas and degus lack an anatomic root (aradicular), grow continuously (elodont), and have a long crown (hypsodont). Each incisor tooth is separated from premolars and molars (commonly named "cheek teeth") by a large diastema, resulting from the loss of the canines and selected mesial (rostral) premolars (P1 through P3). Both species have 4 cheek teeth in each dental quadrant, which are morphologic identical. The dental formula is 2 (I 1/1, C 0/0, P1/1, M 3/3) for a total of 20 teeth (16 cheek teeth). These features are shared among all hystricomorph rodents, which include the guinea pig (*Cavia porcellus*), chinchilla (*Chinchilla lanigera*), degu (*Octodon degus*), and Patagonian cavy (*Dolichotis patagonum*) as well as the old world and new world (North American) porcupines (*Hystricidae* and *Erethizontidae*), the nutria (*Myocastor coypus*) and the capybara (*Hidrochoerus hydrochaeris*), which are occasionally kept as companion animals.

The term *reserve crown* is used to describe the part of the tooth below the gingival level and within the alveolus. The portion above the gingival margin visible within the oral cavity is termed the *clinical crown*.[3]

Incisor Teeth

Rodents are some of the most highly specialized mammals with regard to their feeding apparatus. The labial surface of the incisor teeth is pigmented yellow-orange in chinchillas (**Fig. 1**) and degus. Chinchillas have maxillary incisor apices that reach to approximately one-half of the diastema, with mandibular incisor apices that end near the mesial–lingual aspect of the premolar (mandibular first cheek tooth). In degus, the maxillary incisors apices extend two-thirds of the diastema with mandibular incisor apices that end distal to the last molar.

The incisors have enamel only on the full length of their labial surface, extending from the apical area to the occlusal edge. The enamel of the incisor teeth of *Hystricognathi* have multiple serial Hunter–Schreger bands with an angular arrangement of the interprismatic matrix to the prism long axes, which strengthens the enamel and provides a higher wear resistance.[4] As a result these teeth wear to a chisel-shaped cutting edge owing to the rostral–caudal gliding movement of the jaw during normal feeding.[5] Upper lip skin folds are pushed inward through the diastema and meet behind the upper incisor and above the tongue to close off the oral cavity, so that the incisors occlude outside the mouth.[5]

Cheek Teeth

Premolars and molars have a similar structure and represent a uniform functional grinding unit in each quadrant. They are commonly named "cheek teeth." The crowns of the cheek teeth in chinchillas and degus diverge from rostral to caudal, however, to a much lesser extent than in guinea pigs.[5] The occlusal surface of the cheek teeth is horizontal and consists of ridges of enamel alternating in between exposed surface of

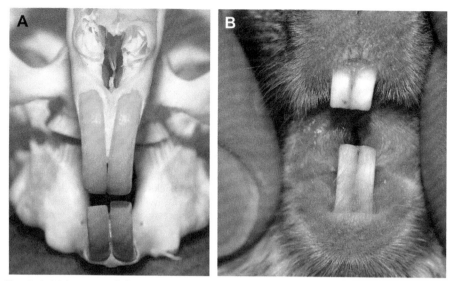

Fig. 1. Labial aspect of the incisor teeth in chinchillas. (*A*) Normal appearance shown in a bony specimen. Note the physiologic yellow-orange coloration of the enamel covering only the labial aspect. (*B*) Abnormal appearance. Note the depigmentation of the enamel. (*Courtesy of* Christoph Mans, Madison, WI; with permission.)

dentin and cementum (**Figs. 2–4**). As a consequence of a strictly herbivorous nutrition, the occlusal surfaces are rough and uneven, with a series of enamel folds and dentinal grooves. Each mandibular cheek tooth is in occlusion with the opposite maxillary cheek tooth. In resting jaw position, their occlusal planes are almost in contact. The occlusal surface of degus cheek teeth resembles the shape of the "8" number, giving the name of their genus (*Octodon*: octo = 8; don(t) = tooth, see **Figs. 3** and **4**).

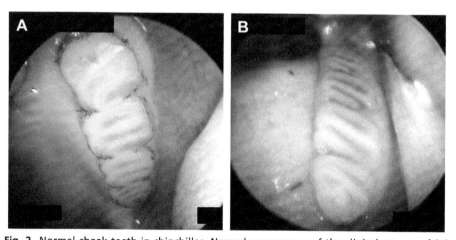

Fig. 2. Normal cheek teeth in chinchillas. Normal appearance of the clinical crowns of (*A*) maxillary and (*B*) mandibular cheek teeth. Note the short clinical crowns, the flat occlusal planes and the lack of interproximal spaces. (*Courtesy of* Christoph Mans, Madison, WI; with permission.)

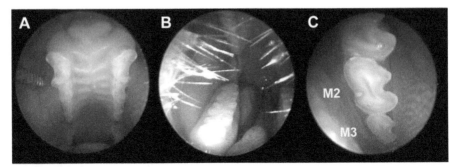

Fig. 3. Normal cheek teeth in degus. The occlusal surfaces of the maxillary (*A*) and mandibular (*B*) cheek teeth are flat. The clinical crowns of the cheek teeth are of the same height. (*C*) Detailed view of the right mandibular cheek teeth with whitish enamel ridges, displaying the typical shape, which resembles a figure of 8. (*Courtesy of* Vladimir Jekl, Brno, Czech Republic; with permission.)

Chewing

The natural diet of strictly herbivorous species is rich in crude fiber, and its low energy content requires a high intake and thorough chewing. This results in the proper wear of the elodont cheek teeth. The incisor and cheek teeth (separated by the diastema) represent 2 distinct functional units used for gnawing and chewing. Because of the anatomic mismatch between the length of the maxilla and the mandible, the incisors and molars are not in occlusion at the same time. The 2 chewing modes are mutually exclusive: the mandible must be moved rostrally and caudally with respect to the cranium (propalineal) to accomplish both these tasks.[6] In adult octodontids, 2 combined chewing movements are present: propalineal bilateral (primarily associated with rostrocaudal displacement of the mandible and simultaneous occlusion) and oblique unilateral feeding (associated with rostrolingual jaw displacement and alternate occlusion of left and right cheek teeth).[7]

In hystrichomorph rodents, both chewing modes are associated with specific muscle and temporomandibular joint anatomy. The deep part of the masseter muscle has a broad extent cranial to the zygomatic arch and attaches on the muzzle just rostrally to the eye. This provides the very powerful gnawing action typical of this rodent group.

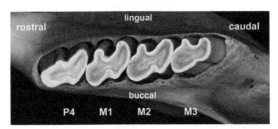

Fig. 4. Close up of the left mandible of a degu from a 3-dimensional rendering of microcomputed tomography, displaying the occlusal surface of cheek teeth. Premolar and molar teeth have a similar structure, and in each quadrant they form a uniform functional grinding unit. The occlusal surface resemble a figure of 8. Note the whitish enamel ridges and yellow to brown color of dentinal grooves. This illustration adheres to the standard numbering system naming the first premolar as P4. (*Courtesy of* Vladimir Jekl, Brno, Czech Republic; with permission.)

The lateral masseter muscle is only used in closing jaw, and the temporalis muscle is small. Like other rodents, chinchillas and degus have a specific temporomandibular joint anatomy with a deep and long longitudinal sulcus, the glenoid fossa. The articular process of the mandible slides along the fossa, allowing jaw movements either forward to the rostral position (where the incisors are in occlusion but the cheek teeth are not), or to the backward position (where the cheek teeth are in occlusion but the incisors are not).[8]

Because of the orthogonal disposition of the enamel bands with respect to mandibular chewing movements, *Octodontidae* focus chewing pressure onto fewer enamel cutting edges.[9] This adaptation, together with the enamel reinforcement after the repeated secondary acquisition of radial enamel, would improve grinding of the more abrasive vegetation present in the southwest of South America. Even more, the grinding performance could be enhanced by an oblique chewing mode.

PATHOPHYSIOLOGY OF DENTAL DISEASE AND DENTAL DISORDERS
Disorders of the Incisor Teeth

Disorders of the incisor teeth, in particular coronal elongation, is often secondary to cheek teeth disorders. Pathologies of enamel, dentin, and cementum (such as depigmentation, horizontal enamel ridges, rough enamel surface, and cementum and dentin demineralization) are owing to germinal tissue disorders, especially in cases of metabolic imbalance (eg, high phosphorus diet, hypocalcaemia, systemic diseases) or chronic trauma (biting in the cage bars; **Figs. 5** and **6**). Primary incisor diseases are associated primarily with trauma and less often with developmental disorders (see **Fig. 5**C).[10]

Disorders of the Cheek Teeth

Nutritional and genetic causes have been proposed as the predisposing factors for the development of dental disease in chinchillas.[3] Captive-bred chinchillas tend to have significant longer cheek teeth when compared with their wild counterparts. It has been hypothesized that reduced chewing of a less abrasive diet in captivity would

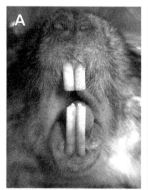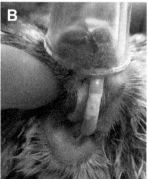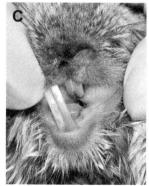

Fig. 5. Disorders of the incisor teeth in chinchillas. (*A*) Enamel depigmentation, coronal elongation, and malocclusion. (*B*) Severe coronal elongation and malocclusion of the maxillary incisor teeth. The clinical crown of both mandibular incisors is missing. (*C*) Enamel depigmentation, coronal elongation, and malocclusion of mandibular incisor teeth in a 3-month-old chinchilla owing to congenital maxillary brachygnathism. ([*A*] *Courtesy of* Vladimir Jekl, Brno, Czech Republic; with permission; [*B*] *Courtesy of* Christoph Mans, Madison, WI; with permission.)

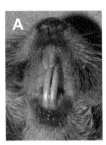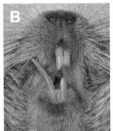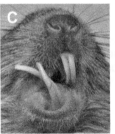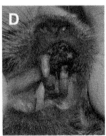

Fig. 6. Disorders of the incisor teeth in degus. (*A*) Elongation and enamel depigmentation of the clinical crowns. (*B*) Severe malocclusion and deviation of the right mandibular incisor tooth after a traumatic injury. (*C*) Iatrogenic right lateral deviation of mandibular incisor teeth and overall coronal elongation after trimming of clinical crowns with pliers. (*D*) Displacement and malocclusion of incisor teeth secondary to a maxillary melanoma. (*Courtesy of* Vladimir Jekl, Brno, Czech Republic; with permission.)

diminish tooth wear, leading to elongation of continuously growing cheek teeth.[3] However, less abrasive diets also have an undesirable high phosphorus content and inappropriate Ca:P ratio, which may induce secondary dietary hyperparathyroidism and dental disease. In degus, a resulting Ca:P dietary imbalance by feeding a high phosphorus and normal calcium (1:1) diet has been shown to induce dental disease of all teeth (incisor depigmentation, enamel hypoplasia, disruption in dentin and cementum formation, and apical and coronal cheek teeth elongation) within 6 months, in addition to significantly reduction in mandibular bone density.[11]

Tooth elongation affecting the reserve and/or the clinical crown is the cause for most clinical signs and symptoms associated with dental disease in chinchillas and degus. Apical cheek tooth elongation can result in pain associated with apical tooth pressure onto the nerve endings, growth through the periosteum, and intrusive pressure of the tooth to the germinal tissue associated with ischemia. The apices of affected mandibular teeth commonly perforate adjacent bone, resulting in the presence of palpable surface irregularities on the ventral mandibular surface. In chinchillas, the apices of maxillary cheek perforate the maxilla on the lateral surface, in the preorbital/infraorbital and orbital area (**Fig. 7**). In degus, the reserve crowns of the maxillary premolars are elongated dorsorostrally (apical–mesially) and last the molars caudally (apical–distally). Reserve crowns of the maxillary first and second molars (second and third cheek teeth) are elongated apically in straight direction and can perforate the nasal or frontal bone.

As a consequence of a disrupted chewing pattern, orthodontic tooth movement within a jaw and improper dental wear, clinical crowns become elongated and can cause pronounced dysphagia. In chinchillas, maxillary cheek teeth curve buccally and mandibular teeth slightly lingually and the formation of spurs leads to soft tissue trauma. Gingiva surrounding the maxillary cheek teeth is commonly hyperplastic. As the disease progresses in severity, the mandible is displaced more and more distally with an increasing intraoral elongation of the cheek teeth. The angle between the jaws becomes wider so that the incisors become elongated secondarily. Because the maxillary incisors are more markedly curved, their elongation results in the teeth growing distally into the oral cavity. In degus, the clinical crowns of the maxillary cheek teeth do not commonly bend buccally, but elongate more coronally in the direction of the long axis of the tooth. Mandibular cheek teeth elongate lingually. Mandibular premolars (first cheek teeth) elongate below the tongue or above with typical formation of a "bridge" and subsequent entrapment of the tongue.

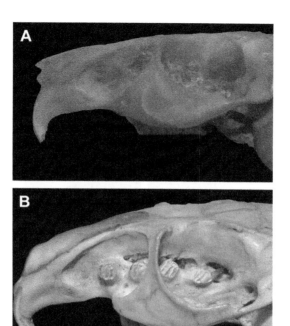

Fig. 7. Lateral view of the chinchilla skull. (*A*) Normal dentition of the maxillary left quadrant. (*B*) Advanced dental disease and severe apical elongation of maxillary cheek teeth. The apices of check teeth 1 and 2 can be palpated in the preorbital region. (*Courtesy of* Vladimir Jekl, Brno, Czech Republic; with permission.)

PERIODONTAL DISEASE AND TOOTH RESORPTION

Periodontal disease is very common in chinchillas. The evaluation of 181 skulls in 1 study reported a periodontal disease rate of 63%.[12] Although the etiology remains unknown in chinchillas, it is suspected that the same pathophysiology occurs as in other species, such as secondary to dental disease, genetic factors, age, oral microflora, and nutrition.[10,12] In chinchillas, tooth resorption leads to loss of clinical crowns of the cheek teeth, followed by food impaction within the widened interproximal spaces and frequently development of periodontal disease (**Figs. 8–10**). Thorough cleaning of retained food material in the oral cavity and assessment of each tooth for mobility and associated periodontal abnormalities is critical for diagnosis of periodontal disease in chinchillas (see **Fig. 10**). Untreated periodontal disease will progress, and will result in bone and tooth resorption. This condition is a source of chronic intraoral pain, leading to reduced and insufficient food intake followed by weight loss and potential metabolic complications such as ketoacidosis and hepatic lipidosis. Therefore, any chinchilla or degu showing clinical signs and symptoms suggestive of periodontal disease should be assessed and treated appropriately.

CARIES

Dental caries (synonyms: cavities, tooth decay) is defined as demineralization and destruction of tooth substance after bacterial infection. Demineralization of the tooth

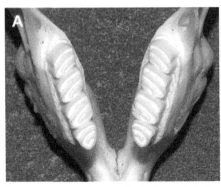
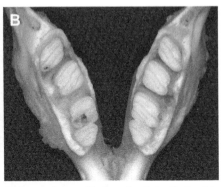

Fig. 8. Bony specimens displaying normal and diseased mandibular cheek teeth in chinchillas. (*A*) Normal appearance of clinical crowns, periodontal bone, and lack of interproximal space. (*B*) Mandibles and cheek teeth of a chinchilla affected by severe periodontal disease and secondary bone and tooth resorption. Widening of the alveolar space, widened interproximal spaces, shifting of the cheek teeth, and caries lesions of the occlusal surfaces are present. (*Courtesy of* Christoph Mans, Madison, WI; with permission.)

substance follows production of lactic acid by the cariogenic bacteria.[13] A combination of gram-positive and gram-negative bacteria have been reported in caries of chinchillas. Caries are common in chinchillas and have been reported to be present in 52% among 181 skulls of captive chinchillas.[10,12]

Caries can be detected as brown-to-black colored lesions affecting the occlusal and interproximal surfaces of the cheek teeth clinical crowns (see **Fig. 10**F; **Fig. 11**).[10,12,13] It is unknown why dental caries is more common in chinchillas as compared with other rodent species and rabbits. Feeding high sucrose supplements and reduced attrition owing to low-fiber diets (which may lead to increased plaque formation and reduced salivation) have been proposed as possible predisposing factors

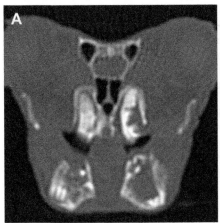
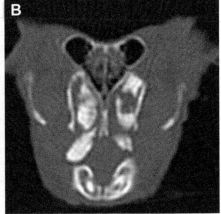

Fig. 9. (*A, B*) Computed tomography of the head of 2 chinchillas with severe periodontal disease, axial views. Tooth resorption of the clinical and reserve crowns, as well as widening of the alveolar spaces secondary to bone resorption and remodeling are present. (*Courtesy of* Christoph Mans, Madison, WI; with permission.)

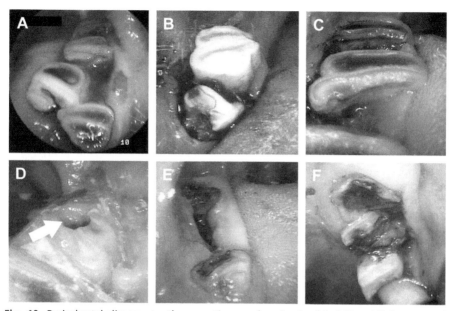

Fig. 10. Periodontal disease, tooth resorption, and caries in chinchillas. (*A*) Severe periodontal disease of the left mandibular cheek teeth and lingual displacement of cheek tooth 2. Abnormal position and displacement of the reserve and clinical crowns are commonly caused by periodontal abscessation. (*B*) Periodontal disease and tooth resorption of the mesial aspect of the right mandibular cheek tooth 1. (*C*) Periodontal disease and partial tooth resorption of the clinical crown of the right mandibular cheek tooth 3. (*D*) Resorptive tooth lesion (*arrow*) of the clinical crown of the left mandibular cheek tooth 4. (*E*) Resorption of the clinical crowns of check tooth 2 and cheek tooth 3 on the right mandibular arcade. Note the discoloration and presence of caries, and the gingival hyperplasia lingual to cheek tooth 4. (*F*) Severe caries affecting the clinical crown of the left maxillary check tooth 1 and check tooth 2. Marked gingival hyperplasia is also present. (*Courtesy of* Christoph Mans, Madison, WI; with permission.)

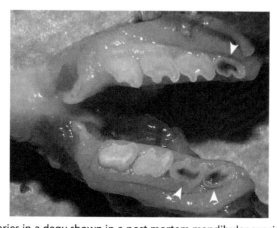

Fig. 11. Dental caries in a degu shown in a post mortem mandibular specimen. The occlusal surface of right cheek tooth 4 and left cheek tooth 3–cheek tooth 4 (*arrows*) shows brownish to black discoloration of the dentin. (*Courtesy of* Vladimir Jekl, Brno, Czech Republic; with permission.)

for development of dental caries in chinchillas.[13] Dental plaque formation is a predisposing factor for development of dental caries in other species as well. In chinchillas, elongation of the clinical crowns of the cheek teeth results in the accumulation of large amounts of bacterial plaque, predisposing those species to develop caries lesions.[12]

NEOPLASIA AND PSEUDONEOPLASTIC LESIONS OF THE ORAL CAVITY

The most common tumor associated with the oral cavity and dentition in degus are elodontomas (**Fig. 12**).[2,14,15] Elodontomas are defined as a hamartoma of continuously developing odontogenic tissue and alveolar bone at the periapical bud of elodont teeth.[16] The exact pathophysiology of elodontomas in pet rodents is not clear, but proposed etiologies include trauma, inflammation, age related changes, acquired dental disease, and subsequent impaired (arrested) eruption owing to apical elongation and germinal tooth tissue damage. Base on one of the authors experience (V.J.), the survival time of degus receiving palliative treatment (meloxicam, assist-feeding if necessary, intranasal oxymetazoline drops) following the diagnosis of elodontoma, is 1 day to 1.5 years (median 6 months).

Other tumors seen in oral cavities of degus include melanoma and fibrosarcoma (**Fig 6**D and **13**).[3]

Pseudoodontomas (pseudoneoplastic lesions) are associated with continued deposition of dysplastic tooth structure at the apices of the incisors and premolars, which is responsible for the formation of a space-occupying mass, which in case of maxillary teeth often obstructs the middle or caudal part of the nasal cavity in these species causing intermittent or chronic mild to severe respiratory distress.[14,15]

THE CLINICAL EXAMINATION

Presenting complaints for chinchillas with dental disease include reduced activity or lethargy, reduced food intake, change of food preferences in favor of more easily chewable items, weight loss, and reduced fecal output of smaller irregular fecal pellets. Additional signs and symptoms are wetting and crusting of the fur around the mouth and chin and forefeet (**Fig. 14**). Epiphora, poor fur condition, and fur chewing are also abnormalities commonly associated with dental disease in chinchillas.[1] The presentation in degus is similar to chinchillas, with a lesser incidence of fur chewing, but with a greater incidence of inspiratory dyspnea owing to elodontoma formation or

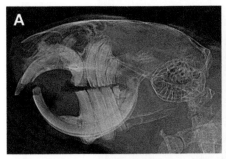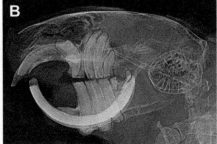

Fig. 12. (*A, B*) Lt 10° V - Rt D oblique lateral skull radiographs of a degu with incisor malocclusion (*mandibular incisors highlighted in yellow*), apical elongation of the mandibular incisors and cheek teeth (*apices highlighted as red lines*). In this case, respiratory problems were associated with a radiodense mass consistent with an elodontoma (*blue*), which obstructed the nasal cavity. (*Courtesy of* Vladimir Jekl, Brno, Czech Republic; with permission.)

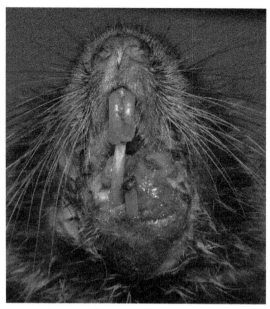

Fig. 13. Fibrosarcoma of the mandible in a 5-year-old degu with displacement of the mandibular left incisor tooth. (*Courtesy of* Vladimir Jekl, Brno, Czech Republic; with permission.)

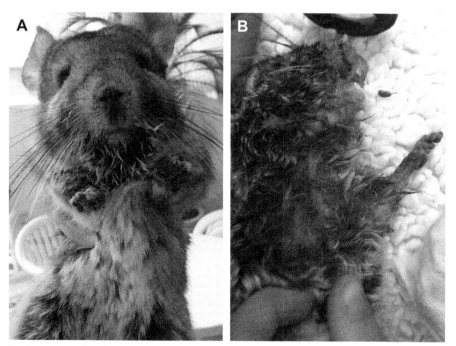

Fig. 14. Hypersalivation secondary to intraoral dental disease in 2 chinchillas. (*A*) Matted fur under the chin. (*B*) Dermatitis, matted fur and alopecia of the lateral aspect of the chin, ventral neck and forelimbs. (*Courtesy of* Christoph Mans, Madison, WI; with permission.)

owing to apical elongation of the first 3 maxillary cheek teeth.[2,14] However, despite severe elongation of reserve and clinical crowns of the cheek teeth, animals may often be able to eat almost normally, and can maintain a good body condition until severe changes and complications (such as soft tissue trauma from sharp dental spikes and/or periodontal infection) have occurred.

The most common clinical findings at physical examination include poor body condition, palpable deformities of the ventral border of the mandible, depigmentation of the normal yellow-orange labial aspect of the incisor teeth (see **Figs. 1** and **5**), overgrowth and abnormal occlusal surface wear of the incisors (see **Figs. 5** and **6**), epiphora, poor fur condition, and saliva-stained skin and fur with crusting and alopecia of the perioral area, the chin, and the forefeet (see **Fig. 14**).[1,2] In chinchillas, apical elongation of maxillary premolars and first molars can in some cases be palpated in the preorbital fossa in a form of bulging areas (see **Fig. 7**). Facial abscesses of periodontal origin are not seen frequently in chinchillas and degus, but may occur (**Fig. 15**).

DIAGNOSTIC IMAGING

Diagnostic imaging of the head is essential for a complete evaluation of dental disease in chinchillas and degus, in particular for the assessment of the reserve crowns. Radiography or computed tomography should be performed whenever possible, because clinical and subclinical stages of dental disease can be missed easily without imaging of the bony structures and of the reserve crowns. However, radiologic modalities do not replace a complete intraoral examination in an anesthetized patient, preferably using an endoscope.

A diagnostic set of radiographs of the head consists of a laterolateral, 2 oblique, and a dorsoventral (or ventrodorsal) projection. The rostrocaudal view is also diagnostic for the temporomandibular joint, the mandibular symphysis, the tympanic bullae, the occlusal plane of cheek teeth and the presence of abnormal spikes, especially maxillary. Also, it may be helpful for imaging of disorders of the nasal cavities. Optimal head positioning is of paramount importance for symmetric projections, because any obliquity could result in misinterpretation of radiographic findings (**Figs. 16–19**). Anatomic reference lines for objective interpretation of skull radiographs and staging of dental disease in chinchillas have been published.[17] Changes in the clinical crown, reserve crown, tooth apex, and alveolar bone need to be recorded as well.

Computed tomography is the preferred imaging technique for evaluation of the skull and teeth in chinchillas and degus (see **Fig. 9**) because it avoids the superimposition of

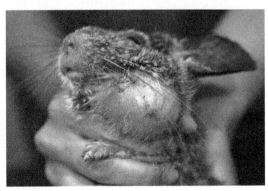

Fig. 15. Odontogenic mandibular abscess in a chinchilla. (*Courtesy of* Christoph Mans, Madison, WI; with permission.)

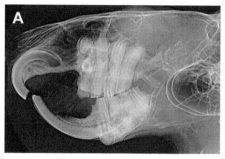
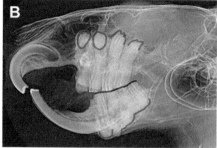

Fig. 16. (*A, B*) Lateral skull radiograph of a chinchilla with advanced stage of dental disease. All cheek teeth show apical elongation (*red lines*), have abnormal structure (loss of radio-dense enamel folds), and have uneven occlusal plane (*blue line*). The reserve crowns of the maxillary cheek teeth are elongated laterally and perforate the cortical bone and the periosteum. Radiographically, this is visible as the presence of a radiolucent line around the apex (*red circles*). The occlusal plane of the incisors is uneven (*yellow lines*) and apical elongation of the mandibular incisors is present. (*Courtesy of* Vladimir Jekl, Brno, Czech Republic; with permission.)

anatomic structures on a single plane, which makes diagnostic interpretation of skull radiographs more challenging. Also, computed tomography is not prone to artifacts caused by positioning of the skull and allows for evaluation of all the structures of the skull including the bones, nasal cavities and ears. However, owing to the small size of degus, the resolution quality of computed tomography imaging might be sub-optimal. Computed tomography should be performed under heavy sedation or general anesthesia for optimal positioning and to minimize motion artifacts.

DENTAL EXAMINATION
Extraoral Examination

A complete extraoral examination should be performed prior the intraoral examination. The extraoral assessment can be performed as part of the physical examination in the conscious patient, or under sedation or general anesthesia. The integument in the area of the medial canthus of the eyes, around the lips, chin, ventral neck, and forearms

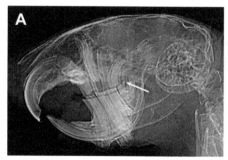
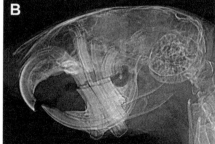

Fig. 17. Left 10° oblique skull radiograph of a degu showing apical and coronal elongation of all cheek teeth and an uneven occlusal plane of the cheek teeth. Bilateral assessment of the occlusal planes of the cheek teeth is possible from this slightly oblique view. (*A*) Spur formation at the distal edge of the mandibular cheek tooth 4 is visible (*arrow*). (*B*) The purple color emphasizes the diseased tooth. Red lines emphasize the location of abnormal apices. (*Courtesy of* Vladimir Jekl, Brno, Czech Republic; with permission.)

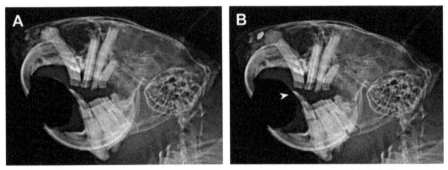

Fig. 18. (*A, B*) Lateral skull radiograph of a degu head that was presented with dyspnea. Radiographs showed severe coronal elongation and apical deformities of cheek teeth with spike formation of the clinical crown of a mandibular check tooth 1 (*arrow*). Diseased apices of all the cheek teeth are clearly visible (*red lines*). The apical radiographic abnormality of a maxillary check tooth 1 was indicative of a dysplastic change (pseudoodontoma, *blue*). The high radiopaque mass within rostral part of the nasal cavity was indicative for chronic inflammatory changes with calcification or for the elodontoma (*green*). Histopathology confirmed the presence of pseudoodontoma of the premolar and elodontoma within the nasal cavity. (*Courtesy of* Vladimir Jekl, Brno, Czech Republic; with permission.)

should be evaluated for alopecia, matted fur, or other abnormalities commonly seen in animals with dental disease. The incisor teeth should be evaluated for normal position, occlusion, and wear, as well as coloration (see **Figs. 1, 5** and **6**). Palpation of the head should focus on asymmetry of the muscles, eye globes, and swelling of hard and soft tissues (see **Figs. 7** and **15**). Special attention should be paid to palpation of the ventral aspect of the mandibles, because apical elongation will result in deformity of the cortices and palpable protrusions. In chinchillas, apical elongation of rostral cheek teeth may be palpated in the preorbital fossa as hard bulging areas (see **Fig. 7**).

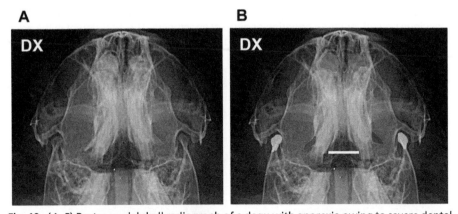

Fig. 19. (*A, B*) Rostrocaudal skull radiograph of a degu with anorexia owing to severe dental disease and dyspnea associated with pseudoodontoma and elodontoma formation. (*B*) Dysplastic reserve crowns and apices of maxillary cheek teeth (*indicative for dysplastic changes, blue*); condyles of the temporomandibular joints (*yellow*) and dental spurs on the maxillary cheek teeth (*red*). The white line displays the normal length (*height*) of the clinical crown in a degu. Histopathology confirmed the presence of a pseudoodontoma (*Courtesy of* Vladimir Jekl, Brno, Czech Republic; with permission.)

Intraoral Examination

General anesthesia

Although inspection of the oral cavity can be performed in the conscious patient using a pediatric laryngoscope, otoscope, or vaginoscope, it does not replace the examination under anesthesia. An intraoral examination in a conscious chinchilla or degu cannot rule out intraoral disease, considering that up to 50% of intraoral lesions can be missed.[1]

Premedication and induction of anesthesia can be performed using the intramuscular administration of the combination of midazolam (0.3–0.4 mg/kg), ketamine (4–5 mg/kg), and butorphanol (0.3 mg/kg). The patient is then maintained on isoflurane (1.5%–2.5%). Alternatively, a combination of dexmedetomidine (0.015 mg/kg) and ketamine (4–5 mg/kg) administered intramuscularly can be used to induce anesthesia in chinchillas, which is suitable for an intraoral examination and treatment of approximately 45–60 minutes.[18] No isoflurane supplementation is required for this protocol, but oxygen supplementation should be provided (eg, by face mask). During anesthesia, the patient should be provided supplemental heat and closely monitored.

Equipment for intraoral examination

Dedicated equipment is necessary in order to perform a complete intraoral examination in chinchillas and degus. The table top mouth gag (**Fig. 20**) is the preferred instrument for positioning the patient. If a standard mouth gag is used, an assistant is needed to position and hold the patient in place throughout the intraoral examination and treatment. Delicate lightweight mouth gags are preferred for chinchillas and degus. Although standard small cheek dilators with short wings can be used, the authors prefer the use of mouth gags with tapered or open wings (**Fig. 21**), which are easier to place into the mouth of chinchillas and degus. A small metal spatula (**Fig. 22**A) or a tongue depressor split in half should be used to manipulate the tongue and other soft tissues. A small dental probe is used to assess the cheek teeth for mobility, to remove entrapped debris and to probe gingival pockets. Standard sized cotton-tipped applicators can be used to remove food and saliva from the oral cavity, but smaller applicators are preferred (**Fig. 22**B). A more efficient way to remove debris and saliva is by use of a suction unit. Small plastic suction tips (**Fig. 22**C) can be used

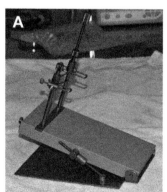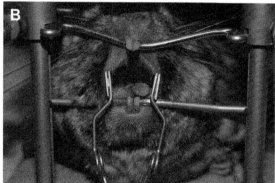

Fig. 20. (*A*) Table top mouth gag for rabbits and rodents. This dental table has adjustable horizontal bars acting as a mouth gag. (*B*) Chinchilla under general anesthesia positioned on the table top mouth gag with a cheek dilator in place. The face mask used for delivery of oxygen has been removed for demonstration purpose. (*Courtesy of* Christoph Mans, Madison, WI; with permission.)

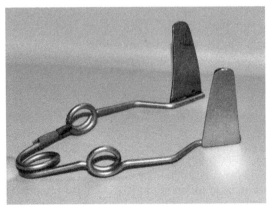

Fig. 21. Small cheek dilator with tapered wings, suitable for chinchillas and degus. (*Courtesy of* Christoph Mans, Madison, WI; with permission.)

in the narrow oral cavity. Suction allows for thorough cleaning of the oral cavity and of gingival pockets in particular, as well as removal of fluids used for rinsing.

Stomatoscopy

Endoscopy-guided intraoral examination (stomatoscopy) provides superior visibility and increases the chance for detection of pathologic lesions, by providing illumination and magnification of the intraoral structures (see **Figs. 2**, **3**, and **10**). Stomatoscopy also greatly simplifies intraoral treatment, and allows for documentation of intraoral findings. Stomatoscopy is considered mandatory by the authors for a complete intraoral examination in chinchillas and degus, and should be considered the standard of care.

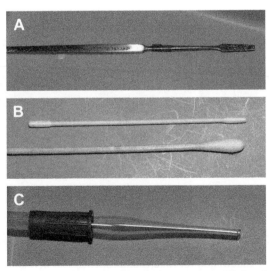

Fig. 22. Equipment for intraoral examination and treatment. (*A*) Small metal spatula. (*B*) Cotton-tipped applicators. Note the small applicator, which is more suitable for chinchillas and degus. (*C*) Small suction tip. (*Courtesy of* Christoph Mans, Madison, WI; with permission.)

Different rigid endoscopes are suitable for stomatoscopy (**Fig. 23**). Telescopes with a 30° viewing angle are more versatile, but telescopes or videootoscopes with a straight nonangled view can also be used, but they do not allow detailed examination of occlusal surfaces of the cheek teeth or gingival pockets. For examination of these structures and to examine cheek tooth extraction sites, a 70° endoscope is most well-suited. The authors prefer using telescopes with a diameter of 4 mm, which can be used safely without the need for a protective sheath.

The intraoral examination includes thorough evaluation of the soft tissues (lips, tongue, gingiva, and oropharynx). Common abnormalities include cheilitis or ulceration of the buccal mucosa, gingival hyperplasia, and gingival pockets (**Fig. 24**) with associated periodontal disease (see **Fig. 10**). The next step is to verify that all clinical crowns of cheek teeth are present (see **Figs. 2** and **3**; **Fig. 25**). A missing cheek tooth can be congenital (see **Fig. 25A**) or secondary to tooth resorption (see **Fig. 25B**). Any food material and impacted food debris in between interproximal spaces should be removed before evaluation of the cheek teeth. The most common acquired dental disease is represented by tooth resorption leading to fractures of the clinical crowns (especially in degus). Periodontal disease leads to widened interproximal spaces (see **Figs. 10** and **25B**) followed by impaction of food debris. All cheek teeth should be examined carefully for elongation of clinical crowns, malocclusion, mobility, and presence of fractures of other pathologies such as dental caries (see **Figs. 10** and **24**; **Figs. 26** and **27**). The clinical crowns of cheek teeth in chinchillas are very short and almost at level of the gingival sulcus with a nearly horizontal occlusal plane (see **Fig. 2**). They should also be assessed for mobility, periodontal disease, caries and resorptive lesions (see **Fig. 11**). Sharp dental spikes, in particular those arising from the maxillary cheek teeth and directed buccally, may be easily overlooked if they are covered by the buccal mucosa (see **Figs. 24B, 26**, and **27E**). The authors recommend sliding a spatula along the buccal aspect of the maxillary cheek teeth to ensure that no buccal spurs are present (see **Fig. 25A**). All findings of the oral examination should be recorded for each patient. If the endoscopy unit is equipped with a recording system, photographs of intraoral findings can be included in the medical records.

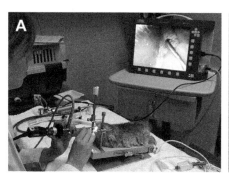 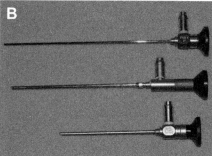

Fig. 23. (*A, B*) Endoscopy-guided intraoral examination (stomatoscopy) in a chinchilla under general anesthesia. The face mask used for delivery of oxygen has been removed for demonstration purposes. (*B*) Different types of rigid endoscopes suitable for stomatoscopy. Note the different lengths and viewing angles (top to bottom: 0°, 30°, and 70°). The 30° viewing angle is the most versatile viewing angle, although a 70° viewing angle allows for better visualization of the occlusal surfaces, interproximal spaces, and periodontal pockets. (*Courtesy of* Christoph Mans, Madison, WI; with permission.)

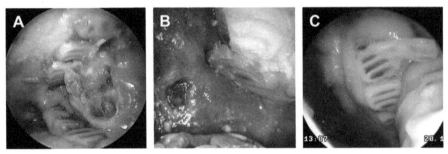

Fig. 24. Soft tissue disorders of the oral cavity secondary to dental disease in chinchillas. (*A*) Large and deep ulceration of the buccal mucosa secondary to buccal spurs of the left maxillary cheek tooth 2 and 3. (*B*) Deep ulceration of the buccal mucosa after a spur of the fourth right maxillary cheek tooth. (*C*) Gingival hyperplasia of the left maxillary cheek teeth. Note the large buccal spur of the first cheek tooth. (*Courtesy of* Christoph Mans, Madison, WI; with permission.)

TREATMENT

Any hyporexic or anorexic patient will likely progress to dehydration, ketoacidosis, and may frequently develop hepatic lipidosis. Stabilization of the patient is therefore of paramount importance before planning and performing any dental procedure under general anesthesia.

The primary goal of any dental treatment in chinchillas and degus is to restore the patients' ability to chew and eat sufficient amounts of food. This is accomplished by reducing coronal elongation, which prevents normal wear and causes soft tissue trauma. Complications such as infections associated with the teeth should be addressed as well. Prognosis should be discussed extensively with the owners because long-term or definitive cure of diseased elodont teeth is rarely achieved in

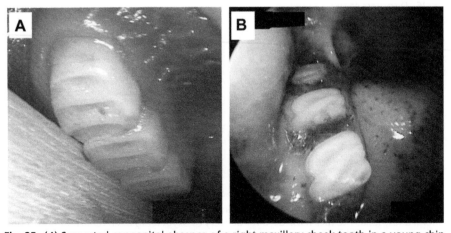

Fig. 25. (*A*) Suspected congenital absence of a right maxillary cheek tooth in a young chinchilla. Note that the interproximal spaces are not wider than normal. (*B*) Widened interproximal spaces and food impaction after acquired loss of the of a right mandibular cheek tooth in a chinchilla secondary to complete tooth resorption. (*Courtesy of* Christoph Mans, Madison, WI; with permission.)

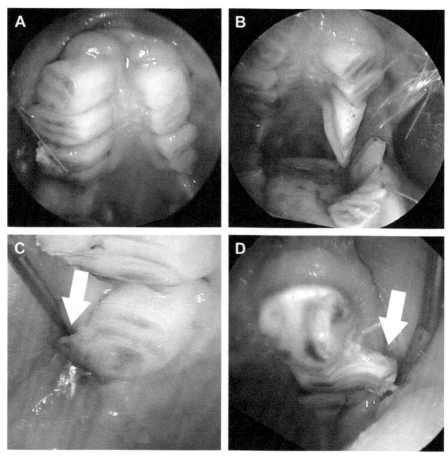

Fig. 26. Disorders of the cheek teeth in chinchillas. (*A*) Coronal elongation and malocclusion of the maxillary cheek teeth and gingival hyperplasia. (*B*) Excessive coronal elongation and malocclusion of the left maxillary (in particular cheek tooth 3 and cheek tooth 4) and mandibular cheek teeth (in particular cheek tooth 4). (*C*) Sharp buccal spur of the right maxillary cheek tooth 4 (*arrow*). These spurs are easily missed and cause trauma to the buccal mucosa. (*D*) Buccal spur of the left maxillary check tooth 2 (*arrow*). (*Courtesy of* Christoph Mans, Madison, WI; with permission.)

these species. Repeated dental treatments, usually for the remainder of the patients' life, are necessary to successfully manage most dental diseases in chinchillas and degus.

Intraoral always require general anesthesia and should never be performed in awake or inadequately anesthetized animals. Minor dental procedures, such as coronal reduction of incisor teeth, can be performed in the patient under heavy sedation.

Treatment of Incisor Teeth Disorders

Coronal reduction of incisor teeth and correction of the occlusal plane can be performed with a diamond or carbon cutting disc (**Fig. 28**) mounted on a low-speed straight dental hand piece (~30,000 rpm). A safety shield to protect the rotating burr (see **Fig. 28**) should be used whenever possible. Adjacent tissues should also be protected using a lingual spatula or a tongue depressor.

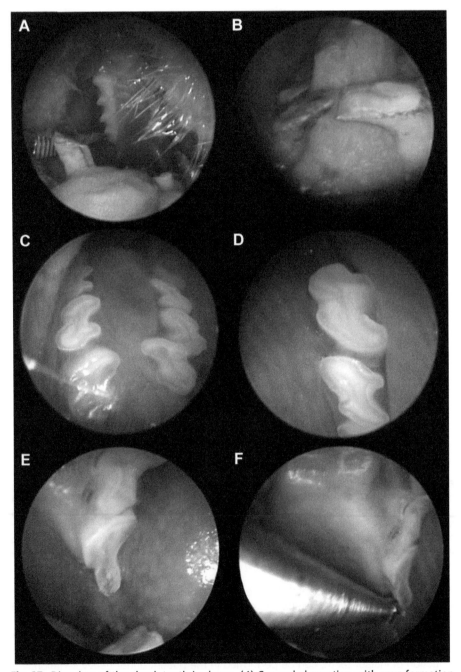

Fig. 27. Disorders of the cheek teeth in degus. (*A*) Coronal elongation with spur formation of the right mandibular first cheek tooth. (*B*) Bilateral coronal elongation of mandibular check tooth 1, with typical formation of a "bridge" and subsequent entrapment of the tongue. (*C, D*) Coronal elongation and lingual displacement of the clinical crowns of mandibular check tooth 1 with widening of the interproximal spaces (*D*). (*E*) Spike formation at the distal aspect of the left maxillary cheek tooth 4. (*F*) These spikes should be removed carefully, using a fine burr to prevent the risk of soft tissue injury and severe bleeding. (*Courtesy of* Vladimir Jekl, Brno, Czech Republic; with permission.)

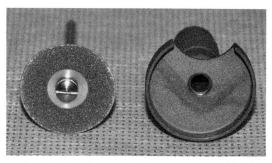

Fig. 28. Diamond cutting disc (*left*) and soft tissue protector (*right*) suitable for coronal reduction of the incisor teeth. (*Courtesy of* Christoph Mans, Madison, WI; with permission.)

Extraction of incisor teeth is rarely indicated in chinchillas and degus. Periapical infection, severe malocclusion, and elodontomas in degus are possible indications for the extraction of the incisor teeth. Extraction should only be performed after diagnostic imaging of the skull has been completed, in order to assess the shape of the incisor teeth as well as to evaluate for lytic or osteoproliferative changes. Luxators for incisor teeth suitable for rabbits are too large to be used in most rodent species; therefore, contoured needles (18-G) are preferred. Extraction of mandibular incisors can be facilitated by lateral osteotomy of the mandible, especially when periapical infection is present. The location of the skin incision is lateral to the incisive portion of the mandible and the bone over the apical (distal) part of the reserve crown is drilled out using dental burr. Particular attention must be paid during luxation of mandibular incisors to avoid iatrogenic displacement of the mandibular symphysis, especially in degus.

Treatment of of Cheek Teeth Disorders

Coronal reduction of the cheek teeth and correction of the occlusal plane from spurs and other irregular shapes can be performed using a diamond or silicon carbide burr (see **Fig. 27**F; **Fig. 29**) mounted on a low-speed straight dental hand piece

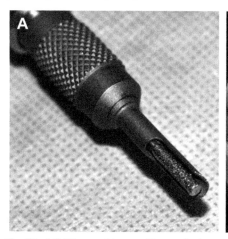
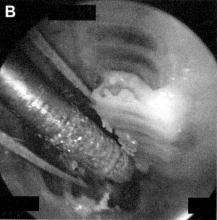

Fig. 29. (*A*) Diamond burr with a soft tissue protector mounted on a straight hand piece. This instrument is suitable coronal reduction of the cheek teeth. (*B*) Diamond burr with soft tissue protector used to remove buccal spurs of the right maxillary cheek teeth in a chinchilla. Note that the soft tissue protector prevents iatrogenic damage of the buccal mucosa. (*Courtesy of* Christoph Mans, Madison, WI; with permission.)

(~30,000 rpm). High-speed hand pieces are not recommended, because they are angled and cannot be placed in the oral cavity properly. A soft tissue protector is available and should be used whenever possible (see **Fig. 29**). However, care should be taken to avoid entrapment of the tip of the tongue between the burr and the protector, because this can lead to severe injury. Fissure cut burrs may be required if a large amount of coronal substance needs to be removed, but the risk of iatrogenic soft tissue trauma and tooth fracture is greater compared with the use of diamond burrs. In case of the degus' small oral cavity, the standard dental equipment may not be suitable. Even if the table top mouth gag can be used in the degus, standard forceps or a hemostat can replace the mouth gag. Forceps can also be used as cheek dilator or tongue depressor. The soft tissue protector is usually too big, so the use of the naked burr may be the only option.

The elongated clinical crowns should be reduced in height to a physiologic length whenever possible (**Fig. 30**). Sharp spurs should be removed to promote healing of soft tissue (see **Figs. 24, 26, 27, and 29B**). Gingival hyperplasia surrounding the maxillary cheek teeth is typical of chinchillas suffering from dental disease (see **Figs. 10F and 24C; Fig. 31**). It makes coronal reduction more difficult or suboptimal, because shortening of the clinical crowns at the gingival level is not sufficient. Resection of the hyperplastic gingival tissue using an electrocautery (gingivectomy) might be an option to allow adequate adjustment of the maxillary cheek teeth (see **Fig. 31**B). Coronal reduction below or to the gum level is not recommended because chewing over the gum is painful, discouraging the patient to chew. Any soft tissue trauma could lead to unnecessary pain; excessive salivation and prolonged recovery, so care must be taken when using dental burrs. Moreover, there should be no contact of the burr shank/hand piece with the lips or soft tissues because heat and abrasion produced by the rotating instrument causing local inflammatory and/or ulcerative reactions could result.

Extraction of cheek teeth may be indicated in cases of severe dental disease, but complete extraction is challenging because of apical elongation and frequently present ankylosis to the surrounding bone. These cases frequently need a combined intraoral and extraoral approach for complete extraction. Extraoral approach consists of the skin incision over the affected area, exposure of the bone, periosteum elevation, drilling of the hole in the affected bone, removal of the affected tooth and surrounding tissue, alveolar debridement, and wound marsupialization. In the case of maxillary premolars/molars, the rostral part of the zygomatic arch need to be removed

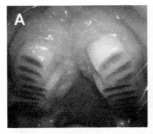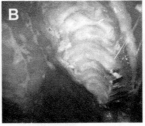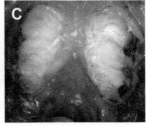

Fig. 30. Coronal reduction of the maxillary cheek teeth in a chinchilla. (*A*) Abnormal coronal elongation and malocclusion of the cheek teeth, with gingival hyperplasia and abnormal bending of the occlusal planes. (*B*) Intermediate step of incomplete coronal reduction of the left maxillary cheek teeth. (*C*) Occlusal plane after coronal reduction of the elongated maxillary cheek teeth. Note the iatrogenic gingival trauma, which can occur if gingival hyperplasia is present. (*Courtesy of* Christoph Mans, Madison, WI; with permission.)

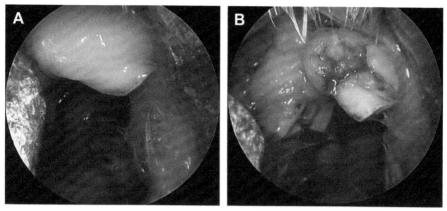

Fig. 31. Resection of hyperplastic gingiva in a chinchilla to allow adequate coronal reduction of the maxillary cheek teeth. (*A*) Gingival hyperplasia surrounding the left maxillary check tooth 1 (*B*) Appearance after gingivectomy using monopolar electrosurgery. (*Courtesy of* Sue Chen.)

(ostectomy) first. When retrobulbar abscessation is present, enucleation needs to be considered.

Treatment of Periodontal Disease

Intraoral treatment of periodontal disease is challenging owing to the small size of the oral cavity and the advanced stage often present at the time of diagnosis. Treatment aims to reduce periodontal infection resulting in reduced intraoral pain, followed by increased food intake. Therapy of periodontal disease consists of both local and systemic treatment.

Local treatment

During the intraoral examination, retained food debris should be removed, and any interproximal spaces cleaned and probed (**Fig. 32**). If periodontal pockets or periodontal infection are present, the lesions should be carefully flushed with an antiseptic solution. One of the authors (C.M.) prefers the use of 3% hydrogen peroxide owing to its foaming action (see **Fig. 32**C), which leads to superior retention (minimizing the risk of aspiration) and debriding action at the site of application compared with other products such as chlorhexidine solution. Moreover, hydrogen peroxide has specific antimicrobial properties so it may help to control periodontal infection and dental plaque formation. Another option is to use a mechanical scaler to remove as much as plaque as possible, followed by flushing with diluted chlorhexidine (0.125%) after packing the oropharynx with gauze. The local application of sustained-release antibiotics is common both in human and small animal dentistry for treatment of periodontal disease (see **Fig. 32**E, F).[19] Biodegradable antibiotic formulations are available, administered subgingivally in deep pockets, and provide high antimicrobial concentrations for several weeks.[19] Doxycycline (Doxirobe, Pfizer Animal Health, New York, NY) is the most commonly used local antibiotic in veterinary dentistry, and is available as a commercial product for veterinary use. This product is a biodegradable liquid, which solidifies on contact with fluids, providing a physical barrier and thereby aiding to prevent reimpaction of gingival pockets with food material and related bacteria. Through its antimicrobial efficacy, it promotes gingival healing (see **Fig. 32**). Doxirobe should be applied within deep periodontal pockets to increase the chance of long-term retention.

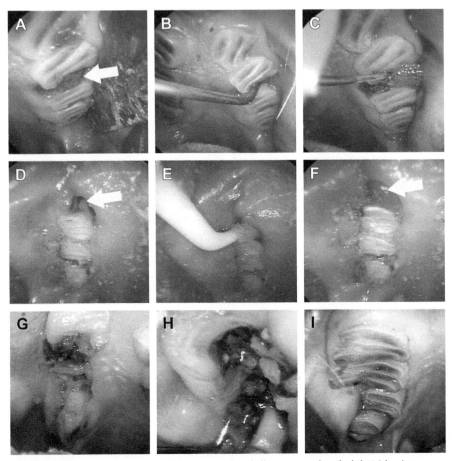

Fig. 32. Treatment of periodontal disease in chinchillas. Case 1 (*A–C*). (*A*) Wider interproximal space between left maxillary cheek teeth 2 and cheek tooth 3 leading to food impaction and predisposition to periodontal disease (*arrow*). (*B*) Removal of food debris using a probe (*C*) Application of 3% hydrogen peroxide for lavage and disinfection of the periodontal pocket. Case 2 (*D–F*). (*D*) Missing crown of right maxillary check tooth 1 of the right resulting in a deep periodontal pocket (*arrow*). (*E*) Subgingival instillation of a doxycycline-containing sustained-release biodegradable liquid (Doxirobe) into the periodontal pocket. (*F*) Appearance after application of Doxirobe. The initially liquid hardens and prevents impaction of the periodontal pocket with food debris. Case 3 (*G–I*). (*G*) Severe periodontal disease, partial tooth resorption, food impaction, and gingival hyperplasia of the right maxillary arcade. (*H*) Gingival and periodontal disease after extraction of mobile and diseased clinical crowns, and lavage of the periodontal pockets with 3% hydrogen peroxide. (*I*) Follow-up 4 months after local and systemic treatment of periodontal disease. The cheek teeth have regrown and periodontal disease is no longer present. Note the reduction of gingival hyperplasia. (*Courtesy of* Christoph Mans, Madison, WI; with permission.)

Systemic treatment

Periodontal pathogenic bacteria in rodents and lagomorphs are usually mixed aerobic/anaerobic populations.[20] Antimicrobial drugs should be chosen based on their efficacy against anaerobic bacteria after culture/sensitivity tests and the ability to reach high concentration in bones. Systemic antimicrobial treatment should be considered for any chinchilla affected by periodontal disease at advanced stage as an adjunct to local antibiotic treatment. Parenteral long-acting penicillin G benzathine/procaine combination (50,000 IU/kg subcutaneously every 3-5 days) has been used extensively by one the authors (C.M.). It has shown to be effective and safe in chinchillas. Penicillin G provides excellent coverage against anaerobic bacteria and reaches high levels in bones.[20] The duration of treatment depends on severity of periodontal disease. One author (V.J.) routinely uses a combination of doxycycline (5 mg/kg every 12 hour) and metronidazole (30 mg/kg every 24 hours) orally for 10 to 14 days. However, the duration of treatment is variable and depends on severity.

Other antibiotic drugs, effective against anaerobic bacteria and safe in chinchillas and degus, include chloramphenicol and azithromycin. Trimethoprim-sulfonamide (30 mg/kg every 12 hours for 7–12 days) and enrofloxacin (10 mg/kg every 12 hours for 7–14 days) should not be used unless administered as an adjunct to antibiotic treatment effective against anaerobic bacteria.

Treatment of Caries

No treatment guidelines for dental caries in chinchillas have been established. Diseased tooth substance should be removed using a burr, to a level where healthy tooth substance is apparent (**Fig. 33**), followed by restoration of the normal occlusal surface. A ball-tipped diamond burr works best for this treatment (see **Fig. 33**B). Application of diluted chlorhexidine to the tooth surfaces, using cotton-tipped applicators, is also recommended to remove plaque.

Treatment of Pseudoodontomas and Elodontomas

Surgical treatment of maxillary pseudoodontoma is very challenging and includes lateral or dorsal rhinotomy and removal of the affected tooth. In the case of elodontoma, complete removal (if possible) of the tumor is indicated. In most cases, gentle tumor debulking is an alternative treatment of choice.

SUPPORTIVE TREATMENT

After dental treatment, patients should receive nutritional support of syringe-fed critical care formula and parenteral fluid therapy, as well as pain management. Monitoring urine pH and ketones is a noninvasive and inexpensive method to assess if nutritional support is adequate.

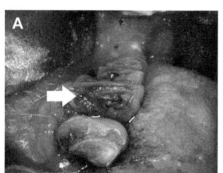 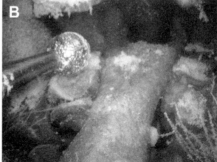

Fig. 33. Treatment of caries in a chinchilla. (*A*) Periodontal disease and caries lesion of the second right mandibular cheek tooth (check tooth 2, *arrow*). (*B*) Removal of the diseased tooth substance using a ball-tipped diamond burr. Note the appearance of healthy tooth substance after removal of the caries lesion. (*Courtesy of* Christoph Mans, Madison, WI; with permission.)

After dental treatment, nutrition should be adjusted to provide optimal Ca:P ratio (about 1.5:1), a high-quality and high-fiber diet (such as grass hay, a combination of meadow and alfalfa hay, fruit tree branches) and intake of sufficient amount of nutrients by feeding optimal pelleted food. Chinchillas and degus may remain anorexic after the treatment of dental disease, because hepatic lipidosis and ketoacidosis are very common sequelae of anorexia in these species. Therefore, ensuring sufficient food intake is critical to allow animals to recover and resume normal food intake.

If the underlying dental pathology prevents ingestion of hay, then the long-term management of animals with chronic dental disease should include provision of a diet that is easier to chew, such as soaked alfa-alfa pellets. In some cases, daily assisted feeding of small amount of commercially available convalescence diet for herbivores (Oxbow Critical Care, Lafeber/Emeraid Critical Care, Supreme Recovery, etc) is necessary. Analgesia should be provided if a painful condition is present. However, limited information is available on the efficacy of analgesic drugs in chinchillas and degus.

REFERENCES

1. Jekl V, Hauptman K, Knotek Z. Quantitative and qualitative assessments of intraoral lesions in 180 small herbivorous mammals. Vet Rec 2008;162(14):442–9.
2. Jekl V, Hauptman K, Knotek Z. Diseases in pet degus: a retrospective study in 300 animals. J Small Anim Pract 2011;52(2):107–12.
3. Crossley DA, Miguelez MM. Skull size and cheek-tooth length in wild-caught and captive-bred chinchillas. Arch Oral Biol 2001;46(10):919–28.
4. Martin T. Phylogenetic implications of glires (Eurymylidae, Mimotonidae, Rodentia, Lagomorpha) incisor enamel microstructure. Zoosyst Evol 1999;75(2):257–73.
5. Crossley DA. Clinical aspects of rodental dental anatomy. J Vet Dent 1995;12(4): 131–5.
6. Cox PG, Rayfield EJ, Fagan MJ, et al. Functional evolution of the feeding system in rodents. PLoS One 2012;7(4):e36299.
7. Olivares AI, Verzi DH, Vassallo AI. Masticatory morphological diversity and chewing modes in South American caviomorph rodents (family Octodontidae). J Zool 2004;263(2):167–77.
8. Humme ID. Gut morphology, body size and digestive performance in rodents. In: Chivers DJ, Langer P, editors. The digestive system in mammals. 1st edition. Cambridge (United Kingdom): Cambridge University Press; 1994. p. 315–23.
9. Becerra F, Vassallo AI, Echeverria AI, et al. Scaling and adaptations of incisors and cheek teeth in caviomorph rodents (Rodentia, Hystricognathi). J Morphol 2012;273(10):1150–62.
10. Crossley DA. Dental disease in chinchillas in the UK. J Small Anim Pract 2001; 42(1):12–9.
11. Jekl V, Gumpenberger M, Jeklova E, et al. Impact of pelleted diets with different mineral compositions on the crown size of mandibular cheek teeth and mandibular relative density in degus (Octodon degus). Vet Rec 2011;168(24):641.
12. Crossley DA. Dental disease in chinchillas. Manchester (United Kingdom): Department of Dental Medicine and Surgery, University of Manchester; 2003.
13. Crossley DA, Dubielzig RR, Benson KG. Caries and odontoclastic resorptive lesions in a chinchilla (Chinchilla lanigera). Vet Rec 1997;141(13):337–9.
14. Jekl V, Zikmund T, K. H. Dyspnea in a degu (Octodon degu) associated with maxillary cheek teeth elongation. J Exotic Pet Med 2016;25(2):128–32.

15. Jekl V, Hauptman K, Skoric M, et al. Elodontoma in a Degu (Octodon degus). J Exot Pet Med 2008;17(3):216–20.
16. Boy SC, Steenkamp G. Odontoma-like tumours of squirrel elodont incisors–elodontomas. Journal of comparative pathology 2006;135(1):56–61.
17. Boehmer E, Crossley D. Objective interpretation of dental disease in rabbits, guinea pigs and chinchillas. Use of anatomical reference lines. Tieraerztliche Praxis 2009;37(K)(4):250–60.
18. Fox L, Snyder L, Mans C. Comparison of dexmedetomidine-ketamine with isoflurane for anesthesia of chinchillas (Chinchilla lanigera). J Am Assoc Lab Anim Sci 2016;55:312–6.
19. Zetner K, Rothmueller G. Treatment of periodontal pockets with doxycycline in beagles. Veterinary therapeutics: research in applied veterinary medicine 2002;3(4):441–52.
20. Tyrrell KL, Citron DM, Jenkins JR, et al. Periodontal bacteria in rabbit mandibular and maxillary abscesses. J Clin Microbiol 2002;40(3):1044–7.

Anatomy and Disorders of the Oral Cavity of Rat-like and Squirrel-like Rodents

 CrossMark

Elisabetta Mancinelli, DVM, CertZooMed, DECZM (Small Mammal)[a,*],
Vittorio Capello, DVM, DECZM (Small Mammal), DABVP-ECM[b,c]

KEYWORDS

• Myomorphs • Sciuromorphs • Dental disease • Pseudo-odontoma • Elodontoma

KEY POINTS

• The order *Rodentia* is the largest and most diversified mammalian group, comprising approximately 40% of all mammalian species, differing widely in size, behavior, feeding habits, anatomy, and physiology.
• All rodent species have 2 well-developed maxillary and mandibular aradicular incisor teeth, which represent the most distinguishable dental feature of this order.
• Myomorphs and sciuromorphs have elodont incisors and anelodont cheek teeth, whereas hystrychomorphs have full anelodont dentition.
• Odontogenic tumors and tumor-like lesions (odontomas, complex odontomas and elodontomas) affecting incisor teeth are frequently seen in sciuromorph rodents, including pseudo-odontoma in prarie dogs. Challenging surgical approaches may be required for treatment.
• The use of computed tomography is particularly useful and has great advantages compared with standard radiography.

INTRODUCTION

The order *Rodentia* represents the largest and most diverse mammalian group, comprising approximately 40% of all mammal species. These animals differ vastly in habitat, body size, feeding habits (omnivore to specialized herbivore), dietary requirements, behavior, anatomy, and physiology. The past decade has seen an exponential increase in the number of certain rodent species, such as rats, mice, hamsters, gerbils, prairie dogs, and squirrels, being owned as pets. Rodent owners are increasingly expecting the same high-quality veterinary care to be afforded to their valued

The authors have nothing to disclose.
[a] Bath Referrals, Rosemary Lodge Veterinary Hospital, Bath, Wellsway, Somerset BA2 5RL, UK;
[b] Clinica Veterinaria S.Siro, Via Lampugnano, 99, Milano 20151, Italy; [c] Clinica Veterinaria Gran Sasso, Via Donatello, 26, Milano 20134, Italy
* Corresponding author.
E-mail address: eli2705@gmail.com

vetexotic.theclinics.com

companion as is provided to dogs and cats. The approach to oral disorders in these animals can be in part extrapolated from other more common rodent species such as guinea pigs, and from rabbits; however, specific information regarding their natural feeding habits along with a knowledge of their dental and oral anatomy and physiology is essential. Appropriate diagnostic testing and imaging techniques are also necessary to obtain a definitive diagnosis, formulate a prognosis, and develop a treatment plan. In particular, pseudo-odontomas of prairie dogs require an intimate understanding of their anatomy, as they pose a unique challenge regarding anesthetic protocols and surgical treatment.

TAXONOMY OF RODENT SPECIES

The order *Rodentia* (from the Latin word *rodere*, ie, "to gnaw")[1] is the largest and most diversified mammalian group, comprising approximately 40% of all mammalian species (more than 2000) differing widely in size, behavior, feeding habits, anatomy, and physiology.[2] These hundreds of species are grouped in 3 suborders based on the anatomic and functional differences of the masseter muscles: the *Caviomorpha* or *Hystrichomorpha* (otherwise named "porcupine-like", "cavy-like" or "guinea pig–like" rodents, such as the guinea pig, chinchilla, and degu), the *Myomorpha* ("rat-like" or "mouse-like" rodents), and the *Sciuromorpha* ("squirrel-like"rodents).[3]

Members of the rat-like group include many species commonly kept as pets, such as the rat (*Rattus norvegicus*), the Golden or Syrian hamster (*Mesocricetus auratus*), the Russian hamsters (*Phodopus sungorus, Phodopus campbelli, Phodopus roborovskii*), the Chinese hamster (*Cricetulus griseus*), the mouse (*Mus musculus*), the gerbil (*Meriones unguiculatus*) and the Duprasi or "fat-tailed" gerbil (*Pachyuromys duprasi*). The sciuromorph group includes the prairie dog (*Cynomys ludovicianus*), the European ground squirrel (*Spermophilus citellus*), the Richardson ground squirrel (*Spermophilus richardsonii*), and the chipmunk (*Tamias striatus, Eutamias sibiricus*),[3] which are less commonly kept as pets.[4]

ANATOMY AND PHYSIOLOGY OF DENTITION AND MASTICATION

All rodent species have 2 well-developed maxillary and mandibular elodont aradicular (continually growing and erupting throughout life, which lack an anatomic root) incisor teeth, which represent the most distinguishable dental feature of this order.[1,5] They lack canine teeth, and incisors are separated from premolars by a long toothless space named *diastema*.[3] Unlike rabbits, rodents are monophyodont (having a single set of teeth) and *simplicidentata* (having just 1 pair of maxillary incisors).[1,3,5,6] The incisor teeth have a chisel-shaped occlusal surface and are covered by enamel only over the labial surface. The enamel is characteristically pigmented yellow-orange in most rodents. In cavy-like rodents, all teeth are elodont. Also, premolar and molar teeth are anatomically similar in this group, and are commonly named "cheek teeth".[1,3] A remarkable difference between rat-like and squirrel-like rodent species is that the first group lacks premolar teeth. This is not clinically relevant, but results in diverse dental formulas (**Figs. 1** and **2**). Different from hystrichomorphs, squirrel-like and rat-like rodents have anelodont premolar and/or molar teeth. They are truly rooted (with a limited growth period), single or multiple rooted, and are not worn during normal chewing activity. They are brachyodont (short crowned) with multiple cusps. Depending on species, premolars and molars have more or less different size and shape in the same quadrant. The premolar and molar teeth of prairie dogs and other herbivorous ground squirrels have multiple roots. Molar teeth of myomorphs also have multiple roots. The crown has cusps and ridges that create a rough occlusal surface.[7]

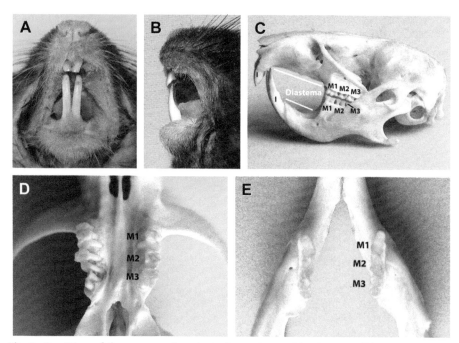

Fig. 1. Dentition of the myomorph rodents shown in a golden hamster *(Mesocricetus auratus)*. (A) Labial aspect of the clinical crowns of incisor teeth. The enamel is yellow-orange. Divergence between mandibular incisors is variable due to the incomplete ossification and the flexibility of the mandibular symphysis. (B) Lateral (distal) aspect of incisor teeth. Clinical crowns are white because the enamel does not cover the distal, mesial, and lingual/palatal aspects of incisor teeth. Note the chisel-shaped occlusal plane and the enognathic appearance of the mandible. (C) Lateral view of the skull and jaws shown on a bony specimen displaying the long diastema and the anelodont, multiple rooted molar teeth. Unlike squirrel-like rodents, rat-like rodents lack premolar teeth. (D) Close up of the maxilla from the ventrodorsal view and (E) of the mandible from the dorsoventral view, displaying the molar teeth. Multiple roots are also visible in (D). (*Courtesy of* Vittorio Capello, DVM, Milano, Italy; with permission.)

Regardless of these differences, the premolar and/or molar cheek teeth of myomorph and sciuromorph rodents are commonly named "cheek teeth" as well.

From an anatomic, physiologic, and clinical standpoint, the rat-like and squirrel-like groups can be merged into a single group, making the 3 suborders of rodents into 2 groups: cavy-like rodents with full elodont dentition (most similar to lagomorphs), and all the other rodents with elodont incisors but anelodont cheek teeth.

The dental formulas of selected rat-like and squirrel-like rodent species are listed in **Table 1**.

Several rodent species, such as hamsters and squirrels, have para-oral structures between the jaws and the cheek, representing an important anatomic feature: the cheek pouches. Cheek pouches are paired, thin-walled, highly vascular, sac-like evaginations of the oral cavity. The pouch actually consists of 4 layers: keratinized stratified squamous epithelium, lamina propria, skeletal muscle, and adventitial connective tissue. The inner surface is covered by mucosa. These distensible, loose cutaneous structures can stretch dorso-caudally along the lateral aspects of the mandible from the mouth over the shoulder regions ventral to the ears.[8,9] Cheek pouches allow

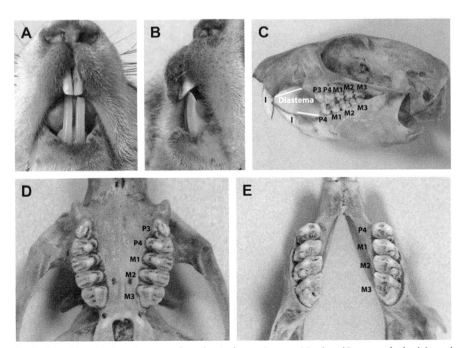

Fig. 2. Dentition of the sciuromorph rodents shown in a prairie dog (*Cynomys ludovicianus*). (*A*) Labial aspect of the clinical crowns of incisor teeth. The enamel is yellow-orange. Divergence or slight separation between mandibular incisors is variable, and due to the incomplete ossification and the flexibility of the mandibular symphysis. (*B*) Lateral (distal) aspect of incisor teeth. The enamel covers the distal and mesial aspects of incisor teeth. Note the chisel-shaped occlusal plane and the enognathic appearance of the mandible. (*C*) Lateral view of the skull and jaws shown on a bony specimen, displaying the long diastema and the crowns with multiple cusps of anelodont premolar and molar teeth. (*D*) Close up of the maxilla from the ventrodorsal view and (*E*) of the mandible from the dorsoventral view, displaying the cheek teeth. The standard system numbering the premolars as P3 and P4 is used in this figure. (*Courtesy of* Vittorio Capello, DVM, Milano, Italy; with permission.)

rapid collection and transport of food. Female hamsters have been known to hide their litter when they perceive the pups are in danger.

Rodents have a highly distinctive anatomic arrangement of the masseter muscle of the jaw (the dominant jaw-closing muscle) and the zygomatic arch of the skull, compared with that of other mammalian groups.[10–12] Researchers have been able to identify 3 distinct layers of the masseter muscle (superficial masseter, deep

Table 1
Dentition and dental formula of selected rat-like and squirrel-like rodent species

Species	Dental Formula	Total No. Teeth
Rat, Golden hamster	2(I 1/1, C 0/0, P 0/0, M 3/3)	16
Prairie dog	2(I 1/1, C 0/0, P 2/1, M 3/3)	22
Eastern gray squirrel (*Sciurus carolinensis*)	2(I 1/1, C 0/0, P 1–2/1, M 3/3)	20–22

Data from Capello V, Gracis M, Lennox AM. Rabbits and rodents dentistry handbook. Lake Worth (FL): Zoological Education Network; 2005. p. 1–274; and Legendre LFJ. Oral disorders of exotic rodents. Vet Clin North Am Exot Anim Pract 2003;6:601–28.

masseter, and *zygomaticomandibularis*, although inconsistencies exist over nomenclature and anatomic details) in all 3 rodent groups.[11]

In hystrichomorphs, an enlarged (as compared with the rat and squirrel) superficial portion of the masseter muscle moves the mandible forward and backward, whereas the reduced deep portion adducts the jaw, thereby closing the mouth.[1,3,11] This propalineal motion (combined lateral and rostrocaudal movement; ie, oblique) results in an effective grinding action by the molars and a reduced gnawing action by the incisors. In the sciuromorphs, the deep masseter expands forward onto the rostrum and it separates into 2 parts (anterior and posterior). In myomorphs, the origins of both parts of the masseter muscle have migrated forward onto the rostrum and work together to move the mandible forward and backward and are therefore equally adapted for both feeding modes (gnawing by the incisors and chewing by the molars).[10,11] In myomorphs, the mandible has a wide range of rostrocaudal movement and can even be subluxated rostrally during gnawing.[1,3] The cheek teeth are in occlusion when the jaw is at rest, giving the mandible a brachygnathic appearance.[1,3] Ultimately, when the incisors are gnawing and the cutting edges of mandibular and maxillary incisors are approximated, the molars are pulled out of occlusion. When chewing of food occurs, it is then that the mandibular incisors move posteriorly to the maxillary ones and the molars occlude again. During crushing of food, upward and forward movements of the mandible become evident.[13]

The dental anatomy reflects into different dietary habits and feeding strategies of the various rodent species as the anatomy of masticatory muscles leads to different stress and strains distributed across the 3 skull morphologies during chewing and gnawing.[11,14] The enlargement of the rostral portion of the deep masseter in sciuromorphs increases the efficiency of biting with the incisors. Conversely, the reduced deep masseter of the guinea pig may indicate this species mostly eats by chewing with the cheek teeth while spending less time gnawing with the incisors compared with squirrels or rats.[15] Actually, rats and squirrels consume more hard food (eg, nuts and seeds) than guinea pigs, which feed primarily on vegetation. Myomorphs are the most versatile, as they merge anatomic features of sciuromorphs and hystricomorphs and are equally efficient at both gnawing and chewing. These 2 feeding modes are mutually exclusive because incisors and molars cannot be in occlusion at the same time due to the mismatch between maxillary and mandibular length. Hence propalineal action is necessary to accomplish these tasks.[16,17]

In some species (eg, rats and squirrels), the cartilaginous tissue between the mandibular symphysis is not ossified, allowing a certain degree of movement between the mandibles[13] visible at the lower incisor teeth.

DENTAL DISEASE AND OTHER ORAL DISORDERS
Incisor Teeth

Primary congenital malocclusion of incisor teeth has been described in growing rats, hamsters, and squirrels.[6] However, this condition may be difficult to distinguish from acquired malocclusion of traumatic origin in adult animals, as often the initial injury is not recognized by most owners. True dwarfism, as recognized in pet rabbits, has not been documented in rodents because these species have not been selectively bred for extreme size variation.[7] However, *brachygnathia superior* (maxillary brachygnathism and enognathism; ie, shortening of the upper jaw) has been reported in myomorphs.[18]

Traumatic injuries of incisor teeth may be uneventful, but severe fractures affecting the pulp canal and/or the germinative tissue are frequently followed by dental disease and malocclusion of clinical crowns (**Fig. 3**). The most common form of acquired

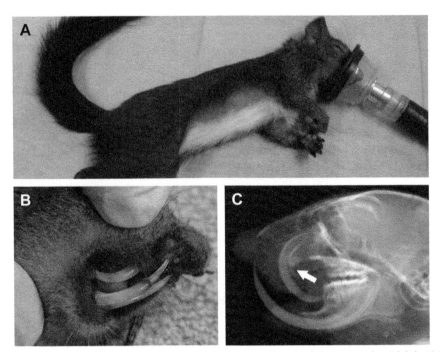

Fig. 3. Malocclusion of incisor teeth in a European red squirrel *(Sciurus vulgaris) (A)*. This young squirrel was rescued with a severe wound of the maxilla. This lesion cause brachignathism of the maxilla, followed by abnormal growth of maxillary incisor teeth. *(B)* Severe malocclusion of incisor teeth creating this lesion was not related to the initial trauma. *(C)* Radiograph of the head, lateral view. Note the severe brachygnathism of the maxilla causing enognathism of the maxillary cheek teeth, the abnormal curvature of the right maxillary incisor, and the hypoplastic left maxillary incisor, not erupting above the gingival level *(arrow)*. *(Courtesy of* Vittorio Capello, DVM, Milano, Italy; with permission.)

malocclusion seen in myomorphs is overgrowth (abnormal coronal elongation of clinical crowns), often accompanied by lateral mandibular shifting (**Figs. 4** and **5**). Because of the flexible symphysis and related movement of each mandible, malocclusion may create abnormal forces capable of slight rotation of the mandibles over the long axis. This allows the mandibular incisors to bypass the maxillary incisors laterally, while the maxillary clinical crowns follow the curvature of the reserve crowns into the oral cavity. In those species with high mechanical pressure at the apical sites of the upper incisors, palatal perforation can occur.[19] Malpositioning after a jaw fracture and age-related loss of clinical crowns in gerbils have also been reported as frequent causes of incisor malocclusion in myomorphs.[18] Abscess formation and osteoresorptive lesions may be seen involving the incisors in these rodent species.[13]

Other types of malocclusion and dental disease of incisor teeth are seen in sciuromorphs (odontomas, complex odontomas, and elodontomas).

Cheek Teeth

Metabolic disease as a predisposing factor for dental disease has not been fully explored or proven for rat-like and squirrel-like rodents.[3,7] Insufficient wearing of cheek teeth following inappropriate diet does not occur in species with anelodont cheek teeth. However, dental problems due to excessive wearing and severe caries

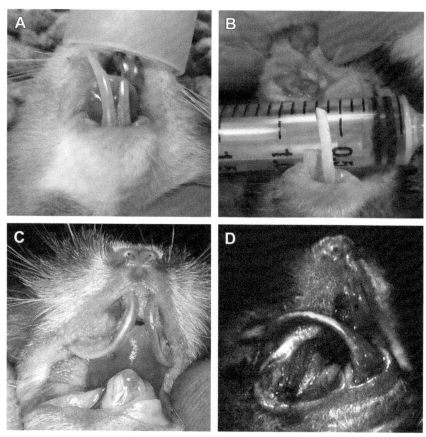

Fig. 4. Dental disease and malocclusion of incisor teeth in golden hamsters. (*A*) Elongation of the right mandibular incisor, and deviation of maxillary incisors. (*B*) Elongation of the left mandibular incisor, and fracture of the other incisors. The clinical crowns of maxillary incisor teeth are fractured at the gingival level. (*C*) Severe malocclusion and elongation with lateral deviation of maxillary incisor teeth. The clinical crowns of mandibular incisors are fractured, and no longer erupting. (*D*) Severe overgrowth and deviation of mandibular incisor teeth, protruding outside the oral cavity and creating a wound of the right cheek pouch. (*Courtesy of* [A, B] Elisabetta Mancinelli, DVM; and [C, D] *Courtesy of* Vittorio Capello, DVM, Milano, Italy; with permission.)

can still occur in these rodents, deeply reducing the crown and resulting in teeth loss[3,7] (**Fig. 6**). Captive myomorphs and sciuromorphs can develop periodontal disease, dental caries, and tooth decay if fed an inappropriate, high-sugar diet.[13,20] Gerbils have been reported to develop spontaneous periodontal disease if fed a standard rat or mouse diet for more than 6 months.[21] These rodents should therefore be fed an appropriate pelleted diet targeted to their specific requirements. Periodontal inflammation stimulates odontoclastic resorption, which creates cavities in the affected tooth. In some cases, repair takes place with granulation tissue moving in, as an attempt to contain the damage but lost dentin is not replaced. Caries lesions in rodents with brachyodont cheek teeth are similar to those seen in humans. Rats, in particular, have been used as animal models for human caries.[22] Hamsters are especially prone to develop periodontal disease, dental caries, and facial abscesses caused by a tooth root abscess.[3,23]

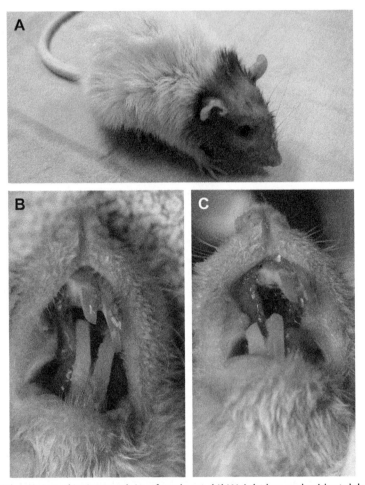

Fig. 5. Malocclusion of incisor teeth in a female rat. (*A*) Weight loss and evident dehydration were associated with mild dyspnea and sneezing. (*B*) Malocclusion of incisor teeth. Unlike the common pattern of malocclusion in which the clinical crown of maxillary incisor teeth can penetrate the palate, this injury is due to elongation of mandibular incisors in this patient. (*C*) A wide oro-nasal fistula is visible after palliative coronal reduction of incisor teeth. (*Courtesy of* Vittorio Capello, DVM, Milano, Italy; with permission.)

Abscesses, possibly involving the masseter muscle, may be seen in rats, mice, hamsters, and other small rodents (**Fig. 7**). They can be secondary to fracture or cavity of cheek teeth, or to endodontic or periapical infections of diseased incisors.[6]

Fractures of the jaws may occur in myomorph and sciuromorph rodents, as well as separation of the mandibular symphysis.[6]

Odontogenic Tumors and Tumor-like Lesions (Odontoma, Pseudo-Odontoma, and Elodontoma)

Odontogenic tumors have long been recognized as uncommon entities in humans and animals of many species.[24] Because most of these tumors are not malignant,[24] the distinction between neoplasms and tumor-like (non-neoplastic) lesions is debatable.

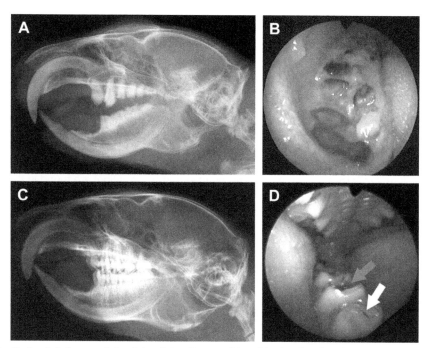

Fig. 6. Dental disease of cheek teeth in a 7-year-old prairie dog (*A*, *B*) and comparison with a normal animal (*C*, *D*). (*A*) Radiography of the head (lateral view), displaying severe damage of most cheek teeth, including the maxillary molar teeth and all the mandibular cheek teeth. Severe and diffuse remodeling of the roots is also present. Note that the incisor teeth are normal. (*B*) Endoscopic view of the right mandibular cheek teeth arcade in the same patient. Crowns are missing, likely following severe caries, and diseased portions of roots are visible at the gingival level. (*C*) Radiography of the head (lateral view), in a normal prairie dog. Note the coronal cusps and the multiple roots of cheek teeth. (*D*) Endoscopic view of the right mandibular cheek teeth arcades in a normal prairie dog with a small caries (*white arrow*) and food debris (*grey arrow*). (*Courtesy of* Vittorio Capello, DVM, Milano, Italy; with permission.)

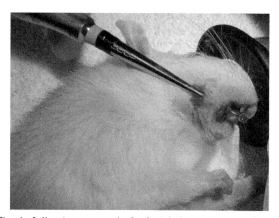

Fig. 7. Extraoral fistula following removal of a facial abscess in a rat. (*Courtesy of* Elisabetta Mancinelli, DVM.)

Several classifications have been proposed to describe these odontogenic abnormalities. Some of them focus on tumors of odontogenic origin,[25] others include hamartomas, congenital malformations, or degenerative or dysplastic lesions.[25–27] Hamartomas are defined as benign tumor-like lesions composed of an overgrowth of mature tissue that normally occurs in the affected part of the body but with disorganization, and often with one element predominating.[28]

Tumors of odontogenic epithelium with odontogenic mesenchyma have been initially reported as *odontomas*.[29] They have been reported in rats,[29] mice,[30] prairie dogs,[23,31–34] and other non-rodent species.[28] Odontomas are further classified as *compound odontomas* and *complex odontomas*, according to their histologic features and degree of organization.[25] All features of normal odontogenesis (ameloblastic epithelium, organized dentin matrix, and enamel matrix formation) are found in these tumors. The compound odontoma (not reported in rodents) is a mass lesion characterized by the presence of numerous fully differentiated, although abnormally shaped, toothlike structures (denticles) originating from within the mass. It is a locally destructive tumor with no metastatic potential.[25] Some consider this lesion more as a hamartoma and not a neoplasia.[25,28]

The complex odontoma (reported in rodents) is a conglomerate mass lesion with fully differentiated dental components that do not form tooth-like structures.[25,28] Histologically, well-differentiated dentinal tissue, enamel matrix, odontogenic epithelium, and cementum are present. Similar to the compound odontoma, it is locally destructive, has no metastatic potential, and may be considered as a hamartoma rather than a neoplasm.[25,28]

An important contribution to the classification and definition of these lesions has been proposed by Boy and Steenkamp.[28] Considering the elodont nature of rodent incisor teeth and the debatable hamartomous versus neoplastic nature of odontomas in brachyodont (and anelodont) teeth, they proposed the term *elodontoma* to replace the term odontoma with respect to hamartomatous jaw lesions in squirrels and similar species with elodont teeth. Elodontoma would therefore be described as a hamartoma of continuously developing odontogenic tissue and alveolar bone at the periapical bud of elodont teeth.[28]

The *odontogenic dysplasia in aging rodents and lagomorphs* has been classified as a tumor-like (non-neoplastic) lesion aside tumors of odontogenic origin. It defines the disorganized development and tumor-like dysplasia at the apex of the continuously erupting incisor teeth of rodents and lagomorphs, following inflammation, trauma, toxicosis, or age alone.[25] Histology reveals disorganized tissue proliferation and dysplastic differentiation of odontogenic elements, including odontogenic epithelium, enamel matrix, or fully mineralized enamel, dentin, cementum, and dental pulp.

Mature prairie dogs, between 2 and 6 years old, are commonly affected by odontoma-like lesions, usually involving the apex and the reserve crown of incisors, particularly the maxillary incisors.[3,5,7,31–35]

This dental abnormality is characterized by abnormal elongation of the reserve crown and the apex. The apical growth causes increased pressure and deformation of the germinal tissue. Apical tooth growth continues, causing primary deformation of the apex and of the reserve crown.[3,6,7,35] This is followed by reduced growth rate, and eventually by arrested eruption, whereas irregular production of new dentine continues.[3,7,35] This results in apical deformity of the apex and part of the reserve crown, and in secondary abnormalities of the surrounding structures (eg, incisive bones, hard palate, and nasal cavities in the case of maxillary incisors). The dental deformity acts as a locally compressive and space-occupying mass, especially with regard to the nasal cavity. Prairie dogs are typically presented with respiratory signs and symptoms.[3,6,7,35]

Nasal obstruction at different anatomic levels occurs, often resulting in severe respiratory compromise to death in this obligate nasal breathing species.[36] Gross anatomy and the longitudinal section of an histology specimen demonstrate folding of new dentine and apex deformity.[3,35] Radiographs show abnormalities consistent with apical dysplasia and display walls of the reserve crowns plicating. Severity can range from mild irregularities due to newly formed folds of dentine (visible in particular at the dorsal border of maxillary incisor teeth), to severe deformity of the reserve crown and apex, with concurrent obstruction of the nasal cavities.[3,5,7,35] This dental abnormality may affect 1 or more incisor teeth, even if the clinical impact is much more severe in the case of diseased maxillary incisor teeth, because of the adjacent nasal passages. If the lesions affect the maxillary incisor teeth, they are usually bilateral, even if their severity can be different between the 2 quadrants.

David Crossley,[35] therefore, proposed the more appropriate term *pseudo-odontoma* for this particular dysplastic, non-neoplastic dental disease of prairie dogs.[3]

The term elodontoma is therefore more specifically a synonym of complex odontoma (locally invasive and destructive lesion with no metastatic potential), not of pseudo-odontoma (locally compressive dysplastic lesion) nor of odontogenic dysplasia, because it does not include dysplastic changes.[37] However, the term elodontoma is sometimes used with a broader meaning (either with regard to complex odontoma and pseudo-odontoma/odontogenic dysplasia) rather than as indication of a specific histologic type.[37] However, the difference carries important clinical implications when formulating a diagnosis, prognosis, and possible treatment plan.

Elodontomas and pseudo-odontomas have been reported affecting elodont incisor teeth of several rodent species. Dental disease with histologic, clinical, and radiological elements consistent with elodontomas or former odontomas have been reported in the guinea pig,[38] degu,[39] pet tree squirrels *(Paraxerus cepapi)*,[28] rats,[29,40–42] and mice.[30,43–45]

Dental disease with histologic, clinical, and radiological elements consistent with pseudo-odontomas have been reported in the prairie dog[3,5,7,31–35,46] (reported also as elodontomas),[47] eastern gray squirrel,[48] and anecdotally in a chinchilla, a chipmunk,[3] and a citellus.[37] Apart from Smith and colleagues[47] and Capello (when those different abnormalities had not yet been identified and classified),[33] elodontoma has not been reported in the prairie dog.

Various etiopathogenetic theories have been proposed for both spontaneously developing and experimentally induced lesions consistent with complex odontomas/elodontomas and pseudo-odontomas. Osteopetrosis is an autosomal recessive disease characterized by abnormal recruitment of osteoclasts. Affected patients may suffer from altered tooth eruption and the formation of odontoma-like masses.[29,30,42,45] Repeated trauma or fractures (from chewing on cage bars, falls from a height, or improper trimming of maloccluded incisors) with resultant acquired dental disease, localized infection near the apical tissue of incisors with damage to the continuously developing odontogenic tissue, its follicle, and to the surrounding alveolar bone have also been suggested as a cause of odontomas, pseudo-odontomas, and elodontomas in prairie dogs and other squirrels.[3,7,28,32] Traumatic damage to the odontogenic tissue may be so severe that it completely disrupts the epithelial cords creating daughter germ cells, each being capable of continuous development forming its own hard and soft tissue components but in a haphazard manner, leading to the formation of hamartomatous masses.[28,30] Whether pseudo-odontomas represent an early stage potentially progressing to elodontoma or the fact that trauma could potentially result in 2 different pathologic processes cannot be determined at this stage.[49]

Other proposed causes considered in laboratory rodents include acquired dental disease, aging changes, hypovitaminosis A, hypomagnesemia, hypophysectomy, and toxin exposure.[23,35,39,50,51]

Other Oral Disorders

Lesions of oral soft tissues with various degrees of inflammation and infection may be seen when seeds, grass, or hay becomes impacted around teeth or in the cheek pouches.[13]

Glossitis ("wooden tongue") due to *Actinobacillus israeli* infection has been diagnosed in rats. The tongue becomes swollen, hard, and painful. Affected animals deteriorate rapidly because they are unable to eat and drink.[13]

Sialodacryoadenitis, caused by a highly contagious rat coronavirus, can result in visible swelling under the mandible and neck due to inflammation and edema of the cervical salivary glands. Concurrent lacrimal gland dysfunction may occur, leading to conjunctivitis, keratitis, corneal ulcers, and hyphema. Cervical lymph nodes also may be enlarged, and rhinitis may be present.[6]

The Syrian hamster is often the preferred species for carcinogenic studies.[36,52,53] This species can be affected by a broad range of tumors, as frequently reported in the literature and many histologic types have been described. However, spontaneous neoplasia of the oral cavity is rare in this and other rodent species.

Impaction, prolapse, abscessation, and neoplasia of cheek pouches have been described in the golden hamster[54] (**Fig. 8**). A spontaneous cheek pouch fibroma has been reported in a Syrian hamster.[55]

Adenomas or adenocarcinomas of the Zymbal gland located at the base of the ear and surrounded by the parotid gland in rats may be locally invasive and should be taken into consideration when assessing skull and facial structures in this species.[52] Tumors of the Harderian lacrimal gland can result in exophthalmos and porphyrin staining of periocular hair. They tend to be highly invasive in mice, leading to infiltration of bone and other structures of the head and should therefore be taken into consideration in the list of differentials. A maxillary osteosarcoma has been reported in a prairie dog[56] and an adenocarcinoma of the buccal salivary gland has been described in a Richardson ground squirrel.[57]

Electrical injuries are not uncommonly seen in domestic rodents, as a result of chewing on power cables and subsequent direct body contact with an electrical source. The hallmark of electrocution is burn marks generally confined to the sites of body contact with the electrical source, especially the lips, oral commissure, and tongue (**Fig. 9**). Paresthesia and drooling may result.[13]

CLINICAL PRESENTATION

The acquired dental disease syndrome in pet rodents often results in a complex of clinical signs and symptoms, both primarily related to dental and/or oral problems and/or secondary to complications affecting other organs. Clinical presentation may therefore vary greatly among individual patients depending on concurrent disease.[7] However, myomorph and sciuromorph rodent species are rarely presented for symptoms and signs specifically related to dental disease.

Patients are frequently presented for reduced activity and reduced food intake, weight loss, emaciation, and ptyalism often accompanied by moist dermatitis. Grooming difficulties and poor coat quality also may be seen. Change of feeding habits or food preferences may be sometimes noted by the owners.

Overgrowth, malocclusion, or other abnormalities of incisor teeth may be immediately evident on visual inspection in rat-like rodents, but often missed by the owners.

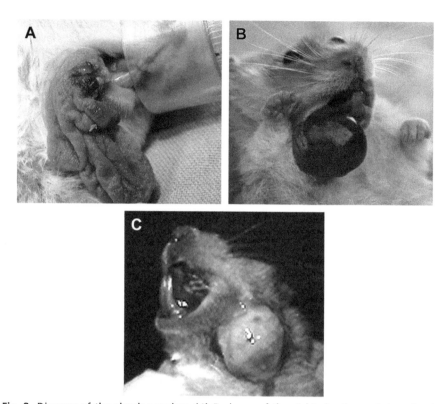

Fig. 8. Diseases of the cheek pouches. (*A*) Prolapse of the right cheek pouch in a Russian hamster *(Phodopus campbelli)*. A small area of necrotic tissue is present. (*B*) Neoplasia of the right cheek pouch in a golden hamster *(Mesocricetus auratus)* after eversion of the mass. Differential diagnosis with impaction (before eversion, or before emptying the food material) and with edema of the mucosa concurrent with prolapse should be considered. (*C*) Abundant pus after rupture of an abscess involving the left cheek pouch in a golden hamster. (*Courtesy of* Vittorio Capello, DVM, Milano, Italy; with permission.)

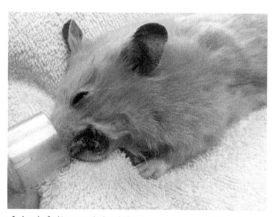

Fig. 9. Skin lesion of the left lips and the labial commissure following an electrocution in a golden hamster. (*Courtesy of* Joanna Hedley, DVM, London, UK; with permission.)

Mild to severe malocclusion may be concurrent with slightly elongated or fractured incisors, and maxillary incisors may be curved toward the palate. Secondary lesions of the tongue, lips, and palate may result. A severe complication is represented by perforation of the palate and oro-nasal fistula.[3,19] Facial swelling or ocular or periocular signs may be seen secondary to periapical infections and abscessation of cheek teeth. In rats, infection with sialodacryoadenitis virus should be considered in case of mandibular and neck swellings. Ocular and periocular structures also may be secondarily involved in both situations.

Hamsters may be presented with a large, persistent unilateral or bilateral swelling of the face. This may be seen when the cheek pouch cannot be emptied by the animal, and food remains impacted. The prolapsed mucosa of a cheek pouch, usually unilateral, presents as a pink mass protruding from the mouth and resembling a tumor. Following self-trauma, the edematous everted mucosa may get dry, inflamed, infected, ulcerated, and necrotic. Abscesses of the cheek pouches may be secondary to lesions and infections of soft tissues, or to dental disease.[3,6,7,54]

Signs and symptoms of dental and oral disorders in captive and free-living squirrels are similar to those encountered in other rodent species[6,58] and may include malocclusion with different types of fractures (especially affecting the incisors); variations in the number, size and shape of teeth; presence of supernumerary teeth; caries; periodontal disease; excessive wearing of cheek teeth in aging patients; periapical infections and abscesses (possibly complicated by osteomyelitis); and traumatic lesions of the oral soft tissues.[58–60]

In captive prairie dogs, fractures of incisor teeth are so frequent following repeated trauma due to poor husbandry, that owners may report "regularly shedding teeth." Fractures may occur either along the clinical crown resulting in visibly shortened tooth or teeth, or along the reserve crown (under the gum line) (**Fig. 10**). In the latter case, the clinical crown may either appear mobile but still attached to the gingiva, or missing. Both lesions are frequently overlooked by owners. In prairie dogs, respiratory signs and symptoms are most common, and are frequently associated with reduced activity, reduced food intake, weight loss, and emaciation.[3,7] Respiratory symptoms may include sneezing, a particular type of snoring (often referred to as "reverse sneezing"), pronounced inspiratory effort, or true dyspnea. They are secondary to the dysplastic changes and apical deformities of diseased maxillary incisors. Because prairie dogs are obligate nasal breathers, these changes may result in reduced nasal air passage to obstruction. A firm swelling of the hard palate caused by the deformed apices may be visible on intraoral inspection of the anesthetized patient[3,7]; however, the size of the lesion above the hard palate does not seem to correlate with the degree of respiratory distress.[23,31] Aging patients, usually older than 5 years, also may be presented for reduced food intake, reduced fecal output, and emaciation in the absence of respiratory signs. Underlying medical issues should be ruled out in these cases, but end-stage dental disease with excessive wearing, caries, and fractures causing flattening of cheek teeth crowns, is usually the primary cause of these presenting signs.[3,5,7]

Mandibular odontomas also have been reported causing dysfunction but not respiratory obstruction, as a space-occupying lesion of the oropharynx, which can lead to starvation and death of the affected animal.[23,47]

DIAGNOSIS OF DENTAL DISEASE AND DIAGNOSTIC IMAGING
Physical Examination

Patients may be presented with a wide variety of symptoms, either specifically related to dental problems and associated complications, or secondary to involvement of

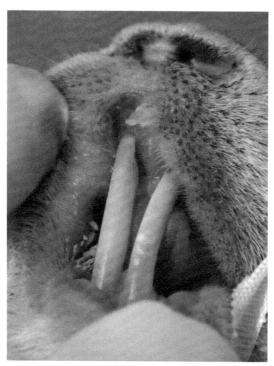

Fig. 10. Malocclusion of incisor teeth in a prairie dog affected by pseudo-odontoma of the right maxillary incisor tooth. History reported several fractures of the clinical crowns of maxillary cheek teeth. The clinical crown of the right maxillary incisor is missing, and the left is shorter than normal. The clinical crown of the right mandibular incisor is elongated; the left is curved, out of occlusion with the opposite maxillary tooth. (*Courtesy of* Vittorio Capello, DVM, Milano, Italy; with permission.)

other organ systems. Therefore, a systematic approach is required. Thorough history, including dietary details, feeding habits, and husbandry with regard to cage construction and design, is of utmost importance. However, the absence of a clear history does not rule out underlying dental problems. In selected rodent species or in calm and adequately restrained individuals, a partial physical and dental examination may be possible without anesthesia. Inspection of incisors may be possible in some prairie dogs. The incisor teeth should be examined from the labial and lateral aspect. Evaluation of the facial symmetry and palpation (including the ventral mandibular borders, and the zygomatic and temporomandibular joint areas) may allow identification of irregularities and swellings. When feasible in the awake patient, lateral and horizontal jaw movement should be assessed. Any discomfort or pain should be noted.[13] Gentle expression of the cheek pouches is necessary to remove stored food, which may hinder examination. They should be examined fully and not mistaken for a pathologic swelling secondary to impaction, prolapse, or neoplasia. An otoscope with appropriately sized plastic cone, or alternatively nasal or vaginal speculum may be used to examine the oral cavity in rodents. The use of a pediatric laryngoscope for examination of the oral cavity of manually restrained small mammals, including prairie dogs, is reported.[61] Eyes, periocular structures, and cheek teeth should be examined as well. Despite the large mouth opening, the oral cavity is small, and the cheek teeth are positioned caudally to the long diastema. Therefore, a complete oral examination may be effectively and safely performed only with the patient under general anesthesia.[3]

The use of specific dental equipment, such as the rabbit and rodent table retractor/restrainer, mouth gags, cheek dilators, adequate lighting, and magnification, greatly enhance a thorough oral cavity examination[3,5] (**Fig. 11**). Gentle and appropriate manipulation is required during the examination. For example, it is imperative to avoid excessive opening of the oral cavity to prevent damage to the temporomandibular joints.[13]

Oral Endoscopy

Oral endoscopy (stomatoscopy) is a relatively simple, noninvasive diagnostic procedure, and should be part of a complete oral examination in rodent species.[3,61–63] Magnification of dental structures allows a more thorough inspection of the oral cavity, facilitating detection of subtle lesions[64] and evaluation of the occlusal surface of the teeth, the mucosal surface of the tongue and hard palate, and the caudal part of the oropharynx. Dental abrasions, fractures, and caries may have fewer symptoms and may be more readily identified on stomatoscopic examination (see **Fig. 6**). A 1.9-mm or 2.7-mm rigid telescope with a 30° viewing angle are generally used for these procedures, because the 30° angle provides a better view of the occlusal surfaces. Each tooth should be examined individually with the use of a periodontal probe. The gingival sulcus should be probed circumferentially to identify the presence of pockets and their depth; purulent discharge; food or hair impaction; and evidence of decay, caries, and any other abnormality.[13] The telescope also can be used periodically to evaluate the intraoperative progress of premolar or molar extractions or to examine the cavity left following extraction.[63]

Endoscopic inspection of the cheek pouches also should be performed.[3]

Radiography

A full radiographic assessment should be done in every rodent species to identify dental abnormalities.[3] General anesthesia and optimal positioning are necessary to

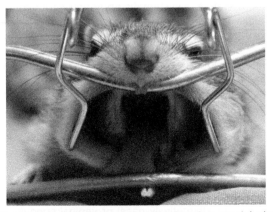

Fig. 11. The rabbit and rodent table retractor/restrainer is a special platform acting as a combined mouth gag and patient positioner. It can be effectively used also for small rodents, such as a chipmunk. In this patient, the cheek dilator is positioned out of the oral cavity to dilate the opening of cheek pouches. The face mask has been temporarily removed for demonstration purpose. (*Courtesy of* Vittorio Capello, DVM, Milano, Italy; with permission.)

obtain good-quality images of diagnostic value. This may be particularly challenging in very small species, such as myomorphs smaller than rats. Multiple views are necessary for full assessment.[65] At least 4 standard views (latero-lateral, 2 obliques, ventro-dorsal, or dorsoventral) are recommended.[3,66] Intraoral views may be useful in larger species, such as the prairie dog, to visualize cheek teeth root tips and the apical incisor area.[3] Among the many dental abnormalities, it is important to discuss those affecting the incisor teeth in case of pseudo-odontomas of prairie dogs and elodonto-mas of other squirrels. In case of dysplastic changes, the apex of maxillary incisor teeth appears enlarged. Both the apex and most of the reserve crown have a dorsal irregular margin, displaying newly formed folds of dentine.[3,5,6,35,66] These radiographic findings are best evaluated at lateral or slightly oblique views. Thirty-degree oblique, ventrodorsal, and rostrocaudal views help to assess if the pseudo-odontoma is unilateral or bilateral, and the stage of severity (**Fig. 12**). Detailed diagnosis is critical for prognosis and the treatment plan. The reserve and/or clinical crown is usually shorter than normal, and the occlusal plane is abnormal as well. Pseudo-odontomas affecting the mandibular incisors show similar radiographic findings, although usually less evident. Similar to radiographic findings in cavy-like rodents affected by elodontoma, such as the degu,[39] radiography of squirrels shows a large radiopaque mass with increased mineral opacity well beyond the apex and the reserve crown, locally invasive and destructive.[28]

Computed Tomography

The use of computed tomography (CT) is particularly useful and has great advantages compared with standard radiography. CT overcomes superimposition on a single plane of adjacent and overlying anatomic structures, and 3-dimensional renderings provide excellent details (even in small mammal species) of bone structures in particular. Superior details and dynamic views allow detection of early changes in tooth structure, evaluation of the involvement of surrounding soft tissue, or extension of osteomyelitic foci. CT therefore enhances the level of diagnostic accuracy, providing more accurate and detailed information than traditional radiographic images. These are critical for accurate prognosis, more tailored surgical planning, and successful treatment.[67] In prairie dogs affected by pseudo-odontomas, CT is particularly useful to assess the extension of the hard mass, the degree of compression of the nasal cavity, the involvement of surrounding tissues, and the most appropriate surgical approach[37] (**Fig. 13**). CT is also particularly useful for assessment of the temporomandibular joint.

Other Diagnostic Testing

A complete blood count and biochemical panel allows evaluation of the general health status of a patient. Bacterial culture and sensitivity is important in cases of periapical infections and abscessation to allow a more targeted antibiotic treatment. Histopathology can be useful when neoplasia or pseudo-odontoma is suspected.[3]

TREATMENT OF DENTAL DISEASE AND OTHER ORAL DISORDERS
Prognosis

The prognosis for dental disease in rodents is generally more guarded than in other small mammal species, such as rabbits[7]; however, it should be formulated for each individual species and case depending on different pathologic patterns. Noncompli-cated incisor malocclusion in myomorphs or sciuromorphs usually carries a fair prognosis. When cheek teeth are involved (in particular with the complication of a facial

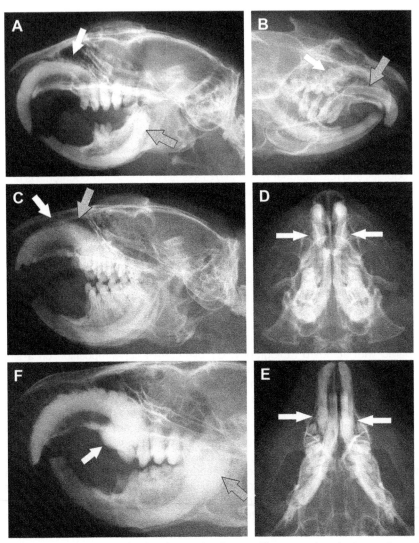

Fig. 12. Standard radiography for diagnosis of a maxillary pseudo-odontomas in prairie dogs. (A) Lateral view displaying the irregular dorsal margin of a maxillary incisor tooth (*white arrow*). Apical deformity is minimal in this patient. The mandibular incisors are affected by similar radiographic abnormalities consistent with pseudo-odontoma (*dotted arrow*). Abnormal and missing crowns of mandibular cheek teeth are also present. (B) A 30° oblique view is useful to evacuate asymmetric abnormalities. In this patient, the apex of the right maxillary incisor is enlarged (*white arrow*), whereas the left is normal (*dotted arrow*). (C) Slight oblique view in a prairie dog affected by bilateral pseudo-odontoma. Obstruction of the dorsal nasal passage (*white arrow*) and reduced nasal cavity (*dotted arrow*) are visible. Evident malocclusion of incisor teeth is also present. Rostrocaudal (D) and ventrodorsal (E) views in the same patient displaying bilateral deformity of the apices of maxillary incisor teeth (*arrows*). (F) Large maxillary pseudo-odontoma in a prairie dog with enlarged and deformed apex (*white arrow*) and typical folds of dentine visible on the dorsal aspect of the clinical and reserve crown. Severe deformity of the mandibular apices is also present (*dotted arrow*). (*Courtesy of* Vittorio Capello, DVM, Milano, Italy; with permission.)

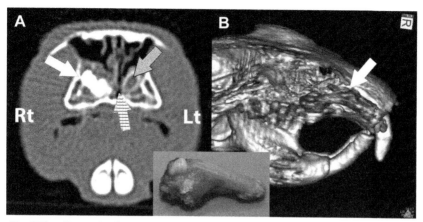

Fig. 13. CT for diagnosis of a maxillary pseudo-odontoma in a prairie dog. (*A*) The axial view depicts the deformity of the reserve crown of the right maxillary incisor tooth (*white arrow*), and the compression of the common nasal meatus (*chiseled arrow*). The pseudo-odontoma is unilateral, facilitating comparison with the transverse section of the normal left maxillary incisor tooth (*dotted arrow*), and with the left, patent, common nasal meatus. (*B*) The 3-dimensional volume reconstruction, after cropping part of the right incisive bone, displays the actual shape of the diseased reserve crown and apex (the grey anatomic structure pointed by the *white arrow*). The CT image compared with the pseudo-odontoma after extraction (inset) is very accurate. (*Courtesy of* Vittorio Capello, DVM, Milano, Italy; with permission.)

abscess), prognosis is guarded to poor, considering the difficulty carried by any surgical approach in such small patients and the extensive involvement of surrounding anatomic structures.[7]

Prognosis for pseudo-odontomas in prairie dogs is strictly related to the presence of unilateral or bilateral disease, the stage of disease at the time of diagnosis, and the degree of compromise of the respiratory system. The overall clinical condition needs to be considered, as well as the feasibility to surgically access and remove the compressive mass. Locally destructive elodontomas in other squirrels carry a poor prognosis, and successful treatment, even if conservative, is not reported. End-stage dental disease of cheek teeth also carries a poor medium to long-term prognosis in prairie dogs.

Treatment of Incisor Teeth

Overgrowth and malocclusion of the incisor teeth is the most common dental disorder of rat-like rodents.[6] Regular coronal reduction may be sufficient to restore an adequate occlusal plane and manage early, uncomplicated cases. However, in most cases, this dental procedure must be repeated for the remainder of the patient's life, unless complications, such as pulp infection or periapical abscessation occur. A cutting burr mounted on a high-speed angled handpiece is used for this procedure. Alternatively, diamond discs mounted on low-speed handpieces are available as well.[6] The soft tissues are protected by placing a tongue depressor or a syringe case caudal to the incisors (**Fig. 14**). Nail clippers or cutters are strongly contraindicated, even under anesthesia, because they can create oblique fractures, lead to pulp exposure, damage the periodontal ligament, and cause soft tissue injuries.

Extraction of incisor teeth can be considered in myomorph and sciuromorph rodents when overgrowth is recurrent and persistent due to severe deviation. Extraction is also an indication for treatment of pseudo-odontomas in prairie dogs. Extraction of

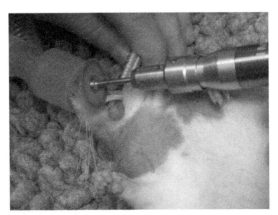

Fig. 14. Coronal reduction of the right mandibular incisor tooth in a golden hamster, using a diamond cutter disc mounted on a straight handpiece. The tongue and other soft tissues are protected using a plastic syringe. The chisel-shaped occlusal plane may be refined after coronal reduction. (*Courtesy of* Elisabetta Mancinelli, DVM.)

incisors does not seem to affect the feeding behavior in captive pets,[6] as they can manipulate food with their forearms. However, diet modification by eliminating hard food items should be considered. The procedure can be performed with careful dissection of the periodontal ligament with the same technique described in rabbits by using small dental luxators[6] or appropriately contoured hypodermic needles[3,7] (**Fig. 15**). However, this is more intricate and difficult due to the small size of the patient, the dental anatomy of these species (mandibular incisors extend within the mandible below the cheek teeth and the apex is located distal to the last molar in hamsters, rats, and squirrels), and possible complications (namely, fracture of the maxillary incisors, fracture of the mandible, and diastasis of the mobile mandibular synchondrosis/symphysis).[7] Radiographs before extraction are recommended to evaluate tooth morphology, curvature, and fracture type, as well as for assessing presence and extension of injuries to the surrounding soft tissues.[13] Post-extraction control radiographs are also important to verify complete extraction. Jekl[13] recommends coronal reduction of the incisors followed by extraction 5 to 7 days later, in cases of failure of correction and excessive regrowth. Regrowth and eruption of a new tooth is a possible complication; therefore, it is recommended to damage the germinative tissue following extraction.

Treatment of Cheek Teeth

Coronal reduction of anelodont cheek teeth in rat-like and squirrel-like rodents must never be performed, as excessive elongation and malocclusion do not occur in these species.[3] Conservative treatment for dental caries and periodontal disease is rarely undertaken in rodent species because of the small size of these patients. When lesions affecting anelodont teeth are extensive or symptomatic, extraction is more appropriate.[6]

Facial abscesses often cause extensive involvement of surrounding anatomic structures. Treatment is usually very challenging and unrewarding; however, the same surgical principles as in other species (eg, thorough debridement, tooth extraction, marsupialization, daily wound care, antibiotic treatment, analgesia, and supportive

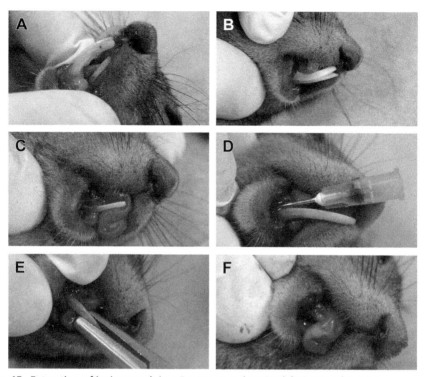

Fig. 15. Extraction of incisor teeth in a European red squirrel *(Sciurus vulgaris)*, same case as in **Fig. 3**. (*A*) Overgrowth and malocclusion of incisor teeth. The nasal wound shown in **Fig.** 3B healed after conservative coronal reduction of mandibular incisor teeth. (*B*) The maxillary incisor tooth has been extracted. (*C*) Appearance of the gingiva after extraction of the right mandibular incisor. (*D*) Luxation of the left mandibular incisor. A contoured 22-G needle is used on the mesial aspect of the tooth as an elevator. Luxation is performed also on the distal, labial, and lingual aspects of the tooth. (*E*) When the tooth is after luxation, the clinical crown is grasped with a small needle holder used as an extraction forceps. (*F*) Appearance of the gingiva after extraction. It may be sutured or left to heal by second intention, in this case. (*Courtesy of* Vittorio Capello, DVM, Milano, Italy; with permission.)

care) should be followed. Abscesses will likely recur if the infected tooth is not addressed and removed.[68]

Treatment of Diseased Cheek Pouches

Impaction of cheek pouches should be treated by emptying the contents adhered to the mucosa, and topical application of antiseptic solutions. If the prolapse of a cheek pouch is recent and the mucosal surface is intact, repositioning can be attempted with the patient under general anesthesia (**Fig. 16**A–C). The mucosa should be rehydrated and lubricated before being replaced. The pouch is repositioned using cotton-tip applicators.[69] A single full-thickness percutaneous mattress suture can be placed into the cheek pouch using 4:0 or 5:0 monofilament nonabsorbable suture material to maintain the pouch in its normal position and prevent reoccurrence.[54,68,69] Amputation of the cheek pouch is indicated in cases of severe mucosal lesions following prolapse, recurrent prolapse, or neoplasia.[54,69] A hemostat is placed at the base of the

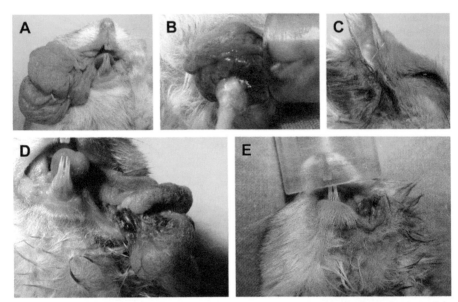

Fig. 16. Treatment of prolapse of cheek pouches in 2 Russian hamsters. Repositioning of the prolapse in a *Phodopus campbelli* (*A–C*) and amputation in a *Phodopus sungorus* (*D, E*). (*A*) Prolapse of the left cheek pouch. (*B*) The prolapse is reduced using a cotton-tip applicator lubricated with lidocaine gel. (*C*) A percutaneous, nonabsorbable suture prevents the relapse. (*D*) Amputation of the cheek pouch is indicated. (*E*) Suture of the mucosa with absorbable suture. (*Courtesy of* Vittorio Capello, DVM, Milano, Italy; with permission.)

prolapsed tissue, and the necrotic pouch is resected. The base of the everted pouch is sutured with absorbable material in a simple interrupted pattern (**Fig. 16**D, E).

Abscesses are best treated with surgical removal of the infected and/or necrotic tissue followed by thorough flushing, marsupialization, and healing by second intention, rather than with a simple incision.

Treatment of Pseudo-Odontoma

Medical, symptomatic treatment (antibiotics, corticosteroids, and decongestants) aimed at relieving respiratory signs and symptoms, as well as providing supportive feeding for these herbivorous species, is considered of little value for the management of patients with pseudo-odontomas. Instead, it is of paramount importance as adjunctive therapy to dental or surgical treatment.

Various dental and/or surgical approaches and techniques have been described for treatment of this condition in prairie dogs.[7,69] These procedures can be classified into symptomatic or palliative (aimed at restoring patency of the upper airways) and causative or primary (aimed at extracting the diseased teeth). Both groups carry advantages and disadvantages, and at this stage none of them can be considered objectively superior to the other. The choice of causative versus palliative treatment should be based on many individual clinical and practical elements, including detailed diagnosis and degree of severity, unilaterality or bilaterality with regard to the diseased maxillary incisors, patient's age and overall clinical conditions, patient's behavior, surgeon's experience and skills, and owner's expectations. Palliative treatment even may be considered as a preliminary surgical step to improve the overall condition of the patient before extraction of diseased teeth.

Anesthesia

The anesthetic procedure for treatment of pseudo-odontoma is challenging, especially in patients in which compression and subsequent obstruction of the nasal passages are severe, and respiratory function is compromised. Two surgical aspects to consider before planning an anesthetic protocol are the surgery time (which may vary significantly depending on the kind of treatment and the surgical approach/technique) and anticipated hemorrhage at the maxillary and nasal surgical sites.

The gold standard of anesthetic maintenance for this surgery is orotracheal intubation. The procedure for the orotracheal intubation in the prairie dog has been reported.[70,71] It is challenging due to anatomic features, such as the fleshy tongue and the presence of the oropharyngeal ostium, but may be less difficult with specialized equipment. Alternative techniques to assess patency of upper or lower airways during surgery are nasal intubation via rhinotomy/rhinostomy (which is actually part of the palliative technique), and direct tracheal intubation via tracheotomy (feasible, but more invasive).[37,71] In selected patients with milder respiratory distress, oxygen and inhalant anesthetics delivered via a face mask, preferably coupled with an extranasal approach to the diseased tooth, may be sufficient in cases in which intubation attempts fail. In these circumstances, the surgical procedure time should be as short as possible, and special attention should be paid to hemostasis at the surgical site. Monitoring oxygen saturation via pulse oximetry is mandatory for these surgical procedures.

Palliative procedures

The goal of palliative procedures is restoration of sufficient air flow creating an alternative nasal passage via a stoma on the dorsal aspect of the nasal cavities. Even if this procedure can be combined with extraction procedures, the standard palliative approach is aimed at alleviating the obstruction without extraction of affected tooth/teeth. Reported variations of this permanent rhinostomy technique via a dorsal approach may or may not include the use of a stent.[31,34] The patient is placed in sternal recumbency with the head slightly elevated. The skin is incised over the midline with a linear incision or with a biopsy punch, as the rhinostomy site and the stent opening will be round. Rhinotomy of the nasal bones is performed with a 2.5-mm or 3-mm intramedullary pin, and the nasal cavity is exposed. A small, plastic catheter is cut to proper length and inserted into the nasal cavity, just dorsal to the mass if the goal is to keep the rhinostomy site open,[37] or beyond (caudally) the pseudo-odontoma to allow passage of air into the rhinopharynx[31,34] (**Fig. 17**). The use of a metal stent has been reported.[46] The stent can be removed or exchanged for a smaller one a few weeks postoperatively to keep the skin from closing over the bony rhinostomy opening. Advantages include short anesthesia and surgery time, simplicity, rapid recovery, and quick improvement of respiratory symptoms. However, it should be noted that this surgical option does not stop the dysplastic process; therefore, the rhinostomy site and/or the stent may eventually no longer be sufficient. Another disadvantage is that postoperative management of the rhinostomy site includes removal of mucus and debris. This may or may not be easy depending on the patient's temperament.

Surgical debulking of the mass also has been reported in conjunction with more invasive surgical approaches.[35,37] Temporary tracheostomy is a viable alternative, although often not successful for long-term management of these cases.[23]

Causative procedures

Causative dental and surgical techniques instead pursue extraction of the diseased tooth/teeth compressing the upper airways.[3,5,7,23,33,37,47,69,72,73]

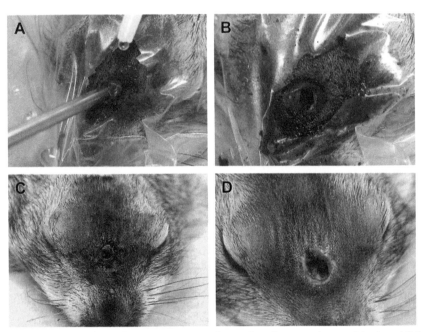

Fig. 17. Rhinostomy for palliative treatment of pseudo-odontoma in a prairie dog. (*A*) The anesthetized prairie dog is placed in sternal recumbency. The area over the nasal bones is surgically prepared and draped with a transparent adhesive drape. A circular portion of the skin is removed using a biopsy punch, and the nasal bone is exposed. A 2.5-mm intramedullary pin is used to drill a small rhinotomy access. (*B*) The rhinotomy site is then enlarged using a small bur. (*C*) A plastic stent, consisting a of a 1-mL syringe, is placed within the rhinotomy access and sutured to the skin, to keep the rhinostomy site patent. (*D*) The plastic stent is removed 10 days after the surgical procedure. (*Courtesy of* Vittorio Capello, DVM, Milano, Italy; with permission.)

The goal of a primary treatment is extraction of the affected maxillary incisor tooth or teeth. Mandibular incisors can be extracted during the same surgery, or at a later time as a second procedure to decrease initial anesthesia.[5]

Standard intraoral extraction The standard technique for extraction is technically similar to that described for rabbits, but it is much more challenging in prairie dogs because of apical deformities and dental ankylosis that are always present to some extent.[3,33,69] Also, affected teeth may have a very short clinical crown, making the use of extraction forceps difficult. The most frequent complication is fracture of the tooth while attempting removal, which represents a treatment failure.[69] Contoured 19-gauge needles are recommended to luxate the incisor teeth. However, if severe deformity and/or ankylosis are present, this technique is not practical and not effective because the reserve crown would invariably fracture.

Transpalatal intraoral approach Indications for the transpalatal approach[7,35,67,69] are represented by complete fracture of the clinical crown below the gingival level, and in cases in which the apex is deformed with a ventral prominence, causing an evident deformity of the hard palate. With the patient placed in dorsal recumbency and a mouth gag positioned to keep the mouth wide open, an incision is performed over the mucosa of the hard palate. The mucosa is then bluntly dissected free from the underlying hard tissue to expose the ventral aspect of the deformed apex, which is ankylotic with the incisive bone (**Fig. 18**). The apex and the proximal aspect of the reserve crown are then meticulously separated from the ankylotic attachment. Complete extraction or debulking is performed depending on the case. The mucosa is then sutured over the defect.

Rhinotomy extraoral technique The rhinotomy technique with a dorsal approach has been reported.[35,47,73]

The reserve crowns do not actually perforate the incisive bones penetrating the nasal cavities. However, this approach is effective to access the dorsal aspect of the reserve crown of the maxillary incisor teeth affected by pseudo-odontoma, which protrude making the nasal meatuses much narrower. This technique is also effective to create a temporary or permanent rhinostomy site, usually larger than the palliative rhinostomy. The procedure is performed with the patient in sternal recumbency and the head slightly elevated. After a skin incision on the midline and proper retraction of soft tissues, the rhinotomy is performed by burring the nasal bones. The reserve crowns and the apex of diseased teeth are then manipulated for complete extraction or debulking.

Lateral approach through the incisive bone Originally described by one of the authors (V.C),[49,72] this technique is completely extraoral and extranasal, and has the advantage to approach the reserve crown and the apex on their lateral aspect, therefore approaching the "shell" of the pseudo-odontoma, which is the incisive bone (**Fig. 19**). Because the ipsilateral nasal cavity is not entered, excessive bleeding is usually not a concern. The patient is placed in lateral recumbency, and the lateral aspect of the upper lip is shaved, aseptically prepared, and surgically dressed. A skin incision is performed over the incisive bone, and hemostasis is controlled with cotton-tip applicators. Blunt dissection of the underlying soft tissues allows exposure of the lateral aspect of the incisive bone, and a specialized retractor (eg, the Lone Star Retractor; Lone Star Medical Products, Inc. Stafford, TX) is positioned. Osteotomy of the incisive bone is performed with a small 2-mm ball-tipped bur, until the reserve crown of the pseudo-odontoma becomes visible with the typical folds of dentine. The reserve crown is then meticulously worked with small dental elevators or contoured needles,

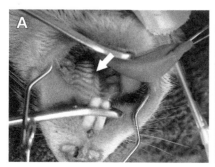 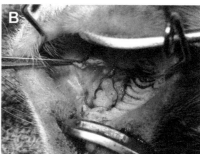

Fig. 18. Transpalatal approach for extraction of pseudo-odontoma in a prairie dog. (*A*) The patient is placed in dorsal recumbency with a mouth gag and a cheek dilator. Direct tracheal intubation via tracheotomy was performed in this case. Note deformity of the hard palate due to the pseudo-odontoma affecting the left maxillary incisor (*white arrow*). (*B*) The mucosa has been incised, dissected free, and retracted by a small hemostat to expose the deformed apex of the pseudo-odontoma ankylotic with the incisive bone. (*Courtesy of* Vittorio Capello, DVM, Milano, Italy; with permission.)

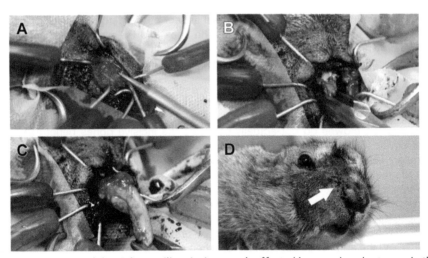

Fig. 19. Extraction of the right maxillary incisor tooth affected by pseudo-odontoma via the lateral approach to the incisive bone. (*A*) With the patient anesthetized and placed in lateral recumbency, the lateral aspect of the incisive bone is exposed. Osteotomy is performed with a small 2-mm ball-tipped bur to expose the lateral aspect of the reserve crown of the diseased incisive tooth. (*B*) Extraction of the rostral portion of the reserve crown. (*C*) Complete extraction of the diseased tooth, including the deformed apex. (*D*) Suture of the skin (*arrow*) and postoperative cosmetic appearance of the surgical access. (*Courtesy of* Vittorio Capello, DVM, Milano, Italy; with permission.)

to resolve ankylosis. However, the bone fenestration may not be sufficient to extract the pseudo-odontoma in one whole piece. Therefore, the reserve crown may be intentionally cut to allow retrograde extraction of the rostral portion of the reserve crown and the clinical crown (when present), and the anterograde extraction of the proximal portion of the reserve crown and the deformed apex. The skin is sutured over the site as routine.

The lateral approach also has been reported with the patient in sternal recumbency, creating a bone window between the nasal and the incisive bone.[74] However, it reports debulking via extraction only of the apical portion of the pseudo-odontoma, whereas the rostral portion of the reserve crown and the clinical crown remain in place.[74]

SUMMARY

The order *Rodentia* is divided into 3 groups based on anatomic and functional differences of the masseter muscle. Myomorph and sciuromorph species have elodont incisors and anelodont cheek teeth, unlike hystrichomorph species, which have full anelodont dentition. Diseases of incisors and cheek teeth of rat-like and squirrel-like rodents result in a wide variety of symptoms and clinical signs. Appropriate diagnostic procedures are essential to a definitive diagnosis, prognosis, and treatment plan. Pseudo-odontomas of prairie dogs are challenging and require surgical expertise for effective treatment.

REFERENCES

1. Crossley DA. Clinical aspects of rodent dental anatomy. J Vet Dent 1991;8:131–4.

2. Nowak R, Paradiso J. Walker's mammals of the world. 4th edition. Baltimore (MD): The Johns Hopkins University Press; 1983.

3. Capello V, Gracis M, Lennox AM. Rabbits and rodents dentistry handbook. Lake Worth (FL): Zoological Education Network; 2005. p. 1–274.

4. Lennox AM, Bauck L. Sections four: small rodents. Basic anatomy, physiology, husbandry and clinical techniques. In: Quesenberry KE, Carpenter JW, editors. Ferrets, rabbits and rodents clinical medicine and surgery. 3rd edition. St Louis (MO): Elsevier Saunders; 2012. p. 339–53.

5. Capello V, Lennox AM. Section VI: general topics. Small mammal dentistry. In: Quesenberry KE, Carpenter JW, editors. Ferrets, rabbits and rodents clinical medicine and surgery. 3rd edition. St Louis (MO): Elsevier Saunders; 2012. p. 452–71.

6. Legendre LFJ. Oral disorders of exotic rodents. Vet Clin North Am Exot Anim Pract 2003;6:601–28.

7. Capello V. Diagnosis and treatment of dental disease in pet rodents. J Exotic Pet Med 2008;17(2):114–23.

8. Chiasson RB. The phylogenetic significance of rodent cheek pouches. J Mammal 1954;35:425–7.

9. Goshal NG, Bal HS. Histomorphology of the hamster cheek pouch. Lab Anim 1990;24:228–33.

10. Cox PG, Jeffery N. Reviewing the morphology of the jaw-closing musculature in squirrels, rats, and guinea pigs with contrast-enhanced microCT. Anat Rec 2011; 294:915–28.

11. Cox PG, Rayfiel EJ, Fagan MJ, et al. Functional evolution of the feeding system in rodents. PLoS One 2012;7(4):1–11.

12. Druzinsky RE. Functional anatomy of incisal biting in *Aplodontia rufa* and sciuromorph rodents—Part 1: masticatory muscles, skull shape and digging. Cells Tissues Organs 2010;191:510–22.

13. Jekl V. Rodents: dentistry. In: Keeble E, Meredith A, editors. BSAVA manual of rodents and ferrets. Gloucester (United Kingdom): British Small Animal Veterinary Association; 2009. p. 86–95.

14. Yarto-Jaramillo E. Respiratory system anatomy, physiology and disease: guinea pigs and chinchillas. Vet Clin Exot Anim 2011;14:339–55.

15. Druzinsky RE. Functional anatomy of incisal biting in *Aplodontia rufa* and sciuromorph rodents—Part 2: sciuromorphy is efficacious for production of force at the incisors. Cells Tissues Organs 2010;192:50–63.

16. Becht G. Comparative biologic-anatomical researches on mastication in some mammals. Proc K Ned Akad Wet C 1953;56:508–27.

17. Hiiemae K, Ardran GM. A cinefluorographic study of mandibular movement during feeding in the rat (*Rattus norvegicus*). J Zool 1968;154:139–54.

18. Reese S, Fehr M. Small mammals. In: Krautwald-Junghanns ME, Pees M, Reese S, et al, editors. Diagnostic imaging of exotic pets. Hannover (Germany): Schlütersche Verlagsgesellschaft mbH & Co; 2011. p. 143–307.

19. Zuri I, Terkel J. Reversed palatal perforation by upper incisors in ageing blind mole-rats (*Spalax ehrenbergi*). J Anat 2001;199:591–8.

20. Robinson M, Hart D, Pigott GH. The effects of diet on the incidence of periodontitis in rats. Lab Anim 1991;25:247–53.

21. Vincent AL, Rodrick GE, Sodeman WA Jr. The pathology of the Mongolian gerbil (*Meriones unguiculatus*): a review. Lab Anim Sci 1979;29:645–51.

22. Yankell SL. Oral disease in laboratory animals: animal models of human dental disease. In: Harvey CE, editor. Veterinary dentistry. Philadelphia: WB Saunders Co; 1985. p. 281.
23. Bennet RA. Odontomas in prairie dogs. In: Proceedings of the North Am Vet Conference. Orlando (FL): 2007. p. 1707–10.
24. Losco PE. Dental dysplasia in rats and mice. Toxicol Pathol 1995;23(6):677–88.
25. Head KW, Cullen JM, Dubielzig RR, et al. Histological classification of tumors of the alimentary system of domestic animals. In: WHO histological classification of tumors of domestic animals, second series. Washington, DC: Armed Forces Institute of Pathology; 2003. p. 46–57.
26. Thoma KH, Goldman HM. Odontogenic tumors: a classification based on observations of the epithelial, mesemchymal, and mixed varieties. Am J Pathol 1946; 22:443–9.
27. Walsh KM, Denholm LJ, Cooper BJ. Epithelial odontogenic tumours in domestic animals. J Comp Pathol 1987;97:503–21.
28. Boy SC, Steenkamp G. Odontoma like tumours of squirrel elodont incisors-elodontomas. J Comp Pathol 2006;135:56–61.
29. Jang DD, Kim CK. Spontaneous complex odontoma in Sprague-Dawley rat. J Vet Med Sci 2002;64(3):289–91.
30. Ida-Yonemochi H, Noda T, Shimokawa H, et al. Disturbed tooth eruption in osteopetrotic (op/op) mice: histopathogenesis of tooth malformation and odontomas. J Oral Pathol Med 2002;31(6):361–73.
31. Wagner RA, Garman RH, Collins BM. Diagnosing odontomas in prairie dogs. Exotic DVM Magazine 1999;1(1):7–10.
32. Phalen DN, Antinoff N, Fricke ME. Obstructive respiratory disease in prairie dogs with odontomas. Vet Clin Exot Anim Pract 2000;3:513–7.
33. Capello V. Incisor extraction to resolve clinical signs of odontoma in a prairie dog. Exotic DVM 2002;4(1):9.
34. Wagner R, Johnson D. Rhinotomy for treatment of odontoma in prairie dogs. Exotic DVM 2001;3:29–34.
35. Crossley DA. Small mammal dentistry (part I). In: Quesenberry KE, Carpenter JW, editors. Ferrets, rabbits and rodents clinical medicine and surgery. 2nd edition. St Louis (MO): Elsevier Saunders; 2004. p. 370–9.
36. Greenacre CB. Spontaneous tumours of small mammals. Vet Clin Exot Anim 2004;7:627–51.
37. Capello V. Dentistry of prairie dogs and other squirrels. In: American board of veterinary practitioners symposium 2014 proceedings. Nashville (TN): 2014. p. 1–4.
38. Capello V, Lennox AM, Ghisleni G. Elodontoma in two guinea pigs. J Vet Dent 2015;32(2):111–9.
39. Jekl V, Hauptman K, Skoric M, et al. Elodontoma in a degus (Octodon degus). J Exotic Pet Med 2008;17:216–20.
40. Barbolt TA, Bhandari JC. Ameloblastic odontoma in a rat. Lab Anim Sci 1983; 33(6):583–4.
41. Ernst H, Rittinghausen S, Mohr U. Ameloblastic odontoma in a Sprague-Dawley rat. Dtsch Tierarztl Wochenschr 1989;96(4):207–9.
42. Philippart C, Arys A, Dourov N. Experimental odontomas in osteopetrotic op/op rats. J Oral Pathol Med 1994;23(5):200–4.
43. Dayan D, Waner T, Harmelin A, et al. Bilateral complex odontoma in a Swiss (CD-1) male mouse. Lab Anim 1994;28(1):90–2.
44. Nyska A, Waner T, Tal H, et al. Spontaneous ameloblastic fibro-odontoma in a female mouse. Oral Pathol Med 1991;20(5):250–2.

45. Lu X, Rios HF, Jiang B, et al. A new osteopetrosis mutant mouse strain (ntl) with odontoma-like proliferations and lack of tooth roots. Eur J Oral Sci 2009;117(6): 625–35.
46. Bulliot C, Mentré V. Original rhinostomy technique for the treatment of pseudoodontoma in a prairie dog (Cynomys ludovicianus). J Exotic Pet Med 2013;22: 76–81.
47. Smith M, Dodd JR, Hobson P, et al. Clinical techniques: Surgical removal of elodontomas in the black tailed prairie dog (Cynomys ludovicianus) and eastern fox squirrel. J Exotic Pet Med 2013;22:258–64.
48. Mitchell SC. Rhinotomy for treatment of odontoma in an Eastern gray squirrel. In: AEMV Proceedings. Oakland (CA): 2012. p. 71.
49. Capello V. Odontomas in rodents: surgical treatment of pseudo-odontomas in prairie dogs. In: AEMV Proceedings. Oakland (CA): 2012. p. 105–9.
50. Slootweg PJ, Kuijpers MHM, van de Kooij AJ. Rat odontogenic tumors associated with disturbed tooth eruption. J Oral Pathol Med 1996;25:481–3.
51. Berman JJ, Rice JM. Odontogenic tumours produced in Fischer rats by a single intraportal injection of methylnitrosourea. Arch Oral Biol 1980;25:213–20.
52. Percy DH, Bathold SW. Pathology of laboratory rodents and rabbits. Oxford (United Kingdom): Blackwell Publishing; 2007. p. 3–309.
53. Harness JE, Wagner JE. Specific diseases and conditions. In: Harness JE, Wagner JE, editors. The biology and medicine of rabbits and rodents. 4th edition. Philadelphia: Williams ad Wilkins; 1995. p. 171–322.
54. Capello V. Surgical techniques in pet hamsters. Exotic DVM 2003;5(3):32–7.
55. West WL, Gaillard ET, O'Connor SA. Fibroma (myxoma) molle in a hamster (Mesocricetus auratus). Contemp Top Lab Anim Sci 2001;40(6):32–4.
56. Mouser P, Cole A, Lin TL. Maxillary osteosarcoma in a prairie dog (Cynomys ludovicianus). J Vet Diagn Invest 2006;18:310–2.
57. Yamate J, Yamamoto E, Nabe M, et al. Spontaneous adenocarcinoma immunoreactive to cyclooxygenase-2 and transforming growth factor-beta1 in the buccal salivary gland of a Richardson's ground squirrel (Spermophilus richardsonii). Exp Anim 2007;56(5):379–84.
58. Sainsbury AW, Kountouri A, DuBoulay G, et al. Oral disease in free-living red squirrels (Sciurus vulgaris) in the United Kingdom. J Wildl Dis 2004;40(2):185–96.
59. Miles AEW, Grigson C. Colyer's variation and diseases of teeth of animals. Cambridge (United Kingdom): Cambridge University Press; 1990. p. 672.
60. Wiggs RB, Lobprise HB. Dental and oral disease in rodents and lagomorphs. In: Wiggs RB, Lobprise HB, editors. Veterinary dentistry principles and practice. Philadelphia: Lippincott-Raven; 1997. p. 518–37.
61. Jekl V, Knotek Z. Evaluation of a laryngoscope and a rigid endoscope for the examination of the oral cavity of small mammals. Vet Rec 2007;160:9–13.
62. Taylor M. Endoscopy as an aid to the examination and treatment of the oropharyngeal disease of small herbivorous mammals. Semin Avian Exot Pet 1999;8: 139–41.
63. Hernandez-Divers SJ. Exotic mammal diagnostic endoscopy and endosurgery. Vet Clin Exot Anim 2010;13:255–72.
64. Hernandez-Divers SJ. Clinical technique: dental endoscopy of rabbits and rodents. J Exotic Pet Med 2008;17:87–92.
65. Silverman S, Tell LA. Radiology of rodents, rabbits and ferrets. An atlas of oral anatomy and positioning. St. Louis (MO): Elsevier Saunders; 2005.
66. Capello V, Lennox AM. Clinical radiology of exotic companion mammals. Ames (IA): Wiley Blackwell; 2008. p. 1–486.

67. Capello V, Lennox AM, Widmer WR. The basic of radiology. In: Capello V, Lennox AM, editors. Clinical radiology of exotic companion mammals. Ames (IA): Wiley-Blackwell; 2008. p. 2–51.

68. Bennet RA. Soft tissue surgery. In: Quesenberry KE, Carpenter JW, editors. Ferrets, rabbits and rodents clinical medicine and surgery. 3rd edition. St Louis (MO): Elsevier Saunders; 2012. p. 373–91.

69. Capello V. Common surgical procedures in pet rodents. J Exotic Pet Med 2011; 20(4):294–307.

70. Johnson DH. Over-the-endoscope endotracheal intubation of small exotic mammals. Exotic DVM 2005;7(2):18–23.

71. Capello V. Intubation techniques for exotic companion mammals. In: Proceedings of the North Am Vet Conference. Orlando (FL): 2009. p. 1829–31.

72. Capello V. We are not smaller rabbits, either. Dentistry of other rodent species and ferrets. In: Proceedings of the North Am Vet Conference. Orlando (FL): 2011. p. 1681–4.

73. Johnson DH. Rhinotomy approach for the removal of pseudo-odontoma in sciuromorphs. In: Proceedings of the AEMV Conference. Indianapolis (IN): 2013. p. 42.

74. Pelizzone I, Vitolo GD, D'Acierno M, et al. Lateral approach for excision of maxillary incisor pseudo-odontoma in prairie dogs (Cynomys ludovicianus). In Vivo 2016;30:61–8.

Anatomy and Disorders of the Oral Cavity of Ferrets and Other Exotic Companion Carnivores

Cathy A. Johnson-Delaney, DVM*

KEYWORDS

- Ferrets • Dental disease • Oral disease • Exotic carnivores • Dental treatment

KEY POINTS

- Carnivore dental and oral anatomy is similar in the species discussed and the ferret serves as a model for description and function.
- Common carnivore dental diseases include plaque and calculus, malocclusion, tooth extrusion, wear, fractures, loss and necrosis, gingival hyperplasia, gingivitis and periodontal disease, and abscesses.
- Ferret oral disorders in addition to dental disease include cleft lips and/or palate, ulcers, fracture of the jaw, tonsillitis, salivary microliths and mucocele, and neoplasia.
- Dental care should include annual or biannual dental examination under anesthesia, and cleaning.
- Treatment of dental and oral disease in exotic carnivores is similar to that used in dogs and cats.

INTRODUCTION

Exotic carnivores share similar dental anatomy, function, and diseases. Dental and oral diseases are most commonly described in ferrets (*Mustela putorius furo*), which serve as the model for the rest of the category. Dog and cat dentistry guidelines for veterinary and home care seem to be relevant. Exotic carnivores seen in practice include skunks (*Mephitis mephitis*), fennec foxes (*Vulpes zerda*), and procyonids, including raccoons (*Procyon lotor*), coatimundis (*Nasua* sp) and kinkajous (*Potos flavus*). The most common dental and oral problems are plaque and calculus; teeth fractures; gingivitis and periodontitis; tooth loss caused by a variety of disease processes, such as malnutrition or renal disease; abscesses; and neoplasia. In ferrets, oral

Disclosure: The author has nothing to disclose.
Washington Ferret Rescue & Shelter, 12514 128th Lane NE, Kirkland, WA 98034, USA
* 13813 65th Avenue W #7, Edmonds, WA 98026.
E-mail address: cajddvm@hotmail.com

Vet Clin Exot Anim 19 (2016) 901–928
http://dx.doi.org/10.1016/j.cvex.2016.04.009
1094-9194/16/$ – see front matter © 2016 Elsevier Inc. All rights reserved.

vetexotic.theclinics.com

ulceration and tonsillitis are frequently seen and may accompany systemic disease, whereas salivary microliths and mucoceles are seen occasionally.

THE FERRET
Anatomy and Physiology

The ferret is a strict carnivore and has teeth and jaw structure to accommodate such a diet. It has 28 to 30 deciduous teeth 2(dI 3–4/3: dC 1/1: dM 3/3) (**Fig. 1**). The permanent dental formula is 2(I3/3: C1/1: P3/3: M1/2) = 34 (**Fig. 2**). The mandibular second molar is congenitally missing in some ferrets, which changes the formula to M1/1 = 32.[1] There is speculation that it is in the evolutionary process of becoming lost or vestigial, as has happened in other carnivores. There may also be supernumerary teeth, most commonly found between the first and second maxillary incisors.[2] The ferret, like other mammals, is diphyodont in having 2 distinct sets of teeth: deciduous and permanent.[1] The 3 maxillary incisor teeth of each quadrant are slightly longer than the 3 mandibular incisors. The second incisor of the mandible is set back from the others.[3] (**Fig. 3**A) The mandibular canines close rostrally to the maxillary canines.[3] (**Fig. 3**A, B). Although usually there are 4 premolars in Carnivora, only 3 are present in the ferret. The first premolar has been lost in development.[4] The last maxillary carnassial tooth is the fourth premolar. It has 3 roots.[5] There is a single molar in the maxillary arcade that has 3 roots. It is wider in the buccolingual breadth compared with the mesiodistal length, making it appear to be rooted at right angles to the rest of the teeth. It has a narrow, depressed waist that separates its palatal side from the buccal side of the crown. There are 2 small cusps on the buccal part and a single cusp on the palatal part.[5] This tooth may be overlooked in an awake ferret examination because of its location. The large mandibular carnassial tooth is the first molar. The crown of the first mandibular molar has 3 distinct cusps. Two form the blades of the carnassial tooth. The smaller, lower, and distal cusp, in conjunction with the second molar, interlocks with the cusps of the maxillary molar during occlusion.[5] The first mandibular molar has 2 roots, although sometimes there is an accessory slender central root present. The second mandibular molar, if present, is a small tooth with a single root and a simple crown with a minor ridge and cusplets. It does not occlude with any

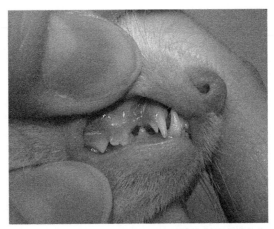

Fig. 1. A 2.5-month-old ferret before complete shedding of deciduous teeth. The smaller deciduous canine tooth, as well as the second and third thin deciduous molars, are still present. The first deciduous molar tooth has already shed. (*Courtesy of* Vittorio Capello, DVM, Milano, Italy; with permission.)

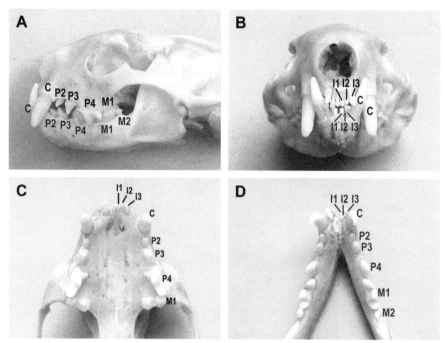

Fig. 2. Dentition of the ferret shown on a specimen carrying minor dental abnormalities such as malalignment of the incisors and blunting of the maxillary canine teeth. (*A*) Lateral view of canine, premolar, and molar teeth. (*B*) Rostral view of canine and incisor teeth. (*C*) Maxillary arcade. Note the large carnassial tooth (P4) and the buccolingual direction of the molar tooth (M1). (*D*) Mandibular arcade. (*Courtesy of* Vittorio Capello, DVM, Milano, Italy; with permission.)

maxillary teeth, but helps with the crushing function of the distal cusp of the first mandibular molar (**Fig. 3**C).

The jaws are short with the well-developed articular condyle of the mandible fitting into a transverse articular fossa.[3] This fossa has a postarticular process preventing dislocation on wide opening for a strong bite.[3] The muscles of mastication include a well-developed masseter muscle that originates at the zygomatic arch and inserts on the masseteric fossa, condyloid crest, and mandibular angular process.[3] The digastric muscle originates on the jugular process and tympanic bulla and passes to the ventral border of the caudal portion of the mandible.[3] It has the action of opening the jaw. The major adductor muscle of the lower jaw is the temporalis, which is well-developed in the male.[3] The deep pterygoid muscles, lateral and medial, assist the masseter and temporalis muscles in the crushing and chewing motion of closing the jaws.[3] The mandibles and the maxillae are approximately equal in length but ferrets are anisognathics, with the mandibles being narrower and fitting medially to the maxillae, which allows the shearing motion during chewing.[3] Mustelids crush their food using the molars distal to the carnassial teeth.[5] Another adaptation is the overlapping and interdigitation of the mandibular arcade with the maxillary arcade by the motions necessary to process plant materials and abrasive food. However, it does allow the dorsoventral movement necessary for the cheek teeth and carnassials to shear tissue-based foods. The temporomandibular joint effectively locks the mandible into the skull, preventing the loss of bite force during predation. The maxillary

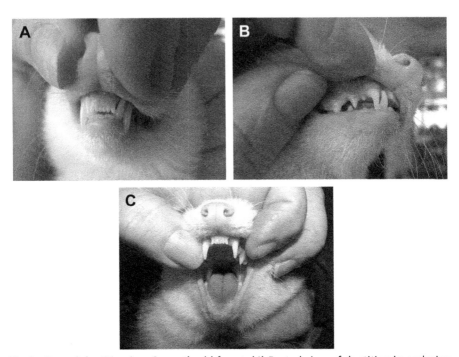

Fig. 3. Normal dentition in a 6-month-old ferret. (*A*) Rostral view of dentition in occlusion, showing the maxillary incisors being slightly longer than the mandibular incisors as well as the slight caudal position of the second mandibular incisors. (*B*) Lateral view. The mandibular canines are close in front of the maxillary canines. (*C*) Rostral view, open mouth. There are only 3 premolars in each arcade because premolar 1 has been lost in development. This ferret is also missing the second mandibular molar, which is absent in many ferrets. (*Courtesy of* Cathy Johnson-Delaney, DVM, Edmonds, WA; with permission.)

canines and cheek teeth are aligned, and effectively become arches, which is a common adaptation of carnivores that strengthens the skull without adding bone mass. The canine teeth form a tight interlock when the mouth is closed. The biomechanics of these adaptations are markedly different from those of herbivores. It is likely that the shift from a whole prey diet to one of dry kibbles may have deleterious impacts on the function of the ferret's specific dental adaptations, although this has yet to be the focus of a published research study. Kibble is crunchy and abrasive, which is a selling point to reduce dental calculus, but chewing kibble may cause structural changes to the teeth and underlying bony support. These changes ultimately cause excessive wear of the teeth and may result in fractures or loss of a tooth or teeth. In short, the ferret's dentition is not well suited to having to grind kibble.[4]

Ferrets, like other carnivores, are capable of widely opening the oral cavity. The labial commissures extend farther caudally than the carnassial teeth. The orbicularis oris muscle is moderately well developed. The lower lip is closely attached to the mandibular gingiva, with little flexibility. Periodontal and gingival tissues and structures are similar to those of other carnivores. The oral microflora of the gingival sulcus and related mucosa at the midbuccal surface of the right upper P4 was investigated. Nearly 100% of the total cultivable flora was composed of facultative anaerobic gram-negative and gram-positive rods. *Pasteurella* spp, *Corynebacterium* spp, and *Rothia* spp were the major components. No anaerobic bacteria were detected.[6]

The ferret has 5 paired salivary glands: parotid, submandibular, sublingual, molar, and zygomatic. The parotid gland secretions are seromucus. The mandibular and sublingual gland's secretions are mucus. The molar and zygomatic glands secrete predominantly mucus but also secrete some serous fluid.[3]

THE DENTAL EXAMINATION

Examination of the ferret oral cavity is an essential part of any physical examination. If the ferret is prone to bite, sedation such as midazolam at 0.25 to 0.4 mg/kg intramuscularly [IM] may be necessary for full examination. Most pet ferrets readily open their mouths for the examination. Teeth and gingiva can be examined using a cotton bud to elevate the lips. The author photographs the teeth before and after the procedure to give the pictures to the owner. These photographs are a good practice builder.

DIAGNOSTIC IMAGING

Standard views for radiography of the ferret head are reported. Laterolateral, ventrodorsal, 2 oblique, and rostrocaudal projections can be taken either closed or open mouth, or both[7] (**Fig. 4**). Small intraoral films can also be used in the ferret for dedicated views of the mandible and the maxilla[7] (**Fig. 5**).

Unlike small herbivore species such as rabbits and cavylike rodents, advanced diagnostic imaging such as oral endoscopy and computed tomography (CT) is less critical, because of the wide opening of the oral cavity and the brachiodont teeth versus elodont teeth of those herbivorous species. However, CT can also be useful for dental diseases in this species. Beside two-dimensional sequential axial, coronal, and longitudinal views, three-dimensional rendering, such as volume renderings, provide details of the anatomy of teeth below the gingival level, as in a bony specimen, or even to their roots within the alveolus (**Fig. 6**).

DENTAL DISEASE
Plaque and Calculus

Calculus (tartar) is defined as the mineralized buildup of plaque on tooth surfaces[2] (**Fig. 7**). Plaque is a buildup of saliva, bacteria, cellular and food debris, epithelial cells,

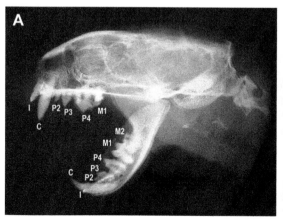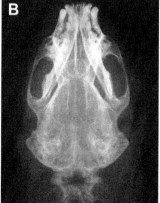

Fig. 4. Radiography of the normal head of a 1-kg male ferret. (*A*) Laterolateral projection, open mouth. (*B*) Ventrodorsal projection. (*Courtesy of* Vittorio Capello, DVM, Milano, Italy; with permission.)

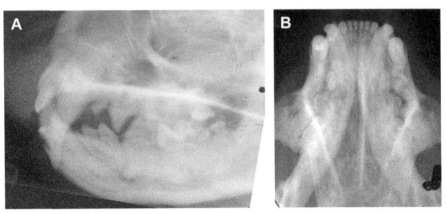

Fig. 5. Radiography of a 2-year-old ferret with normal dentition, intraoral films. (*A*) Latero-lateral projection, in occlusion. (*B*) Dorsoventral projection. (*Courtesy of* Cathy Johnson-Delaney, DVM, Edmonds, WA; with permission.)

and bacterial by-products. It slowly mineralizes. The pH of the saliva as well as enzyme content, enzyme release from bacteria, the content of the diet, and consistency of the diet all influence the degree of plaque buildup. Plaque/calculus in pet ferrets develops whether fed kibble, canned diet, or a liquid diet. Domestic ferrets fed a processed diet seem to lack some of the dietary components that inhibit plaque buildup in wild mustelids.[5] The conformation of the mouth may influence the buildup because the bite may allow pocketing of material. The author has not found studies done on the pH (particularly in periodontal and gingival sulci), and enzyme characterization and levels. In combination with diet content, these would aid in development of effective prophylaxis treatments.

The clinical presentation is plaque and calculus visible on tooth surfaces. It may extend into the gingival pockets where it accumulates and causes gingivitis. There may be periodontitis as well and even abscess associated with the buildup. There may be oral odor. The gums and teeth may be painful. In addition, the ferret may be anorectic, dehydrated, and losing weight.[2] While under anesthesia for removal of the calculus and plaque, radiographs should be taken to assess tooth and bone status. Gingival sulci need also be probed to determine the degree of gingivitis. If teeth are loose or roots are damaged there may need to be extractions. Calculus and plaque should be removed by scaling, either by hand or by ultrasonic methods. Removal of calculus is the most common dental procedure.[8] All scaled teeth should then be polished using a fluoride polish. A fluoride rinse can be applied to the teeth following polish. Prophylactic tooth brushing at home using an enzymatic toothpaste is encouraged. In ferrets that form heavy calculus, biannual dental cleaning under anesthesia may be advised.

Malocclusion

Mismatched bite may be caused by congenital changes such as prognathism, traumatic changes such as jaw fracture, teeth loss, or supernumerary teeth. It is most commonly seen with the mandibular second incisor teeth being caudal to the other incisors.[2] The malocclusive incisors are a common incidental finding. Prognathism is distinctive and may have hereditary factors (**Fig. 8**). Other abnormalities related to

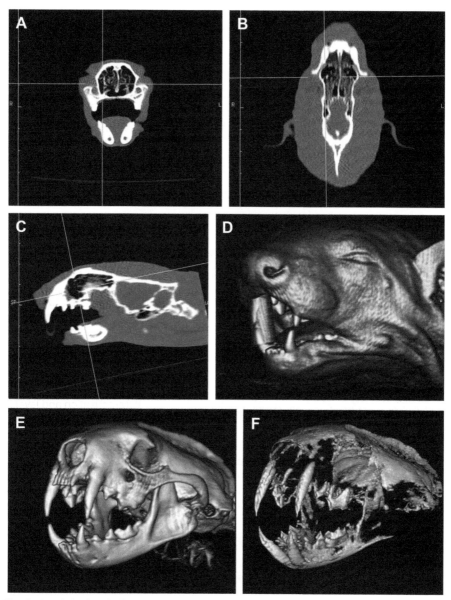

Fig. 6. CT of the head of a 6-year-old ferret, open mouth. Standard two-dimensional axial (*A*), coronal (*B*), and longitudinal (*C*) views. Three-dimensional rendering such as volume renderings are helpful to display details of the anatomy of teeth. Starting from the surface (*D*) and subtracting soft tissues (*E*), teeth can be examined below the gingival level like in a bony specimen. Subtracting part of cortical bone (*F*), they can be examined even to their roots within the alveolus. Extrusion of canine teeth is visible in this ferret. (*Courtesy of* Vittorio Capello, DVM, Milano, Italy; with permission.)

malocclusion found on oral/dental examination are likely asymptomatic or incidental unless there is trauma such as jaw fracture. Prognathism and mandibular second incisor malocclusion do not need treatment unless they would cause ulceration to soft tissues.

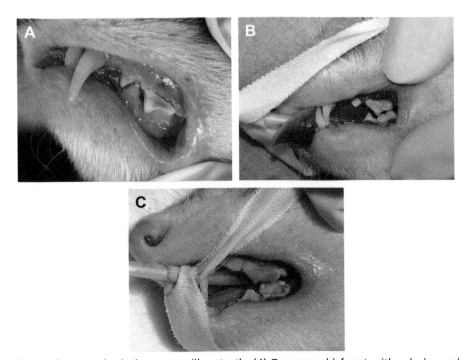

Fig. 7. Plaque and calculus on maxillary teeth. (*A*) Two-year-old ferret with calculus and gingivitis noted during an annual examination. (*B*) Thick calculus and severe gingivitis in a ferret before scaling. (*C*) Thick and extensive buildup of calculus obscuring the interdental spaces. ([*A*] *Courtesy of* Cathy Johnson-Delaney, DVM, Edmonds, WA; with permission; and [*B*, *C*] *Courtesy of* Vittorio Capello, DVM, Milano, Italy; with permission.)

Extrusion of the Canine Teeth

As a ferret ages, the canine teeth extrude, accompanied by gingival recession (**Fig. 9**). There may also be bulging of the gum around the crown. In one study, 93.7% of ferrets were affected by this dental abnormality.[9] Usually the gingiva around the crown appears erythematous and sometimes swollen, but it is not usually painful on probing

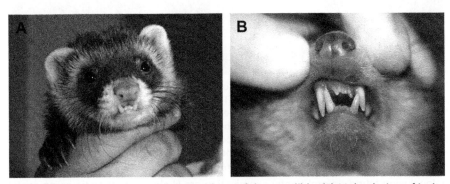

Fig. 8. Malocclusion in ferrets. (*A*) Prognathism of the mandible. (*B*) Malocclusion of incisor and canine teeth. In particular, the tip of the left mandibular canine created an ulceration of the upper lip. ([*A*] *Courtesy of* Cathy Johnson-Delaney, DVM, Edmonds, WA; with permission; and [*B*] *Courtesy of* Vittorio Capello, DVM, Milano, Italy; with permission.)

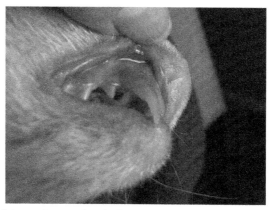

Fig. 9. Extrusion of the canine tooth, which is a normal finding of aging. This ferret also has gingivitis and some calculus buildup. (*Courtesy of* Cathy Johnson-Delaney, DVM, Edmonds, WA; with permission.)

to rule out abscess, gingivitis, and periodontal disease. Dental radiographs are recommended to assess the health of the root and surrounding tissues and bone. No treatment is needed other than normal dental prophylaxis and home oral hygiene if there is no disease found.

Tooth Wear

Teeth may show wear as the ferret ages (**Fig. 10**). If not accompanied by calculus, gingivitis, fractures, or periodontal disease requiring treatment, it is just an incidental finding. It can be noted on any of the tooth surfaces. There is speculation that excessive wear is caused primarily by feeding a kibble diet because the same type of wear is not seen in wild mustelids or ferrets fed a nonkibble diet.[4]

Fractured Teeth

The canine teeth are the most commonly encountered fractured teeth. Most often, the tip is fractured off. Other teeth may be fractured by extensive oral trauma (**Fig. 11**A). In one study, tooth fractures of the ferret were exclusively associated with canine teeth

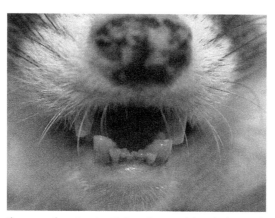

Fig. 10. Severe tooth wear of canine teeth in a 9-year-old male ferret. (*Courtesy of* Vittorio Capello, DVM, Milano, Italy; with permission.)

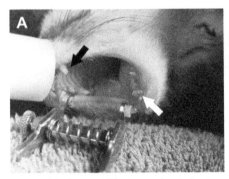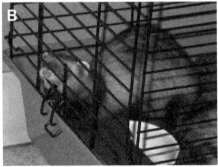

Fig. 11. (A) The mandibular canine is fractured and has become necrotic (*white arrow*). The maxillary canine shows the tip has been fractured (*black arrow*). (B) Ferret biting at the cage bars. (*Courtesy of* Cathy Johnson-Delaney, DVM, Edmonds, WA; with permission.)

and found in 31.7% of the ferrets examined.[9] Pulp exposure was confirmed in 60.0% of these teeth.[9] The author sees the maxillary canine tooth most affected. Pet ferrets frequently bite and pull at their cage bars when they want to get out (**Fig. 11**B). They also fracture teeth during falls and during play when they hit walls and other obstacles. The fractured tooth should be checked for sensitivity to touch or cold. A cotton bud wetted then frozen works well to touch teeth. If sensitive, the tooth may be dying. Many owners do not notice that a tooth is fractured or missing its tip. The affected tooth may be discolored, necrotic, and/or loose. Unless the pulp is exposed and the ferret is painful and/or has associated dental disease, the finding may be incidental. A dental radiograph should be taken to assess the pulp cavity and root even if the fracture seems minor. Probing during anesthesia may be necessary to assess whether the pulp cavity is open. The teeth should be watched closely during subsequent examinations.

If presented immediately after the fracture with the pulp exposed but with the tooth still viable, a superficial pulpotomy can be done in the canine tooth. This procedure involves using a high-speed burr on the pulp a few millimeters below the exposed surface, drying and sterilizing the pulp chamber, and filling with a composite as is done in other species. The danger is in overheating the pulp cavity and damaging the pulp in the process, which would lead to eventual necrosis. A root canal procedure and filling may also be attempted to save the tooth.[10] The author prefers to try to preserve canine teeth if possible, particularly in young ferrets. Despite this salvage dental procedure, many ferrets fracture them again, or the tooth progresses to necrosis. When doing endodontic procedures, parenteral antibiotics should be instigated as well as oral rinses and adequate analgesia. Prognosis is good if the pulp is not exposed. If the pulp is exposed, the long-term prognosis is extraction of the canine tooth at some point, if it becomes abscessed or necrotic.[2]

Tooth Loss

Tooth loss includes noneruptions, such as when the second mandibular molar is congenitally missing. Most tooth loss is caused by trauma or dental disease (**Fig. 12**). It can also be found with a variety of disease processes, such as malnutrition, renal disease, and neoplasia. A thorough dental examination should be done, including dental radiographs, which are important to determine whether a tooth root is still present. A work-up for systemic disease is recommended. If a tooth root

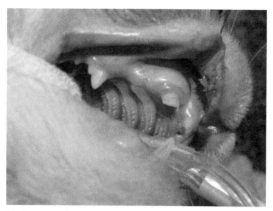

Fig. 12. Tooth loss likely secondary to trauma because the canine tooth is fractured. (*Courtesy of* Cathy Johnson-Delaney, DVM, Edmonds, WA; with permission.)

remains, it should be extracted. Any presence of dental or systemic disease should be addressed per cause.

Tooth Necrosis

A tooth becomes necrotic when the nerve and pulp are no longer viable, and in most cases the tooth is discolored brown or is translucent (**Fig. 13**). It is frequently seen with the canine tooth that had a fractured tip or other trauma. Tooth death can also follow abscess or periodontitis or itself may be a nidus for infection and periodontitis. There is usually a history of trauma to the tooth. The owner may not have noticed the discoloration or any oral symptoms. A thorough oral examination and radiographs should be done to assess the extent of the dental disease. Concurrent disease should be addressed. If the tooth is loose or the radiographs show root, periodontal disease, and/or bone disease, the tooth should be extracted. If the tooth is quiescent, not loose, nonpainful, and there is no abscess or periodontal disease associated with it, extraction may not be necessary. Frequent dental examination should be done to ensure the status does not change.[2]

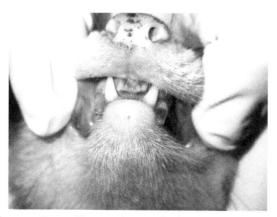

Fig. 13. Bilaterally necrotic maxillary canine teeth. (*Courtesy of* Cathy Johnson-Delaney, DVM, Edmonds, WA; with permission.)

Gingival Hyperplasia

In ferrets, this condition has been associated with administration of phenytoin. However, it can be seen with prolonged, severe gingivitis that proliferates over the teeth, causing deep gingival pockets. Phenytoin for epilepsy administered at a therapeutic oral dosing of 40 mg/kg induced this change within in a month. It is similar to what happens in humans. It is caused by a drug-induced folic acid deficiency and can be prevented by supplementation of folic acid if the ferret is being treated with phenytoin. The dosage of folic acid is unknown because no study was found that has used it to prevent the hyperplasia. Oral hygiene is warranted to avoid complications of gingivitis, calculus, and periodontal disease.[11]

Gingivitis

Simply described, this is inflammation of the gingiva. Plaque and calculus left on tooth surfaces extend into gingival pockets and accumulate causing the gingivitis (**Fig. 14**). As the inflammation increases, the depth of the gingival sulcus increases, which, if untreated, leads to periodontal disease. Periodontal disease includes tissue destruction extending into the periodontal ligaments and the bone. As this process continues, infection and inflammation can involve the tooth root and may involve permanent damage to the tooth.[2] In one study, the normal gingival sulcus depth measured less than 0.5 mm in 87.8% of anesthetized ferrets being screened for dental disease.[9] Gingivitis was defined as probing depths greater than 0.5 mm and less than 2 mm, which is also evidence of periodontal disease.[9] Clinical evidence of periodontal disease was present in 65.3% of anesthetized ferrets (gingivitis or probing depths >0.5 mm).[9] Advanced periodontal disease (ie, periodontal pockets >2 mm or stage 3 furcation exposure) was not found on clinical examination.[9] There is also considerable pain with this process, and many ferrets paw at their mouths and become anorectic. They may lose weight, and gag while eating or drinking. On examination, the gingiva is erythematous and swollen, and it may extend over the tooth surface. There may also be excess salivation and gagging on opening the mouth. Calculus is usually present, sometimes in very large amounts, with halitosis. Tonsils are frequently swollen, although tonsillitis may also be caused by systemic disease. The differential diagnoses include periodontitis, gingival abscess, and neoplasia. Dental radiographs should be taken under anesthesia, and full probing of the gingiva and teeth should be performed. Analgesics should be administered for the pain.

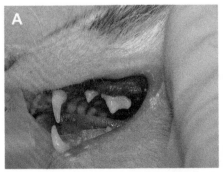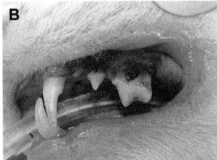

Fig. 14. (*A, B*) Severe gingivitis in the 2 ferrets shown in **Fig. 7**B, C, after scaling. Retraction of the gingiva and exposure of the roots of P3 and P4 are present in (*B*). In both cases, extrusion of canine teeth is present. (*Courtesy of* Vittorio Capello, DVM, Milano, Italy; with permission.)

Antibiotic therapy using a broad-spectrum oral antibiotic should be started before the cleaning and continued for 5 to 7 days following the dental procedure. The teeth should be scaled, sulci flushed, and the teeth polished. If the gingiva has proliferated over the teeth, gingivectomy should be considered, preferably using laser or radiosurgery. Deep sulci can be filled with an antibiotic oral gel (Doxyrobe Gel, Zoetis, Florham Park, NJ), as used in canine dentistry. Oral rinse can be used on a cotton bud applied to the gums and teeth routinely as part of daily prophylaxis. (Listerine Smart Rinse Berry Flavor, McNeill-PPC Inc, Fort Washington, PA) Home brushing using an enzymatic pet toothpaste is recommended.

Periodontal Disease

In cases of periodontal disease, the periodontal ligament is compromised and inflammation/infection usually extends into the periodontal tissues and deeper to the bone, causing an osteomyelitis. The periodontal pocket is deeper than 2 mm when probed under anesthesia.[9] For evaluation of the periodontal disease, the author uses the grading system as listed earlier. The ferrets present with marked calculus and gingivitis that progresses and the inflammation/infection extends into the sulcus, then deepens into the periodontal tissues. If the ligament is compromised, the tooth will become loose. The tooth root may become exposed. Osteomyelitis may be present, particularly with advancing disease. Periodontal disease may involve more than 1 tooth. The patient may be anorectic because of the oral pain. It may also gag, have excess salivation, have halitosis, and paw at its mouth. It may have tonsillitis. Dental radiographs should be taken to assess the degree of periodontal erosion and underlying bone disorder. Treatment starts with scaling of the teeth and treatment of the gingiva. If gingival proliferation is present covering part of the crown, gingivectomy to the normal gingival level should be performed using laser or radiosurgery. The gingival sulcus can be treated with instillation of a dental antibiotic gel used for dogs (Doxyrobe Gel, Zoetis, Florham Park, NJ). If the tooth roots are exposed and/or the tooth is very loose, and if the tooth root and pulp are involved, extraction is usually necessary. A slightly loose tooth may firm up with treatment of the periodontal disease if otherwise the tooth is healthy. Parenteral antibiotics such as amoxicillin (25 mg/kg by mouth every 12 hours) along with a nonsteroidal antiinflammatory drug (NSAID) such as meloxicam (0.2 mg/kg by mouth every 24 hours) are used in treatment. Daily swabbing of the mouth using a cotton bud, with an oral rinse (Listerine Smart Rinse Berry Flavor, McNeill-PPC Inc, Fort Washington, PA) aids in healing. The gum massage with the cotton bud helps to heal the gingiva. Teeth should be brushed daily using an enzymatic pet toothpaste (CET, Virbac, Fort Worth, TX). It is recommended that ferrets more than 3 years of age have biannual thorough dental cleaning under anesthesia.

Abscesses

Dental abscesses may develop because of or following gingival disease, periodontal disease and/or osteomyelitis, or infection[2] (**Fig. 15**A). Infection may also enter the tooth from an exposed pulp cavity caused by fracture. It may also occur after caries, which is rarely seen in ferrets. In general, the tooth root is involved, and this abnormality can be confirmed on radiographs (**Fig. 16**). Abscesses may follow a trauma to an individual tooth or gingival area, or with calculus formation typically in the gingival sulcus. In many cases, by the time the abscess is discovered, the tooth is no longer viable, and there is enough periodontal disease and bone loss to make root canal and tooth retention not an option.

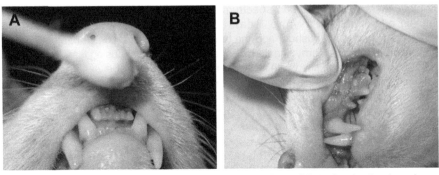

Fig. 15. (*A*) Apical abscess involving the maxillary incisors. (*B*) A fistula developed over maxillary P4. (*Courtesy of* Cathy Johnson-Delaney, DVM, Edmonds, WA; with permission.)

The clinical presentation shows exudate and swelling from the affected site. The tooth may be fractured, discolored, and/or loose. In many cases there is a fistula at the site of the root (**Fig. 15**B). The gingiva may be discolored and regressed over the abscessed tooth. This condition is painful. There may also be odor from the site. The ferret is often anorectic, and in some cases dehydrated, and may have weight loss if the condition is causing oral pain. In some cases, the ferret shows hyperthermia. Dental radiographs are needed to assess tooth roots and surrounding bone. Full probing under anesthesia is needed to determine the extent of the abscess.

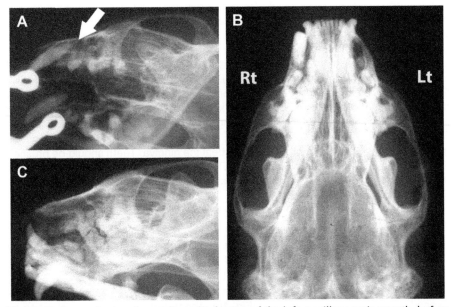

Fig. 16. Radiographs showing periapical infection of the left maxillary canine tooth, before and after extraction. (*A*) Left 30° ventral–right dorsal oblique projection. The root of the affected canine is surrounded by bone lysis (*arrow*). (*B*) Left 30° ventral–right dorsal oblique projection and (*C*) ventrodorsal projection after extraction. (*Courtesy of* Cathy Johnson-Delaney, DVM, Edmonds, WA; with permission.)

If there is a tooth root abscess of the canine tooth, theoretically a root canal proce-dure removing the diseased material from the pulp canal could be performed but, because of the size and curvature of the tooth, it may not be feasible. If a tooth is loose, and particularly if the root is diseased, extraction is necessary. The abscessed tissue should be drained, irrigated, and flushed using saline and/or a dilute chlorhexidine oral solution (2%). If there is a sizeable gap when the tooth is removed and there is enough healthy gum tissue remaining, it is possible to flush the site, then pack it with matrix material (Gelfoam, Pfizer, NY, NY) and loosely suture the gingiva to cover the gap. This procedure holds the gel in place but also prevents food material entering the pocket. If there is a fistula, flushing can also be done through it. Parenteral broad-spectrum oral antibiotics (clindamycin, 5.5–10 mg/kg by mouth every 12 hours) along with an NSAID (meloxicam, 0.2 mg/kg by mouth every 24 hours) and possibly an opioid analgesic should be given (buprenorphine, 0.01–0.03 subcutaneously [SC] every 8–12 hours). Oral swabbing with a dental rinse can be done daily to cleanse the mouth. Prognosis is good for healing of the mouth.

OTHER ORAL DISORDERS
Cleft Lip and/or Palate

Palate and lip malformation have been seen in ferrets[2] (**Fig. 17**). It is a congenital defect, although it may be hereditary There is an open upper lip area and the palate may appear split. There may be secondary abscessation caused by food entering the cleft. Severe cleft palates make nursing difficult. There may be milk in the nasal cavity. Radiographs show the extent of the bone deformation and whether there is interference with the maxillary teeth roots. Surgery to close the tissues is done as in other animals.[12]

Oral Ulceration

Ulcers of the mucosa can occur anywhere in the mouth but most are seen on the buccal mucosa, or the hard or soft palate[11] (**Fig. 18**). There is frequently a history of stress or systemic disease, such as renal disease or lymphoma. However, they may also be present with dental disease. Although they resemble the herpes viral ulcers found in other species, no virus has yet been found. Oral ulceration has been seen following electrocution. Oral ulcers are painful, and ferrets frequently show symptoms such as anorexia, gagging, hypersalivation, and bruxism. There may be concurrent

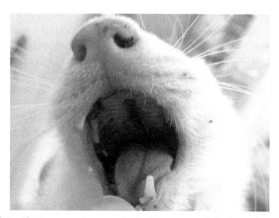

Fig. 17. Cleft palate that was not corrected. (*Courtesy of* Cathy Johnson-Delaney, DVM, Edmonds, WA; with permission.)

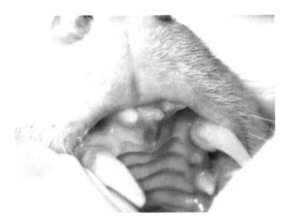

Fig. 18. Oral ulcer on the hard palate. (*Courtesy of* Cathy Johnson-Delaney, DVM, Edmonds, WA; with permission.)

dental disease and tonsillitis. A full work-up should be done, including hematology, chemistries, urinalysis, radiographs, and dental examination. Treatment includes addressing any underlying cause of the ulcer, whether it is local (related to oral disorders) or systemic. Direct soothing of the oral ulcer can be done using sucralfate liquid and a systemic analgesic. A broad-spectrum oral antibiotic may be helpful to prevent secondary bacterial infection. The ferret should be offered a soup made of soaked kibble, although many ferrets prefer to try to eat the hard kibble once on analgesics.

Fractures of the Jaw

When jaw fractures are present, radiographs are useful to examine the skull and tooth roots. Jaw fractures should be treated as they are in other carnivore species. If teeth are loose and bleeding, extraction is indicated. Analgesics are needed for the pain associated with fracture or extraction procedures.

Tonsillitis

On examination of the pharynx, inflamed or infected tonsils may be seen extending from their crypts. They usually appear erythematous and have a surface that looks pitted or rough. The author sees this frequently accompanying other disease, including oral/dental disease and influenza. Systemic lymphoma may also involve the tonsils, which appear enlarged but may not be inflamed or infected. On visual examination this difference may be difficult to discern. *Streptococcus* B infection has been diagnosed in some cases.[2] *Streptococcus* B may be of zoonotic concern, and should be discussed with the owner. A throat swab should be taken for diagnosis of bacterial infection and sensitivity test. A full work-up, including bloodwork, urinalysis, and survey radiographs, should be done to rule out systemic disease. Skull radiographs are indicated if dental and/or other oral disease is seen. In severe cases and/or when the tonsillitis is not responding to standard treatments, a biopsy of the tonsil may be indicated. Treatment depends on the cause of the tonsillitis. If infection includes bacterial upper respiratory infections or dental/oral infection, broad-spectrum oral or parenteral antibiotics (such as amoxicillin, 25 mg/kg by mouth every 12 hours for 10–14 days) may resolve the tonsillitis. Existing dental disease should be treated. If lymphoma is diagnosed, parenteral lymphoma protocols are indicated. Influenza is typically treated with supportive care to alleviate discomfort, such as using an NSAID along with sucralfate (25–100 mg/kg by mouth every 8–12 hours).

Salivary Microliths

Salivary microliths are small mineral concretions usually in the parotid salivary gland.[11] The parotid gland produces secretions that are rich in calcium. The salivary glands contain pockets of inefficient secretion, which may lead to microlithiasis.[11] Microliths may be incidental and asymptomatic, but they can reduce flow and allow ascending bacteria to infect the gland, leading to adenitis. Uncomplicated microliths are found fairly frequently. One study showed that 5 out of 7 ferrets had them with no clinical signs.[11] It is not clear whether they contribute to mucocele development. They can be unilateral or bilateral and may be visible on radiographs, on which they have to be differentiated from neoplasia. Because these are most often incidental findings, they usually do not need treatment unless the gland becomes infected or forms a mucocele. Bacterial adenitis not complicated with mucocele may heal with broad-spectrum antibiotic therapy.

Salivary Mucocele

Damage to a salivary gland leads to leakage of saliva into the surrounding tissue.[11,13] Trauma to the duct openings by other oral disorders or direct trauma to the glands has been implicated (**Fig. 19**). There is swelling in the affected facial area, such as the labial commissures or in the orbital area in the case of a zygomatic mucocele. Aspiration of

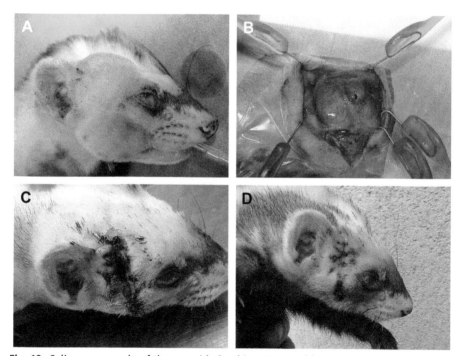

Fig. 19. Salivary mucocele of the parotid gland in a 5-year-old male ferret, likely following trauma affecting the right eye. (*A*) The ferret is prepared for surgery. Large swellings in the parotid and retro-orbital area are evident. (*B*) Surgical exposure of the salivary mucocele. After incision, a very dense and transparent fluid protrudes out of the initial incision. (*C*) Marsupialization of the surgical site with the addition of a tubular drain. (*D*) Follow-up 2 weeks after surgery showing complete resolution of the mucocele and proper healing of marsupialization. (*Courtesy of* Vittorio Capello, DVM, Milano, Italy; with permission.)

the fluctuant mass yields viscous or mucinous and clear or blood-tinged fluid.[13] Cytologic examination should be done and typically yields amorphous debris and occasional red blood cells. Treatment involves surgery. Depending on where the mucocele is located, a scalpel incision may be enough to allow drainage with no recurrence. Marsupialization of the mucocele has been reported as effective if the mucocele has bulged into the oral cavity.[13] Excision of the affected gland is often done to prevent recurrence. It is helpful to inject a contrast medium into the mucocele to define its extent before excision.

Oral Neoplasia

Tumors involving the oral cavity may include bony tumors such as osteoma or osteosarcoma (**Fig. 20**). Source tissue may be any oral anatomic structure, including bones,

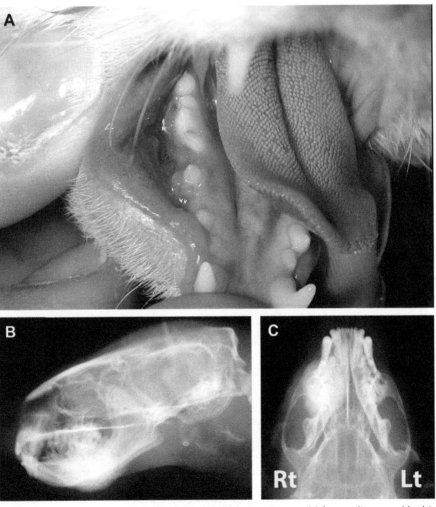

Fig. 20. Osteosarcoma affecting the right mandible in a 5-year-old ferret, diagnosed by histopathology. (*A*) Intraoral appearance of the hard swelling. Lateral (*B*) and ventrodorsal (*C*) projections of the skull with new bone formation and osteolysis. (*Courtesy of* Giorgio Romanelli, DVM, Milano, Italy; with permission.)

teeth, gingiva, and periodontia. Squamous cell carcinoma, osteoma, and lymphoma are the most common in the author's experience. Squamous cell carcinoma typically manifests as a firm swelling of either the maxilla or mandible (**Fig. 21**). They are usually solitary, but multiple sites have been reported.[13] Carcinoma and adenocarcinoma have been found in salivary glands. Fibrosarcoma of the mouth has been reported.[14] Tumors can be benign, such as epulis arising from proliferation of the gingiva, or malignant. Various intraoral or extraoral swellings and proliferations may be seen at the oral examination. Secondary abscessation may be present along with compromised dental structures. The teeth in the affected area may be loose. Radiographs and CT scan define the extent of the mass, whereas biopsy of the tissue allows histopathologic diagnosis of the neoplastic tissue. If the mass is resectable, surgery is indicated. Squamous cell carcinoma excision may require maxillectomy or mandibulectomy. Radiation therapy has also been attempted.[13] Underlying dental structures and teeth may be removed along with the mass. Depending on the histologic type of neoplasia, prognosis is varied.

DENTAL CARE PROGRAM

The author has developed a grading system to assist in determining a dental program for each ferret.[2,5] A healthy mouth has no gingivitis, although there may be a small amount of plaque if the ferret is more than a year of age. No oral ulcers should be present. As a ferret ages, there may be normal extrusion of the canine tooth with gum recession[2] (**Fig. 22**).

Stage 1 includes gingivitis, with inflammation caused by plaque. Some of the plaque may be mineralized (calculus), although buildup is usually minimal. The gingiva is erythematous, and may be slightly swollen along the edge abutting the teeth. The gingiva usually does not bleed when the pockets are probed (**Fig. 23A**).

Stage 2 is early periodontitis. The gingivitis has progressed to infection of the periodontal tissues, although the teeth are still firmly attached, and on radiographs roots are still normal. There may be gingival infection at this point and there may be some gingival recession or periodontal pocket formation. Up to 25% of the dental attachments may have been lost. For oral examination and probing in conscious ferrets at this stage, the author first applies an oral lidocaine 2% gel (Henry Schein, Melville, NY) to the gingival areas (**Fig. 23B**).

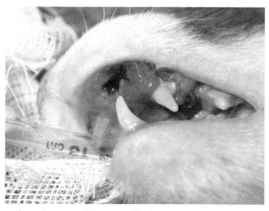

Fig. 21. Squamous cell carcinoma of the maxilla. (*Courtesy of* Cathy Johnson-Delaney, DVM, Edmonds, WA; with permission.)

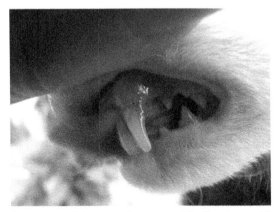

Fig. 22. Extrusion of canine teeth is generally a normal finding in an older ferret. This ferret is 6 years old. (*Courtesy of* Cathy Johnson-Delaney, DVM, Edmonds, WA; with permission.)

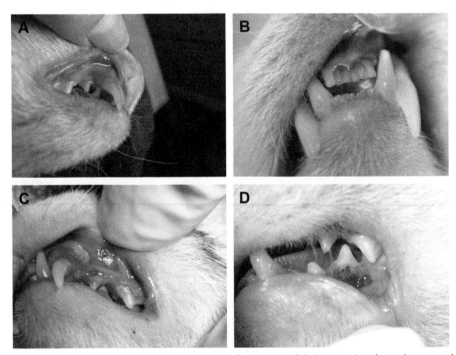

Fig. 23. Grading system to determine a dental program. (*A*) Stage 1 involves plaque and mild gingivitis. Note that this ferret also has some extrusion of the canine tooth. (*B*) Stage 2 showing advancing gingivitis with some periodontal involvement and gingival abscess of the incisors. (*C*) Stage 3 showing gingivitis, periodontal involvement, and calculus buildup. There is a fistula forming from the canine root, and there is an abscess forming under the gingiva of PM3. (*D*) Stage 4. Tooth root exposure along with loosening of the tooth is shown following removal of necrotic debris and abscess. (*Courtesy of* Cathy Johnson-Delaney, DVM Edmonds, WA; with permission.)

Stage 3 is moderate periodontitis. Bleeding usually occurs during dental probing, and affected teeth may have up to 50% loss of attachments. There may be root exposure. Some teeth may be slightly loosened. Abscesses are frequently found around the roots and accumulations of food and debris encountered in the periodontal/gingival pockets. Most ferrets require light sedation (midazolam, 0.25–0.4 mg/kg IM), parenteral analgesia (buprenorphine, 0.01–0.03 mg/kg SC or IM), and a topical dental anesthetic (2% lidocaine gel) for a full oral examination at this stage (**Fig. 23**C).

Stage 4 is advanced periodontitis. There is greater than 50% loss of attachments. Many of the tooth roots are usually exposed because of gingival and bone recession. On radiographs, tooth roots show the lack of attachment and often the degree of abscessation or destruction (lysis), and loss of viability. There is often blood and pus surrounding the tooth. The tooth may also be loose. This condition is painful, and further examination and radiographs require analgesia along with either heavy sedation (such as the combination midazolam, 0.25–0.5 mg/kg and ketamine 5–10 mg/kg; both can be given IM or IV), or inhalant anesthesia. Teeth may be lost at this stage even if periodontal treatment is initiated using protocols used in dogs (including gingival resection, extractions, packing with an antibiotic gel, parenteral/oral antibiotics, scaling, brushing of the teeth as a home care program) (**Fig. 23**D).

Dental instruments used in ferrets include the Nazzy ferret mouth gag (Universal Surgical Instruments, Glen Clove, NY), scalers such as the McColl scaler, double-ended elevator, small feline elevator, dental probe, and regular dental drill and polisher (**Figs. 24** and **25**). Ultrasonic scaling devices, as used in small animal medicine, work well. Note that the Nazzy ferret mouth gag was named after one of the author's ferrets that was used for oral and tooth measurements. Radiographs of the head and ideally dental films should be taken to assess roots and bone. These radiographs should be done at the time of the dental examination and cleaning, and require deep sedation or anesthesia.

Dental Prophylaxis

Cleaning of ferret teeth from plaque or calculus should be done at least annually under anesthesia. The Nazzy ferret mouth gag is used to hold the mouth open. Deep planing of the teeth and removal of calculus can be done using a McColl scaler, which fits under normal ferret gingiva (**Fig. 26**A). After gingival recess planing has been done,

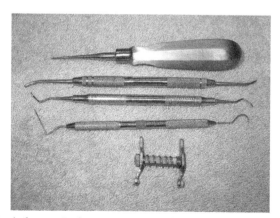

Fig. 24. Dental tools for use in ferrets. From top: feline elevator, double-ended elevator, McColl scaler, probe, Nazzy ferret mouth gag. (*Courtesy of* Cathy Johnson-Delaney, DVM, Edmonds, WA; with permission.)

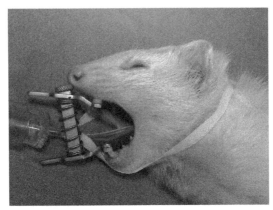

Fig. 25. Nazzy ferret mouth gag in use during oral examination. (*Courtesy of* Vittorio Capello, DVM, Milano, Italy; with permission.)

further removal of plaque can be done using an ultrasonic dental cleaning system or by further hand scaling. Polishing of the teeth can be done using a prophy cup on a low-speed handpiece (3000–5000 rpm) with a mild abrasive polish (Zircon-F, Henry Schein, Melville, NY) (**Fig. 26**B). After rinsing and removal of debris, the teeth can be dried thoroughly and either a fluoride paste, varnish (several brands as used in dogs; Henry Schein, Melville, NY), or a sealant (Oravet, Merial, Duluth, GA) can be applied.[2]

Home Dental Prophylaxis

Home dental care should include the continued application of Oravet (if that was used) on a weekly basis. If teeth are not sealed, then owners should be instructed on how to brush their ferrets' teeth. The author uses cotton buds and an enzymatic toothpaste (CET, Virbac, Fort Worth, TX) in either malt or poultry flavor (**Fig. 27**A). Most pet ferrets easily accept tooth brushing because they like the taste of the toothpaste. They tend to bite down on the cotton bud or small pet brush, which may aid in cleaning between the teeth. Following brushing, the teeth and gingiva can be swabbed with a children's nonalcohol mouthwash (fruit flavored) on a cotton bud (Listerine Smart Rinse Berry

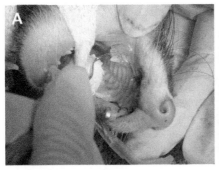
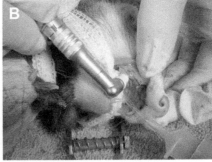

Fig. 26. (*A*) Deep planing of the teeth using a McColl scaler. (*B*) Polishing of the teeth following scaling. (*Courtesy of* Cathy Johnson-Delaney, DVM, Edmonds, WA; with permission.)

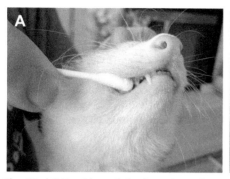
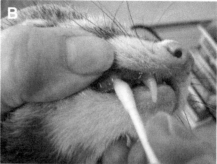

Fig. 27. (*A*) Brushing of the ferret's teeth can be done using a cotton bud with enzymatic toothpaste or using a small pet dental brush. (*B*) Application of a children's nonalcohol mouth rinse to the gums and teeth. (*Courtesy of* Cathy Johnson-Delaney, DVM, Edmonds, WA; with permission.)

Flavor, McNeill-PPC Inc, Fort Washington, PA) (**Fig. 27**B). Follow-up examinations should be done on a regular basis.[2]

DENTAL PROCEDURES

Dental surgery follows the same guidelines as those used in dog and cat dentistry. Infraorbital anesthesia block is routinely used for canine extractions or root canal using lidocaine 2%, approximately 0.05 to 0.1 mL (**Fig. 28**). The injection site is entered at approximately the base of the root of the maxillary canine, at a line just rostral to the second premolar. The needle is advanced parallel to the bone medially to a point rostrally that corresponds approximately with the middle of the orbit. This point corresponds with the exit of the nerve from the infraorbital foramen. It is recommended that practitioners try this technique on a cadaver first to learn the position for the block. The author has found that the lidocaine/epinephrine commercial formulation has caused seizures if used in the infraorbital block. It has not caused this in mandibular blocks.

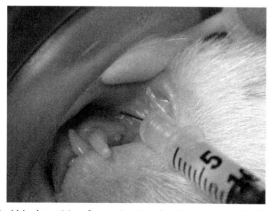

Fig. 28. Supraorbital block position for canine tooth extraction. As the block is taking effect, the ferret is intubated for the surgery. (*Courtesy of* Cathy Johnson-Delaney, DVM, Edmonds, WA; with permission.)

Extraction

The most common dental surgery is tooth extraction. The author advocates locally blocking the area with lidocaine 2% (volume dependent on size of the dental area and weight of the ferret; for most teeth, 0.05–0.1 mL is adequate) in addition to parenteral analgesia, general anesthesia, and intubation, followed by gingivectomy. The periodontal ligaments have to be incised using a #15 scalpel blade around larger teeth or by using an 18-gauge needle around smaller teeth (**Fig 29**A). In some cases it is necessary to remove some alveolar bone. Once the ligamentous tissues have been severed, the tooth can easily be elevated using a fine-tipped elevator or 18-gauge needle (for the smaller teeth), and often can be extracted with just hemostats. If there is an open alveolus, the cavity may be packed with a hydrostatic gel or synthetic bone matrix material (Consil Bioglass, Nutramax, Baltimore, MD). The gingiva can be sutured with 4-0 or 5-0 absorbable suture on a fine swaged-on taper-point needle (**Fig 29**B). Suturing the gingiva closed over the open area encourages healing and decreases the chance of debris being introduced. Analgesics, NSAIDs, and often antibiotics are used postextraction. Owners are usually instructed on how to apply a mild concentration of chlorhexidine rinse (2%) using cotton buds to the sutured area twice daily for up to a week as well. The remaining teeth should be probed, scaled, and polished using commercial prophy cups and paste.

Endodontic Procedures

Superficial pulpectomy can be done in the canine tooth presented with the tip broken off if the tooth is not discolored. This procedure involves using a high-speed burr in the pulp a few millimeters below the exposed surface, drying and sterilizing the pulp chamber with calcium hydroxide, and filling with a composite, as is done in other species. Local anesthetic block is done using lidocaine 2%. Local blocking involves infiltrating the gingival and periodontal tissues surrounding the tooth. The volume to use is usually 0.05 to 0.1 mL, depending on the size of the area to infiltrate. If the tooth is already discolored or necrotic, the tooth cannot usually be preserved by an endodontic procedure and may have to be extracted.

The root canal procedure for removing the diseased material from the pulp canal is sometimes attempted by using a high speed drill into the pulp canal and removing the material. However, this is difficult in the ferret owing to the small size of the canine tooth as well as its curvature. If attempted, the material from the pulp canal is

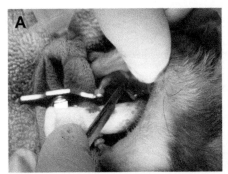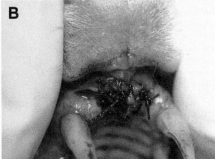

Fig. 29. (*A*) The gingiva and periodontal ligaments can be incised using a #15 blade. (*B*) The gingiva is sutured using 4-0 or 5-0 absorbable suture. (*Courtesy of* [*A*] Vondelle McLaughlin, and [*B*] *Courtesy of* Cathy Johnson-Delaney, DVM, Edmonds, WA; with permission.)

removed, the canal flushed with saline, then air dried, usually using dental points. A dental composite filling is applied as per the manufacturer's instructions. There are many brands available and they are the same as used in canine and feline dentistry (Henry Schein Dental catalogue, www.henryschein.com, Melville, NY).

SKUNKS

There are 11 species of skunks that are classified in the Mephitidae.[15] Older nomenclature classified skunks in Mustelidae. The most common skunk kept as a pet is *M mephitis*, the striped skunk. The dental formula is I 3/3, C 1/1, P 3/3, M 1/1 X 2 = 32.[15,16] Although dentition resembles that of a carnivore, the skunk is considered omnivorous. The natural diet consists of whole prey, insects, and some fruit and vegetable matter.[15] Companion skunks may be fed a diet consisting of premium dog food, canned cat food, fruits, and vegetables; an insectivore diet; or an omnivore diet and treats such as insects, although larval forms of these should be avoided because of their high fat content. Obesity is a major problem in pet skunks.

The dental conditions most commonly seen are fractured tips of the canines and buildup of calculus, predominantly on the maxillary teeth. Treatment is the same as with ferrets. Canine dental chew bones and tartar-controlling treats and foods may help in keeping calculus from accumulating. Skunks generally will use these and they seem to be effective.

FENNEC FOXES

The fennec fox (*V zerda*) has gained popularity as an exotic canid and is in genus *Vulpes*, which also includes the red fox, Arctic fox, and 9 other species.[17] The dental formula is 2(I 3/3, C 1/1, PM 4/4, M 2/3) = 42. Tooth structure is the same as other canines. The diet of wild fennec foxes consists of plant material, fruits, small rodents (gerbils, jerboas), birds, eggs, lizards, and insects such as locusts. Plant roots are a source of water.[17] Pet fennec foxes do well on high-quality dog or cat food, or a zoo diet such as Mazuri Exotic Canine Diet (Mazuri, St Louis, MO, www.mazuri. com). Supplements include vegetables, fruits, rodents, egg, crickets, and mealworms. Raw meat has also been added as a supplement, but should be handled carefully to avoid bacterial contamination.[17]

The most commonly seen dental problems are similar to those of other Canidae: calculus, fractured teeth, with subsequent gingivitis, periodontitis, and tooth abscess. Treatment programs are the same as in ferrets and dogs. Small-dog dental chew toys and supplements can be used to help prevent calculus buildup.

RACCOONS

Raccoons (*P lotor*) are sometimes kept as pets, although they may also be brought into clinics in North America as wildlife. Their dental formula is 2(I 3/3, C 1/1, P 4/4, M 2/2) = 40.[18] The teeth are morphologically similar to those of carnivores. The diet of wild raccoons is omnivorous and contains birds, mice, bird eggs, shellfish, crabs, worms, insects, fish, turtles, frogs, and scavenged pet and human foods left outdoors. Captive raccoons can be fed high-grade dog food kibble along with supplements of fish, chicken, turkey, eggs, fresh fruits, and vegetables. Whole prey items can also be given, such as rodents, day-old chicks, fish, frogs, and crustaceans.[18]

Dental disorders encountered include canine tooth fracture, tooth wear, and calculus. Treatment programs are the same as in ferrets and dogs.

COATIMUNDIS (COATI)

The coatimundi is a member of the Procyonidae. The most common of the 4 species that is encountered in the pet trade is *Nasua narica*, the white-nosed (or brown-nosed) coatimundi, although the others may also be presented.[19] They are native to South and Central America and the southwestern United States. Their dental formula is 2(I 3/3, C 1/1, P 4/4 M 2/2) = 40.[18] The teeth are morphologically similar to those of carnivores. The diet of wild coatimundis is omnivorous, consisting largely of grubs, berries, edible roots, leaves, bird eggs, birds, reptiles, and small mammals.[19] Captive coatimundis can be fed high-grade dog food kibble along with daily supplementation of fresh fruits and vegetables. Poultry, beef, and eggs can be fed as treats along with crickets and mealworms. If allowed ad libitum food they become obese. Whole prey such as rodents, day-old chicks, fish, frogs, crustaceans, and mollusks can be offered occasionally as supplements.[19]

Dental conditions encountered include fractured teeth (particularly canines), tooth wear, and calculus (**Fig. 30**). Treatment of conditions are the same as in ferrets and dogs. Small-dog dental chew toys and supplements can be used to help prevent calculus buildup.

KINKAJOUS

The kinkajou (*P flavus*) is also a member of the Procyonidae and native to Central and South America. The dental formula is 2(I 3/3, C 1/1, P 3/3, M 2/2) = 36.[20] In the wild the diet is more than 90% fruit with less than 10% made up of insects, leaves, and flowers.[20] In captivity, the main portion of the diet is fruit, supplemented with a small amount of high-grade monkey food or dog food kibble that has been soaked in fruit juice. Eggs, insects, cooked chicken, and fresh vegetables may also be offered. Honey can be given as a treat.[20] There is a reference to avoid strawberries, avocado, and dairy products.[20]

Periodontal disease is common because of their soft diet, although calculus buildup, gingivitis, and canine tooth tip fracture has also been seen. Papaya is reported to be used to help prevent periodontal disease.[20]

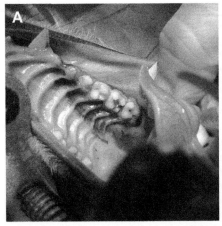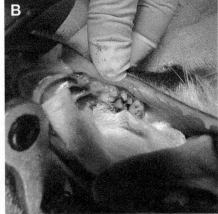

Fig. 30. (*A*) Fractured maxillary molar 1 in a coatimundi. (*B*) Sectioning the tooth in preparation for extraction. (*Courtesy of* Cathy Johnson-Delaney, DVM, Edmonds, WA; with permission.)

REFERENCES

1. Church B. Ferret dentition and pathology. In: Lewington JH, editor. Ferret husbandry, medicine and surgery. 2nd edition. Edinburgh (United Kingdom): Saunders Elsevier; 2007. p. 467–85.
2. Johnson-Delaney CA. Disorders of the oral cavity and teeth. In: Johnson-Delaney CA, editor. Ferret medicine and surgery. Torquay (Devon, UK): CRC Press, Taylor and Francis; 2016.
3. Evans HE, An NQ. Anatomy of the ferret. In: Fox JG, editor. Biology and diseases of the ferret. 2nd edition. Baltimore (MD): Williams & Wilkins; 1998. p. 19–69.
4. Church RR. The impact of diet on the dentition of the domesticated ferret. Exot DVM 2007;9(2):30–9.
5. Johnson-Delaney CA. Diagnosis and treatment of dental disease in ferrets. J Exot Pet Med 2008;17(2):132–7.
6. Fisher RG, Edwardsson S, Klinge B. Oral microflora of the ferret at the gingival sulcus and mucosa membrane in relation to ligature-induced periodontitis. Oral Microbiol Immunol 1994;9(1):40–9.
7. Capello V, Lennox A, Widmer WR. The basics of radiology. In: Capello V, Lennox A, Widmer WR, editors. Clinical radiology of exotic companion mammals. Ames (IA): Wiley-Blackwell; 2008. p. 1–51.
8. Capello V. Ferrets: common surgical procedures. In: Keeble E, Meredith A, editors. BSAVA manual of rodents and ferrets. Quedgeley (United Kingdom): BSAVA; 2009. p. 254–68.
9. Eroshin VV, Reiter AM, Rosenthal K, et al. Oral examination results in rescued ferrets: clinical findings. J Vet Dent 2011;28(1):8–15.
10. Capello V, Lennox AM. Small mammal dentistry. In: Quesenberry KE, Carpenter JW, editors. Ferrets, rabbits and rodents, clinical medicine and surgery. 3rd edition. St Louis (MO): Elsevier Saunders; 2010. p. 452–71.
11. Maurer KJ, Fox JG. Diseases of the gastrointestinal system. In: Fox JG, Marini RP, editors. Biology and diseases of the ferret. 3rd edition. Ames (IA): John Wiley & Sons; 2014. p. 363–75.
12. Pope ER, Constantnescu GM. Repair of cleft palate. In: Bojrab MJ, Waldron D, Toombs JP, editors. Current techniques in small animal surgery. 5th edition. Jackson (MS): Teton NewMedia; 2014. p. 195–201.
13. Hoefer HL, Fox JG, Bell JA. Gastrointestinal diseases. In: Quesenberry KE, Carpenter JW, editors. Ferrets, rabbits and rodents, clinical medicine and surgery. 3rd edition. St Louis (MO): Elsevier Saunders; 2012. p. 27–45.
14. Lewington JH. General neoplasia. In: Lewington JH, editor. Ferret husbandry, medicine and surgery. 2nd edition. Edinburgh (United Kingdom): Saunders Elsevier; 2007. p. 318–45.
15. Kramer MH, Lennox A. Skunk pet care. In: Fisher P, editor. Unusual pet care: the exotic guidebook. Lake Worth (FL): Zoological Education Network; 2005. Skunk section 1–8.
16. Williams CSF. Skunk. In: Williams CSF, editor. Practical guide to laboratory animals. St Louis (MO): The CV Mosby Company; 1976. p. 86–9.
17. Johnson D. Fennec fox pet care. In: Fisher P, editor. Unusual pet care: the exotic guidebook. Lake Worth (FL): Zoological Education Network; 2005. Fennec Fox section 1–6.
18. Johnson D. Raccoon pet care. In: Kottwitz J, Coke R, editors. Unusual pet care volume II: the exotic guidebook. Lake Worth (FL): Zoological Education Network; 2007. p. 90–4.

19. Grant S. Coatimundi pet care. In: Kottwitz J, Coke R, editors. Unusual pet care volume II: the exotic guidebook. Lake Worth (FL): Zoological Education Network; 2007. p. 95–9.
20. Johnson D. Kinkajou pet care. In: Kottwitz J, Coke R, editors. Unusual pet care volume II: the exotic guidebook. Lake Worth (FL): Zoological Education Network; 2007. p. 104–8.

Anatomy and Disorders of the Oral Cavity of Miscellaneous Exotic Companion Mammals

Angela M. Lennox, DVM, DABVP-Avian, Exotic Companion Mammal, DECZM (Small Mammal)[a],*, Yasutsugu Miwa, DVM, PhD[b,c]

KEYWORDS

- Oral cavity • Dentistry • Dental disease • Hedgehog • Sugar glider • Miniature pig

KEY POINTS

- Dentition of sugar gliders, hedgehogs, and miniature pigs varies significantly and must be taken into consideration when diagnosing and treating diseases of the oral cavity.
- Diseases of the oral cavity affect any species; these have been described in unusual exotic companion mammal species as well.
- Thorough evaluation of the oral cavity almost always requires sedation or general anesthesia in these species and is aided by diagnostic imaging.
- The most common disorder of the oral cavity in these species is oral neoplasia in the African hedgehog.

INTRODUCTION

Disease of the oral cavity can occur in any species; although occasionally encountered in exotic mammalian species, it is rarely described in the literature. Anatomy and dentition vary significantly; diagnosis and treatment are often extrapolated from that known in other species. The best-documented disease of the oral cavity in this group of species is oral neoplasia in the hedgehog. This article focuses on more common disease presentations in African hedgehogs, sugar gliders, and miniature pigs.

The authors have nothing to disclose.
[a] Avian and Exotic Animal Clinic, 9330 Waldemar Road, Indianapolis, IN 46268, USA; [b] Veterinary Medical Center, School of Veterinary Medicine, The University of Tokyo, 1-1-1 Yayoi, Bunkyo-ku, Tokyo 113-8657, Japan; [c] Miwa Exotic Animal Hospital, 1-25-5 Komagome, Toshima-ku, Tokyo 170-0003, Japan
* Corresponding author.
E-mail address: birddr@aol.com

ORAL ANATOMY AND DENTITION

Hedgehogs are placental mammals, formerly classified within the order of *Insectivora*. Taxonomy of this now-abandoned biological group has been refined in recent years. The order *Lypotyphla* includes the family *Erinaceidae* and the subfamily *Erinaceinae*, to which spiny hedgehogs belong.[1] Among species, the most common kept as a pet is the African pigmy hedgehog (*Atelerix albiventris*). Spiny hedgehogs normally have 36 teeth with a dental formula of 2(I 3/2, C 1/1, P 3/2, M 3/3).[1-3] However, anomalies in tooth number have been frequently recorded in hedgehogs, including the absence of the second pair of mandibular incisors, and extra incisors.[1] In the African hedgehog, the absence of the second maxillary premolars has been reported[1] as well as a dental formula with 34 teeth and 2 pairs of maxillary incisors: 2(I 2/2, C 1/1, P 3/2, M 3/3).[4,5] Hedgehogs are diphyodont, and molar teeth are absent in the deciduous dentition.[1] Dentition of hedgehog is anelodont (truly rooted). Although classified as insectivores, diet is actually more omnivorous (including plant material and occasional vertebrate prey),[1,3] which is reflected in the dentition. Pairs of incisor teeth have different sizes. The first maxillary pair of incisors is long, sharp, widely spaced and project slightly forward.[1,3] The mandibular first incisors occlude into a space between the maxillary incisors.[3] Incisor teeth resemble canine teeth of other species and are designed to capture small prey. Canine teeth are relatively small and similar to the secondary pairs of incisors, and to the first 2 premolars. The upper third premolar and first 2 molars, and the lower first 2 molars, have well-developed cusps, a typical 4-sided appearance, and multiple roots.[1] The third maxillary premolar shears against the first mandibular molar, a feature resembling the carnassial tooth pattern of carnivores[1] (**Fig. 1**).

Sugar gliders (*Petaurus breviceps*) are arboreal marsupial mammals native to Australia and New Guinea, with highly specialized dentition.[6] They have sharp and well-developed first (primary) mandibular incisor teeth[4] designed for peeling bark to obtain insects and plant resins. The rest of the diet consists of gums, saps, and other local and seasonal items.[6] Limiting shearing action allows compression of insects, as opposed to biting into smaller pieces. Therefore, gliders tend to extract hemolymph and soft tissues of insects and discard the exoskeleton.[7]

Despite a superficial resemblance to selected rodent species such as the hamster, primary mandibular incisor teeth of sugar gliders are anelodont (truly rooted),[6] as is the rest of dentition. Maxillary primary incisors are also present, but less developed than the corresponding mandibular. Additional pairs of incisor teeth are much smaller. Maxillary canine are small, and the mandible lacks canine teeth. Dental formula is 2(I 3/2, C 1/0, P 3/3, M 4/4) for a total of 40 teeth[4,5] (**Fig. 2**).

All domestic pigs descend from the wild boar (*Sus scrofa*), belonging to the placental mammal order of *Artiodactyla*. After domestication and inbreeding, the skull became foreshortened, and the frontal profile more concave (**Fig. 3**) Although the skull is smaller and shorter in miniature pigs, the oral cavity and dentition are the same as in other species of swine. Dentition reflects a more omnivorous diet. Although most teeth are anelodont and brachyodont (short crowned), the maxillary and mandibular canine teeth are hypsodont (long crowned) and elodont (continuously growing).

In the boar, growth of these teeth, also referred to as tusks, can be extensive. Growth of the tusks is limited in castrated males and in females.[8] When developed, they wear and self-sharpen against each other. Dental formula of adult pigs is 2(I 3/3, C 1/1, P 4/4, M 3/3) for a total of 44 teeth, whereas the deciduous teeth are 28 2(I 3/3, C 1/1, P 3/3, M 0/0)[9] (see **Fig. 3**).

A careful understanding of comparative oral anatomy is important, and dental formulas for all 3 species are listed in **Table 1** (see **Figs. 1–3**).

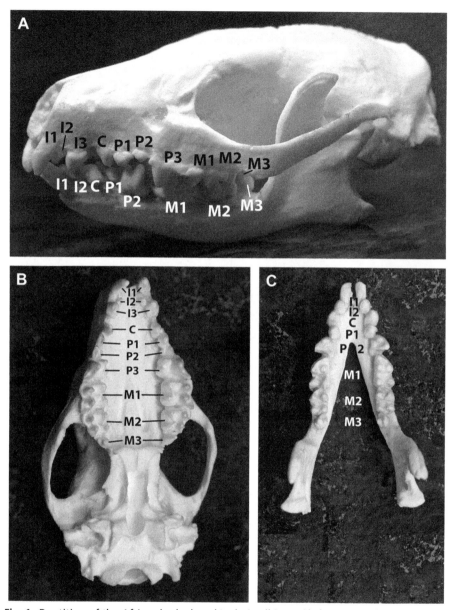

Fig. 1. Dentition of the African hedgehog (*Atelerix albiventris*) shown on a bony specimen with the standard dental formula of 2(I 3/2, C 1/1, P 3/2, M 3/3). (*A*) Lateral view of the skull with the mouth in occlusion. (*B*) Ventrodorsal view of the maxilla displaying the maxillary arcade. (*C*) Dorsoventral view of the mandible displaying the mandibular arcade. Note the primary incisor teeth resembling canine teeth of other species. Maxillary P3, M1, M2 and mandibular M1, M2 have well-developed cusps, a typical 4-sided appearance, and multiple roots.[1] The maxillary P3 shears against the mandibular M 1, a feature resembling the carnassial tooth pattern of carnivores.[1] (*Courtesy of* Angela Lennox, DVM; with permission. Photos by Katie Lennox, graphics by Vittorio Capello, DVM.)

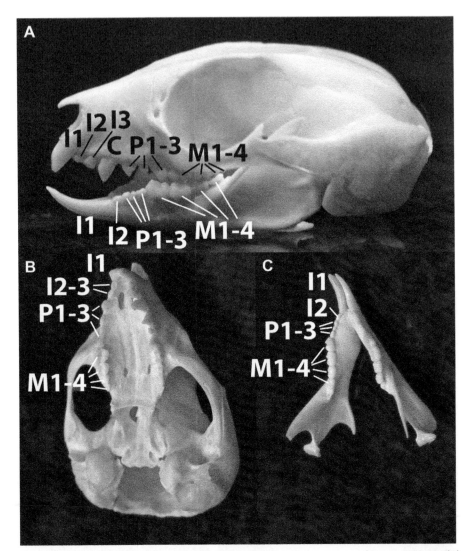

Fig. 2. Dentition of the sugar glider (*Petaurus breviceps*) shown on a bony specimen. (*A*) Lateral view of the skull with the mouth in occlusion. (*B*) Ventrodorsal view of the maxilla displaying the maxillary arcade. (*C*) Dorsoventral view of the mandible displaying the mandibular arcade. Note the sharp and well-developed primary mandibular incisor teeth. (*Courtesy of* Angela Lennox, DVM; with permission. Photos by Katie Lennox, graphics by Vittorio Capello, DVM.)

PRESENTATION OF PATIENTS WITH DISEASES OF THE ORAL CAVITY

Clinical signs and symptoms in any animal with disease of the oral cavity can range from subclinical to those typically seen in other species, including changes in food preference, reduced food intake, dysphagia, anorexia, orofacial swellings, presence of blood, and foul breath. Severe oral disease can produce debilitation and a host of secondary disease conditions.

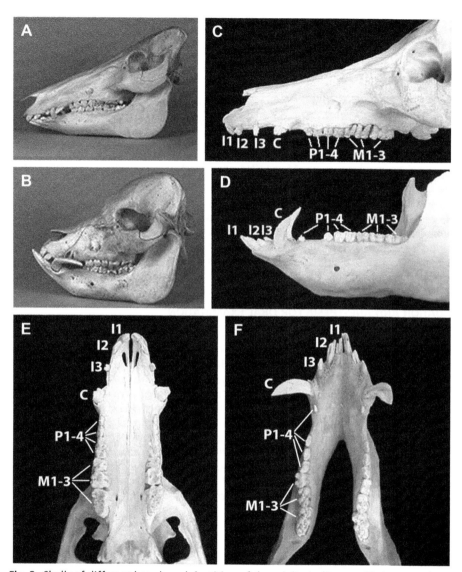

Fig. 3. Skulls of different breeds and dentition of the adult pig (*Sus scrofa*) shown on bony specimens. (*A*) Skull of a domestic hybrid of wild boar. (*B*) Skull of a Vietnamese potbellied pig. Note the foreshortened skull with a more concave profile of the miniature breed. This morphologic difference does not affect the dentition and the dental formula. (*C*) Lateral view of the maxilla displaying the maxillary quadrant. (*D*) Lateral view of the mandible displaying the mandibular quadrant. (*E*) Ventrodorsal view of the maxilla displaying the upper arcade. (*F*) Dorsoventral view of the mandible displaying the lower arcade. Note the well-developed mandibular canines ("tusks") and the gap of the first mandibular premolar from the second. (*From* [*A*, *B*] Will's skull page—*Sus Scrofa*. Available at: http://www. skullsite.co.uk/pig/pig_gen.htm; and [*C–F*] Pathophysiology of the Digestive System, Dental Anatomy of Pigs, Colorado State University. Available at: http://www.vivo.colostate.edu/ hbooks/pathphys/digestion/pregastric/pigpage.html. Accessed February 15, 2016.)

Table 1
Dental formulas of African hedgehogs, sugar gliders, and miniature pigs

Species	Dental Formula	Total Number of Teeth
African hedgehog (variation)	2(I 3/2, C 1/1, P 3/2, M 3/3)	36
	2(I 2/2, C 1/1, P 3/2, M 3/3)	34
Sugar glider	2(I 3/2, C 1/0, P 3/3, M 4/4)	40
Miniature pig	2(I 3/3, C 1/1, P 4/4, M 3/3)	44

Data from Chaprazov T, Dimitrov R, Stamatova Yovcheva K, et al. Oral and dental disorders in pet hedgehogs. Turkis J Vet Anim Sci 2014;38:1–6; and Wolff CF, Corradinia PRM, Cortes G. Congenital erythropoietic porphyria in an African Hedgehog (Atelerix albiventris). J Zoo Wildl Med 2005;36(2):323–5.

The most commonly reported symptoms of dental disease in gliders and hedgehogs are reduced food intake and weight loss. In these small, difficult-to-handle species, owners seldom note an abnormality of dentition itself. However, oral neoplasms in hedgehogs often increase in size and eventually become readily apparent (**Fig. 4**). Owners of miniature pigs will occasionally report visibly abnormal teeth, including fractures and discoloration.

SEDATION AND ANESTHESIA FOR ORAL EXAMINATION

With the exception of very sick or debilitated patients, thorough evaluation of the oral cavity requires deep sedation to general anesthesia. Most sugar gliders and hedgehogs do not tolerate invasive handling, and both are difficult to restrain, the sugar glider due to size and agility, and the hedgehog due to the tendency to roll into a defensive ball. Even very tame patients may tolerate a cursory evaluation of the lateral aspects of the teeth and gingiva; however, thorough examination of the oral cavity, including beneath the tongue, requires some form of chemical restraint. Miniature pigs are powerful enough to make a thorough oral examination challenging as well.

Sedation as an alternative to general anesthesia is gaining acceptance in exotic pet medicine and can be beneficial for a thorough brief oral examination. Although potentially safer than general anesthesia, patient condition should always be optimized before sedation. Suggested dosages as shown in **Table 2** are anecdotally derived.

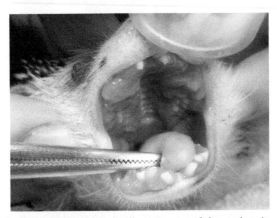

Fig. 4. African hedgehog with squamous cell carcinoma of the oral cavity confirmed via histopathology. Same case as in **Fig. 13.** (*Courtesy of* Yasutsugu Miwa, DVM, Tokyo, Japan; with permission.)

Table 2
Drug dosages and combinations suggested by the authors for intramuscular sedation or premedication of hedgehogs and sugar gliders to facilitate oral examination

	Drug	Dosage (mg/kg)	Comments
Gliders and hedgehogs	Midazolam plus	0.5–1.0	Midazolam/opioid/ketamine can be combined into a single syringe Reversible with flumazanil
	An opioid: Butorphanol Buprenorphine With the addition of: Ketamine	— 5–7	Midazolam/opioid/ketamine can be combined into a single syringe Reversible with naloxone Midazolam/opioid/ketamine can be combined into a single syringe
	OR Alfaxalone	1–2	Administer alfaxane separately after giving midazolam and opioid
Miniature pigs	Midazolam Hydromorphone Dexmedetomidine OR	0.3 0.10 0.02	Combine into a single syringe and inject IM — —
	Midazolam	0.25	Intranasally as a single agent

Patients in less than optimal condition may require lower dosages, whereas healthy patients often require higher dosages. One author (A.M.L.) and others prefer intramuscular (IM) injection of a combination of midazolam plus an opioid, with the addition of ketamine for sedation of hedgehogs and sugar gliders (see **Table 2**). These agents can be combined into one syringe and carefully injected into the hind limb musculature of the glider, or the epaxial musculature of the hedgehog (**Fig. 5**).

A promising alternative is the use of alfaxalone IM in place of ketamine, which may be beneficial in patients with cardiac insufficiency, or other conditions where ketamine is contraindicated. Because the manufacturer does not recommend combining alfaxalone with other drugs, this necessitates a second IM injection, which is often easier after administration of midazolam and an opioid.

One author (A.M.L.) prefers a combination of midazolam, an opioid, and dexmedetomidine for premedication of miniature pigs (see **Table 2**). Drugs are combined into a

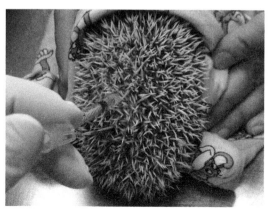

Fig. 5. IM injection into the epaxial musculature of a hedgehog. Drugs for sedation are combined into a single syringe. (*Courtesy of* Angela Lennox, DVM, Indianapolis, Indiana; with permission.)

single syringe and administered IM. Johnson recently described a practical alternative to IM injection in the pig: intranasal midazolam at 0.25 mg/kg is often adequate for brief sedation of the miniature pig for cursory handling and physical examination (Dan Johnson, personal communication, 2015). The pig is tipped upwards balancing on the haunches, and the drug is dripped into the nares without touching the nose **(Fig. 6)**.

If oral examination reveals a condition requiring general anesthesia for diagnostics or treatment, the sedated patient can be induced and maintained with inhalant agents.

Simple facemask or chamber induction is commonly performed, but requires much higher concentrations of inhalant agents; handling and anesthetic gas odor can produce stress and anxiety, and veterinary staff exposure to waste gas is increased.

THE ORAL EXAMINATION

Examination must be thorough and involve evaluation of the entire oral cavity, including the most caudal molar teeth and under the tongue. Small wire mouth gags, hemostats, or even gauze strips are useful for gliders and hedgehogs, as are cotton-tipped applicators and small dental spatulas **(Fig. 7)**. Evaluation of the oral cavity of the pig can be performed with large metal speculums or gauze strips and an assistant.

DIAGNOSTIC IMAGING

Radiographs of the head are extremely important for evaluation of dental structures, especially of those of bone or the tooth roots. Examples of normal radiographs have been published for the hedgehog, the sugar glider, and the miniature pigs[10–12] **(Figs. 8–10)**.

Important abnormalities that may be detected include fractured teeth, bony changes including fractures and osteomyelitis, and potentially periapical changes. However, detecting subtle abnormalities is extremely difficult in small species such as the hedgehog and the sugar glider.

Advanced diagnostic imagining modalities such as computed tomography (CT) should be strongly considered as well; however, small patient size may make interpretation difficult using standard equipment. Micro-CT has recently emerged in private practice. Originally designed for laboratory animal imaging, it is an outstanding modality for small exotic patients **(Fig. 11)**.

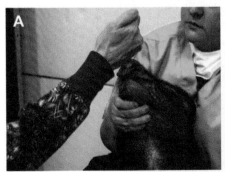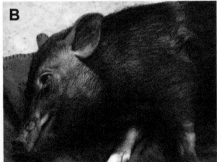

Fig. 6. (*A*) Administration of intranasal (IN) midazolam in a pig. The pig is tipped upwards balancing on the haunches, and the drug is dripped into the nares without touching the nose. (*B*) Effect of sedation a few minutes after IN administration. (*Courtesy of* Angela Lennox, DVM, Indianapolis, Indiana; with permission.)

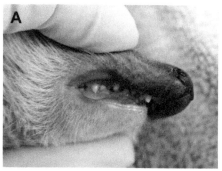
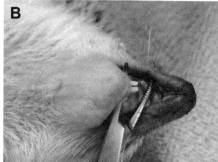

Fig. 7. (*A, B*) Oral examination of the sedated hedgehog. (*Courtesy of* Angela Lennox, DVM, Indianapolis, Indiana; with permission.)

Endoscopy of the oral cavity is well described in rabbits and rodents and is very useful in hedgehogs and sugar gliders as well. Endoscopy may be useful for a complete evaluation of specific structures in the narrow oral cavity of the miniature pig. The magnification provided by smaller rigid or semiflexible endoscopes (typically 1.9–2.7 mm) enhances evaluation of lesions and can allow documentation of lesions. The endoscope may be advanced slightly to allow visualization of the oropharynx.[13]

OTHER DIAGNOSTIC TESTING

Adjunct diagnostic testing is similar to that in other species: culture and sensitivity of abscesses or other sites of infection, and fine-needle aspirates and/or biopsy and histopathology of masses. Biopsy and histopathology are especially important in species prone to oral neoplasia such as the hedgehog. In hedgehogs, early stage oral tumors often present as gingivitis with or without abnormalities of dental structures.

DISORDERS OF THE ORAL CAVITY

Disorders of the oral cavity are likely seen to some degree in virtually every species, including unusual exotic species. Abnormalities include missing, mobile, or fractured

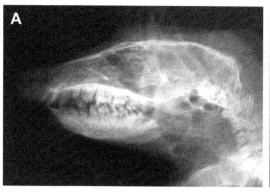
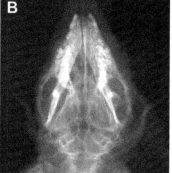

Fig. 8. Radiography of the normal head and dentition of a male African pigmy hedgehog. (*A*) Laterolateral and (*B*) ventrodorsal projection. Note the primary incisor teeth projecting forward, and molar cusps of premolars and molars. Roots of these brachyodont anelodont teeth are also visible. (*Courtesy of* Vittorio Capello, DVM, Milano, Italy; with permission.)

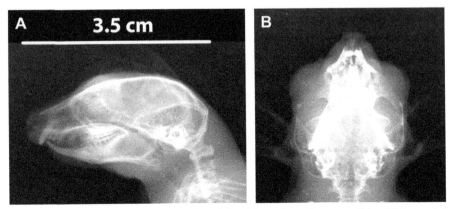

Fig. 9. Radiography of the normal head and dentition of a male sugar glider. (*A*) Laterolateral and (*B*) ventrodorsal projection. Note the well-developed primary incisor teeth. (*Courtesy of* Vittorio Capello, DVM, Milano Italy, and Angela Lennox, DVM, Indianapolis, Indiana; with permission.)

teeth, gingival hyperplasia, gingivitis, periodontal abscesses, and other discrete masses associated with any soft tissues of the oral cavity. Oral neoplasia in the hedgehog may resemble gingival hyperplasia or gingivitis; other masses may be detected under the tongue or affecting other soft tissues.

Trauma affecting the oral cavity soft tissue and dental structure may occur after a fall, blunt trauma, and entrapment of teeth, or from chewing on inappropriate objects. Traumatic injuries to dental structures may result in periodontal infection or endodontic infection.

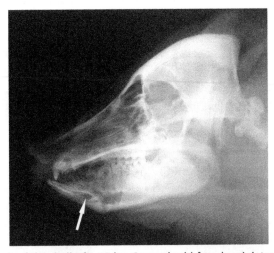

Fig. 10. Radiograph of the skull of a 15-kg, 6-month-old female miniature pig. Eruption of permanent teeth varies as to tooth; therefore, deciduous, permanent, and immature permanent teeth can be present in radiographs of the skull of immature pigs. The gem of the permanent incisor tooth is visible (*arrow*). (*From* Capello V, Lennox AM. Potbellied pig. In: Clinical radiology of exotic companion mammals. Ames (IA): Wiley-Blackwell; 2008; with permission.)

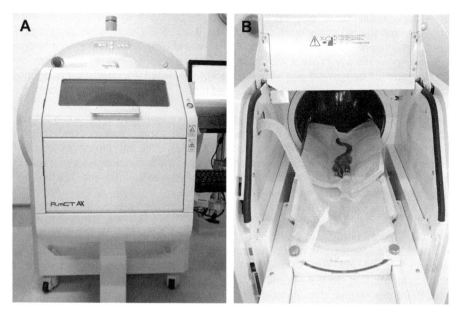

Fig. 11. Micro-CT unit (R_mCT AX, Rigaku Corporation, Tokyo, Japan). The CT unit is mobile, and built-in shielding eliminates the requirements for a designated shielded room. Maximum resolution is 0.06 mm, which is superior to conventional CT for small patients. (*A*) External view of the CT unit. (*B*) Inside of the CT with a sugar glider under anesthesia ready for scanning. (Rigaku Corporation, Tokyo, Japan. *Courtesy of* Yasutsugu Miwa, DVM, Tokyo, Japan; with permission.)

The African hedgehog appears particularly susceptible to gingivitis, periodontitis, and oral neoplasia.[3] One study noted oral squamous cell carcinoma as the most commonly identified neoplasm.[14] Other studies list oral squamous cell carcinoma among the most common neoplasms.[15] A single case report of oral squamous cell carcinoma noted tumor invading the maxilla and protruding into the maxillary sinus and the oral cavity, with no metastasis.[16] Odontogenic fibroma has also been identified.[17] The authors regularly see cases of gingivitis (**Fig. 12**) and tooth loss in African

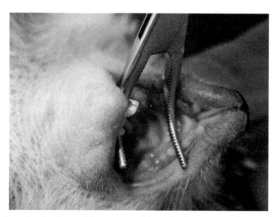

Fig. 12. Gingivitis in a hedgehog. (*Courtesy of* Angela Lennox, DVM, Indianapolis, Indiana; with permission.)

hedgehogs. Proliferative gingival masses must be carefully distinguished from neoplasia with the aid of histopathology (**Figs. 13** and **14**). Calculus resulting in periodontal disease has also been reported.[3,18] Ivey and Carpenter[3] report that hedgehogs may occasionally present with hard food items wedged in the hard palate. An unusual case of congenital erythropoietic porphyria was described in a hedgehog that presented with pink urine and pink-colored teeth.[19] No congenital dental diseases have been reported in either species.

A few sources mention specific dental disorders in sugar gliders, including trauma, periodontal disease, and calculus, but there are no published case reports.[6,20] Some have suggested a link between soft, carbohydrate-rich diets and the development of periodontal disease.[8] The authors have occasional identified incisor trauma (**Fig. 15**), severe periodontitis (**Fig. 16**), and even cases of severe tongue trauma due to penetration of the mandibular incisor teeth (**Fig. 17**).

The miniature pig is a laboratory model for the study of dentition in humans, due to similarities in orofacial/maxillary structures.[21] There are several articles describing experimentally induced dental lesions, but no reports of naturally occurring dental disease in pet pigs. The authors noted traumatic tooth fracture and caries in this species. Tynes notes that older pigs tend to form large amounts of dental calculus that do not appear to lead to severe gingivitis or other complications; therefore, regular dental scaling is not generally recommended (Tynes V, personal communication, 2016). Aging male pigs may form apical abscesses of the large canines (tusks); although not confirmed, this may be a result of repeated trimming throughout the life of the pig. These abscesses are deep and require extraction, which is challenging (Tynes V, personal communication, 2016) due to long reserve crown.

The pig is susceptible to porcine foot and mouth disease, which can present as vesicles of the buccal mucosa; this disease has not been seen in the United States since 1929.[22]

TREATMENT OF DENTAL DISEASE

Gingivitis may respond to appropriate antibiotic therapy. One author (A.M.L.) has seen excellent resolution of gingivitis in hedgehogs with administration of amoxicillin 0.15 mg/kg twice a day orally,[23] which is generally palatable in this species. In one case, gingivitis resolved but a neoplasm developed 8 months later. One author (Y.M.) reported 7 cases of gingivitis in hedgehogs aged 1 year 4 months to 4 years 8 months. All were treated with antibiotics, and one was given short-term prednisone for severe inflammation and salivation. Five of 7 cases responded to therapy; however, in 2 cases that failed to respond, histopathology revealed osteoma and squamous cell carcinoma, respectively.

Indications for oral surgery are the same as for other species. They include repair of traumatic injuries, extraction of fractured or otherwise abnormal teeth and biopsy, and removal of abnormal soft tissue masses. Prophylactic scaling and polishing have been suggested for the sugar glider.[7]

Traumatic disease of the oral cavity (fracture, soft tissue injury) should be treated with analgesics, support feeding, fluids, and antibiotics, if indicated. The authors have encountered traumatic incisor fracture in a sugar glider, which was treated with analgesics and short-term hand-feeding. Ness and Johnson-Delaney[6] describe the use of local lidocaine blocks and extraction and the use of 18- to 22-g needles to extract diseased teeth in the sugar glider. Similar techniques can be used in the hedgehog.

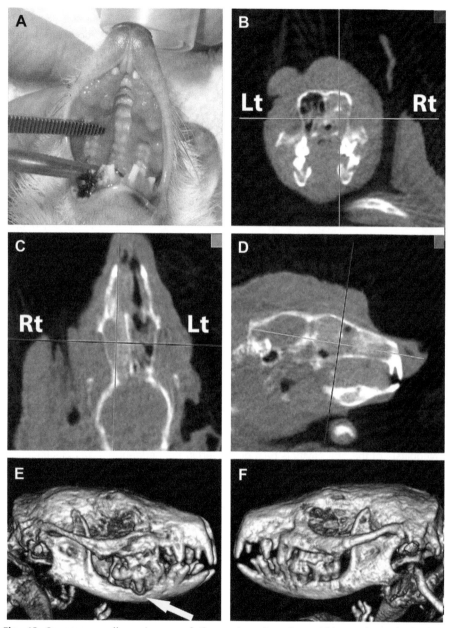

Fig. 13. Squamous cell carcinoma of the oral cavity of an African pigmy hedgehog, confirmed via histopathology. Same case as in **Fig. 4**. (*A*) Clinical appearance of the neoplastic gingival tissue. (*B–D*) Two-dimensional multiplanar reconstruction (2D MPR) displaying axial (*B, purple axis*), coronal (*C, orange axis*), and sagittal (*D, blue axis*) views. In each view, the other 2 corresponding views are indicated with the colored axis. The 2D MPR shows involvement of the right nasal cavity. (*E, F*) Three-dimensional volume reconstruction of the skull, showing bone lysis of the right mandible (*E, yellow arrow*) and comparison with the normal left mandible (*F*). (*Courtesy of* Yasutsugu Miwa, DVM, Tokyo, Japan; with permission.)

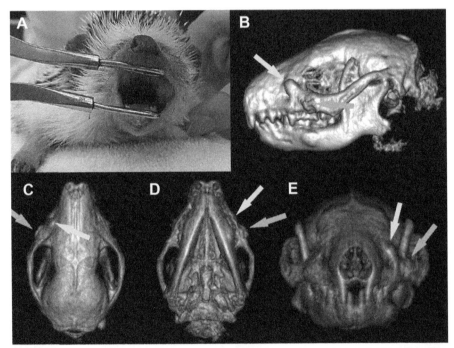

Fig. 14. Oral osteosarcoma in an African pigmy hedgehog, diagnosed after histopathology. (*A*) Clinical aspect of the swelling. Micro-CT displayed bony abnormalities (*arrows*) after 3-dimensional renderings. Lateral (*B*), dorsoventral (*C*), ventrodorsal (*D*), and rostrocaudal (*E*) view. (*Courtesy of* Yasutsugu Miwa, DVM, Tokyo, Japan; with permission.)

A case of a severe traumatic tongue injury in a hedgehog was successfully treated with subtotal glossectomy with an esophagostomy tube to allow time for healing, and for feeding, and administration of medications.[24]

Neoplasia of the oral cavity is best described in the hedgehog. Early identification and removal may be curative; in many cases, complete margins are not achieved

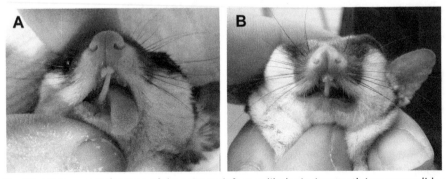

Fig. 15. (*A*) Traumatic fracture of the primary left mandibular incisor tooth in a sugar glider. A lesion of the lower lip is also visible. (*B*) Follow-up 2 weeks after the trauma. The lip lesion has healed. The fractured tooth has not regrown, and the opponent maxillary incisor tooth is not prone to overgrowth and malocclusion because (unlike incisor teeth of rodent species) dentition of sugar gliders is anelodont. (*Courtesy of* Yasutsugu Miwa, DVM, Tokyo, Japan; with permission.)

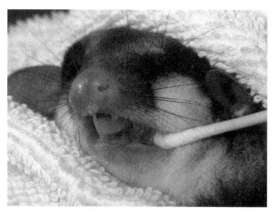

Fig. 16. Severe periodontitis and gingivitis in a sugar glider. The primary left mandibular incisor tooth is missing. (*Courtesy of* Yasutsugu Miwa, DVM, Tokyo, Japan; with permission.)

and disease reoccurs. Oral neoplasms arising from soft tissues may be removed using radiosurgical units, laser, or traditional surgical methods. One author (Y.M.) reports 5 cases of hedgehogs aged 2 years 6 months to 5 years 3 months treated for squamous cell carcinoma using various methods. All were treated with partial excision followed by use of a CO_2 laser (see **Fig. 13**). All received antibiotics, anti-inflammatory medication, and supportive care as needed. Treatment was palliative in all cases, and some underwent repeated laser therapy. One patient received radiation therapy (orthovoltage, 6 Gy, single treatment) followed by hyperthermia therapy in addition to surgery. Although size of the tumor did not appear to increase, the patient lost weight and did not survive. Another patient died because of respiratory distress secondary to invasion of the tumor into the nasal cavity. Overall, short-term quality of life was considered improved in all cases. Three of 5 cases experienced metastasis to adjacent lymph nodes. Survival time was 4 to 24 months.

A single case of multiple odontogenic fibromas was treated with individual resection of the nodules. Tumors appeared as multiple erythematous round masses. Relapse was not noted at recheck 6 months later.[17]

Trimming of the tusks of miniature pigs is occasionally performed, especially when they are used to injure people or other household pets. This dental procedure is often performed during routine hoof trimming and is accomplished under general

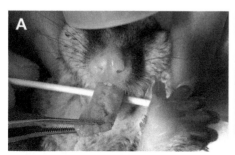
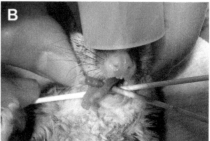

Fig. 17. (*A, B*) Serious injury of the tongue in a sugar glider, apparently caused by perforation of the mandibular incisors. (*Courtesy of* Yasutsugu Miwa, DVM, Tokyo, Japan; with permission.)

anesthesia using a Gigli wire,[8] rotating saw on a dremel tool, or with sharp side cutters. The use of cutters can result in shattering of the tooth. After cutting, the remaining tooth is ground smooth with a dremel tool and burr. Pulp exposure of the canine tooth should be avoided; otherwise, either infection may follow, or an endodontic procedure (pulp capping) should be performed. Preoperative radiographs can help assess the extent of the pulp cavity before coronal reduction.

EVALUATION OF OUTCOME AND LONG-TERM RECOMMENDATIONS

Until there is more information on the treatment and outcomes of diseases of the oral cavity in these species, it is difficult to offer a prognosis. Oral neoplasia carries a guarded to poor prognosis in many species. In both authors' practices, hedgehogs receiving adequate supportive care have lived many months after diagnosis of oral neoplasia.

SUMMARY

Diseases of the oral cavity affect any species; these have been described in unusual companion mammals such as the hedgehog and sugar glider, and anecdotally reported in miniature pigs as well. The most commonly reported and documented disorder of the oral cavity in these species is oral neoplasia in the African hedgehog. As in any species, thorough evaluation is warranted; in these species, thorough oral evaluation almost always requires sedation or general anesthesia.

REFERENCES

1. Reeve N. An introduction to hedgehogs. In: Reeve N, editor. Hedgehogs (Poyser natural history series). Cambridge (MA): T.&A.D. Poyser, Academic Press (imprint of Elsevier); 1994. p. 1–14.
2. Chaprazov T, Dimitrov R, Stamatova Yovcheva K, et al. Oral and dental disorders in pet hedgehogs. Turkis J Vet Anim Sci 2014;38:1–6.
3. Ivey E, Carpenter JW. African hedgehogs. In: Quesenberry KE, Carpenter JW, editors. Ferrets, rabbits and rodents, clinical medicine and surgery 2nd edition. St Louis (MO): Elsevier Saunders; 2012. p. 339–53.
4. Crossley DA. Small mammal dentistry. In: Quesenberry KE, Carpenter JW, editors. Ferrets, rabbits and rodents, clinical medicine and surgery 2nd edition. St Louis (MO): Elsevier Sunders; 2012. p. 370–82.
5. Capello V, Lennox AM. Small mammal dentistry. In: Quesenberry KE, Carpenter JW, editors. Ferrets, rabbits and rodents, clinical medicine and surgery 2nd edition. St Louis (MO): Elsevier Sunders; 2012. p. 452–71.
6. Ness RD, Johnson-Delaney CA. Sugar gliders. In: Quesenberry KE, Carpenter JW, editors. Ferrets, rabbits and rodents, clinical medicine and surgery 2nd edition. St Louis (MO): Elsevier Sunders; 2012. p. 393–410.
7. Hume ID. Omnivorous marsupials. In: Hume ID, editor. Marsupial nutrition. Cambridge: Cambridge University Press; 1999. p. 95–101.
8. Eubanks DL, Gilbo K. Trimming tusks in the Tucatan minipig. Lab Anim (NY) 2005;34(9):35–8.
9. Tucker AL, Widowski TM. Normal profiles for deciduous dental eruption in domestic piglets: effect of sow, litter, and piglet characteristics. J Anim Sci 2009;87: 2274–81.
10. Capello V, Lennox AM. Sugar gliders. In: Clinical radiology of exotic companion mammals. Ames (IA): Wiley-Blackwell; 2008. p. 429–35.

11. Capello V, Lennox AM. Potbellied Pig. In: Clinical radiology of exotic companion mammals. Ames (IA): Wiley-Blackwell; 2008. p. 457–79.
12. Capello V, Lennox AM. African pygmy hedgehogs. In: Clinical radiology of exotic companion mammals. Ames (IA): Wiley-Blackwell; 2008. p. 481–7.
13. Divers S. Making the difference in exotic animal practice: the value of endoscopy. Vet Clin North Am Exot Anim Pract 2015;18:351–7.
14. Pei-Chi H, Jane-Fang Y, Lin-Chiann W. A retrospective study of the medical status on 63 African hedgehogs (Atelerix albiventris) at the Taipei zoo from 2003 to 2011. J Exotic Pet Med 2014;24(1):105–11.
15. Raymon JT, Garner MM. Spontaneous tumours in Captive African hedgehogs (Atelerix albiventris): a retrospective study. J Comp Pathol 2001;124(203): 128–33.
16. Rivera RY, Janovitz EB. Oronasal squamous cell carcinoma in an African hedgehog (Erinaceidae albiventris). J Wildl Dis 1992;28(1):148–50.
17. Wozniak-Biel A, Janeczek M, Janus I, et al. Surgical resection of peripheral odontogenic fibromas in African pygmy hedgehog (Atelerix albiventris): a case study. BMC Vet Res 2015;11(1):145.
18. Hoefer HL. Hedgehogs care and husbandry. Vet Clin North Am Exot Anim Pract 2004;7(2):257–67.
19. Wolff CF, Corradinia PRM, Cortes G. Congenital erythropoietic porphyria in an African Hedgehog (Atelerix albiventris). J Zoo Wildl Med 2005;36(2):323–5.
20. Booth RJ. General husbandry and medical care of sugar gliders. In: Bonagura JD, editor. Kirks' current veterinary therapy XIII. Philadelphia: WB Saunders; 2000. p. 1157–63.
21. Wang S, Liu Y, Fang D, et al. The miniature pig: a useful large animal model for dental and orofacial research. Oral Dis 2007;13(6):530–7.
22. Overview of foot-and-mouth disease. The merck veterinary manual. Available at: http://www.merckvetmanual.com/mvm/generalized_conditions/foot-and-mouth_disease/overview_of_foot-and-mouth_disease.html. Accessed February 15, 2016.
23. Carpenter JW, Marion CJ. Hedgehogs. In: Carpetner JW, editor. Exotic animal formulary. 4th edition. St Louis (MO): Elsevier; 2013. p. 456.
24. Grunkemeyer V. Use of an esophagostomy tube for management of traumatic subtotal glossectomy in an African pygmy hedgehog (Atelerix albiventris). J Exotic Pet Med, in press.

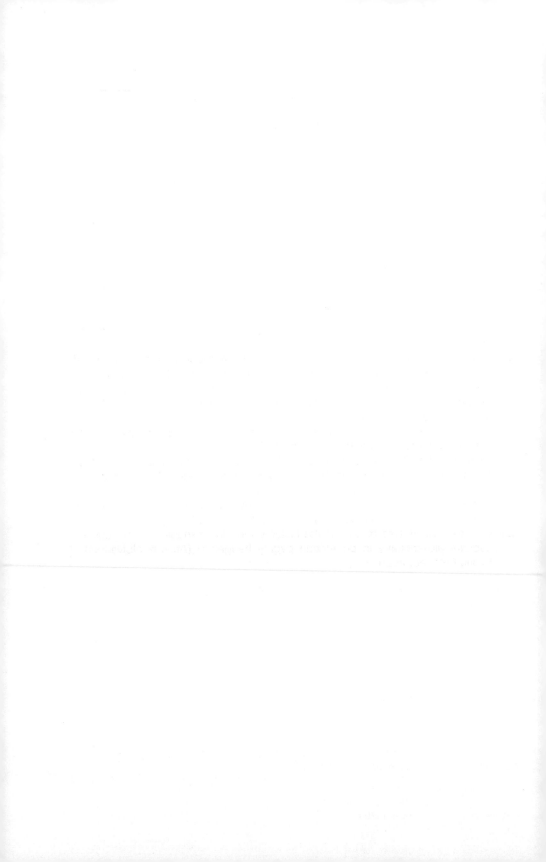

Index

Note: Page numbers of article titles are in **boldface** type.

Vet Clin Exot Anim 19 (2016) 947–997
http://dx.doi.org/10.1016/S1094-9194(16)30026-3
1094-9194/16/$ – see front matter

vetexotic.theclinics.com

Moving?

Make sure your subscription moves with you!

To notify us of your new address, find your **Clinics Account Number** (located on your mailing label above your name), and contact customer service at:

Email: **journalscustomerservice-usa@elsevier.com**

800-654-2452 (subscribers in the U.S. & Canada)
314-447-8871 (subscribers outside of the U.S. & Canada)

Fax number: **314-447-8029**

Elsevier Health Sciences Division
Subscription Customer Service
3251 Riverport Lane
Maryland Heights, MO 63043

*To ensure uninterrupted delivery of your subscription, please notify us at least 4 weeks in advance of move.

Printed and bound by CPI Group (UK) Ltd, Croydon, CR0 4YY

03/10/2024

01040388-0008